Machine Learning and Deep Learning in Efficacy Improvement of Healthcare Systems

Emerging Trends in Biomedical Technologies and Health Informatics

Series Editors

Subhendu Kumar Pani
Orissa Engineering College, Bhubaneswar, Orissa, India

Sujata Dash
North Orissa University, Baripada, India

Sunil Vadera
University of Salford, Salford, UK

Everyday Technologies in Healthcare
Chhabi Rani Panigrahi, Bibudhendu Pati, Mamata Rath, Rajkumar Buyya

Biomedical Signal Processing for Healthcare Applications
Varun Bajaj, G.R. Sinha, Chinmay Chakraborty

Deep Learning in Biomedical and Health Informatics
M. Jabbar, Ajith Abraham, Onur Dogan, Ana Madureira, Sanju Tiwar

For more information about this series, please visit: https://www.routledge.com/Emerging-Trends-in-Biomedical-Technologies-and-Health-informatics-series/book-series/ETBTHI

Machine Learning and Deep Learning in Efficacy Improvement of Healthcare Systems

Edited by
Om Prakash Jena, Bharat Bhushan, Nitin Rakesh,
Parma Nand Astya, and Yousef Farhaoui

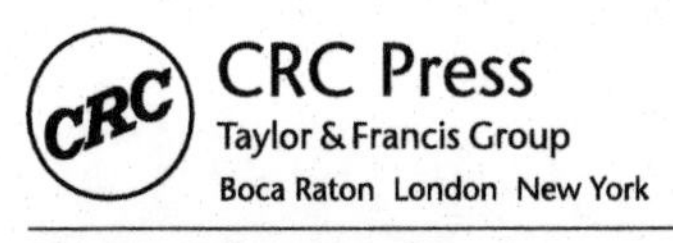

CRC Press is an imprint of the
Taylor & Francis Group, an **informa** business

First edition published 2022
by CRC Press
6000 Broken Sound Parkway NW, Suite 300, Boca Raton, FL 33487-2742

and by CRC Press
4 Park Square, Milton Park, Abingdon, Oxon, OX14 4RN

CRC Press is an imprint of Taylor & Francis Group, LLC

Library of Congress Cataloging-in-Publication Data
Names: Jena, Om Prakash, editor. | Bhushan, Bharat (Software specialist), editor. | Rakesh, Nitin, editor. | Astya, Parma Nand, editor. | Farhaoui, Yousef, editor.
Title: Machine learning and deep learning in efficacy improvement of healthcare systems / edited by Om Prakash Jena, Bharat Bhushan, Nitin Rakesh, Parma Nand Astya, Yousef Farhaoui.
Description: First edition. | Boca Raton : CRC Press, 2022. | Includes bibliographical references and index. | Summary: "This book describes the fundamental concepts of machine learning and deep learning techniques in a healthcare system. The aim of this book is to describe how deep learning methods are used to insure high quality data processing, medical image and signal analysis, and improved healthcare application"-- Provided by publisher.
Identifiers: LCCN 2021031428 (print) | LCCN 2021031429 (ebook) | ISBN 9781032036724 (hardback) | ISBN 9781032037950 (paperback) | ISBN 9781003189053 (ebook)
Subjects: MESH: Machine Learning | Medical Informatics Applications | Deep Learning | Efficiency | Quality Improvement
Classification: LCC R855.3 (print) | LCC R855.3 (ebook) | NLM W 26.55.A7 | DDC 610.285--dc23
LC record available at https://lccn.loc.gov/2021031428
LC ebook record available at https://lccn.loc.gov/2021031429

ISBN: 978-1-032-03672-4 (hbk)
ISBN: 978-1-032-03795-0 (pbk)
ISBN: 978-1-003-18905-3 (ebk)

DOI: 10.1201/9781003189053

Typeset in Times
by MPS Limited, Dehradun

Contents

Preface

Rapid population growth coupled with the evolution of numerous diseases is a matter of concern worldwide. Due to this, the healthcare industry has emerged as an essential service sector. The generation of a large amount of healthcare data and the lack of insight from that data are significant problems in the healthcare sector. Therefore, there is a need for a fully effective and automated system that can help medical stakeholders to take prompt action at the right time. Artificial intelligence (AI) and machine learning (ML) have a very long association with the healthcare sector dating back to 1980s. It gained momentum with the emergence of rule-based systems, hierarchical clustering, and various regression models. ML is an important utility of AI that provides systems with the capacity to automatically examine and enhance action without being specially programmed. However, neither the computers nor the algorithms were efficient enough to enable effective ML based systems. The last five years had seen tremendous rise in the adoption of ML techniques mainly due to emergence of neural network that enhanced the overall computational power. Deep Learning (DL) is a subset of ML where innovations have led to the construction of several novel deep neural network architectures that can be used for the classification of large data sets. AI, ML, and DL techniques can be employed for efficient knowledge discovery from healthcare data. These techniques have shown tremendous results in huge range of tasks such as brain tumor segmentation, medical image reconstruction, lung nodule detection, classification of intestinal diseases, organ recognition, and COVID prediction. Further, ML/DL models have also achieved significant performances in the realm of clinical medicine, radiology, clinical pathology, dermatology, and ophthalmology. It is expected that such models along with intelligent software will revolutionize the medical research and even assist physicians and radiologists in patient examination in the near future. This book aims to integrate several aspects of computational intelligence like ML and DL techniques from diversified healthcare perspectives. This book describes the fundamental concepts of ML and DL techniques and its applications in the healthcare domain. Further, the book is aimed to endow different communities with their innovative advances in theory, analytical approaches, numerical simulation, statistical analysis, case studies, analytical results, computational structuring, and other significant progresses in the healthcare sector.

Editors

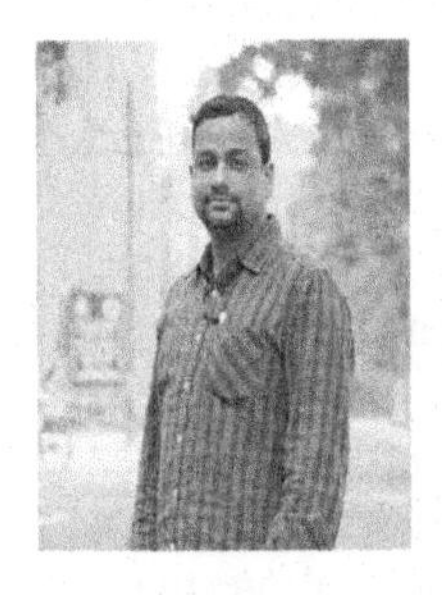

Om Prakash Jena is an assistant professor in the Department of Computer Science, Ravenshaw University, Cuttack, and Odisha. He has 10 years of teaching and research experience in undergraduate and postgraduate levels. He has published several technical papers in international journals/conferences/edited book chapters of reputed publications. He is a member of IEEE, IETA, IAAC, IRED, IAENG, and WACAMLDS. His current research interest includes database, pattern recognition, cryptography, network security, artificial intelligence, machine learning, soft computing, natural language processing, data science, compiler design, data analytics, and machine automation. He has guided many projects and theses at the undergraduate and postgraduate levels. He has many edited books that have been published by Wiley, CRC Press, and Bentham Publication to his credit, and he is also the author of two textbooks with Kalyani Publishers.

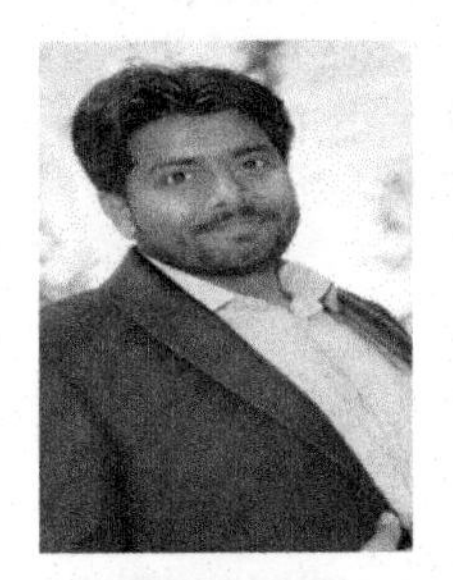

Bharat Bhushan is an assistant professor of the Department of Computer Science and Engineering (CSE) at the School of Engineering and Technology, Sharda University, Greater Noida, India. He earned an undergraduate degree (BTech in computer science and engineering) with distinction in 2012, a postgraduate degree (MTech in information security) with distinction in 2015, and doctoral degree (PhD in computer science and engineering) in 2021 at Birla Institute of Technology, Mesra, India. He also has earned numerous international certifications, such as CCNA, MCTS, MCITP, RHCE, and CCNP. He has published more than 80 research papers at various renowned international conferences and SCI-indexed journals, including *Journal of Network and Computer Applications* (Elsevier), *Wireless Networks* (Springer), *Wireless Personal Communications* (Springer), *Sustainable Cities and Society* (Elsevier), and *Emerging Transactions on Telecommunications* (Wiley). He has contributed more than 25 book chapters in various books and has edited 11 books with the most famed publishers such as Elsevier, IGI Global, and CRC Press. He has served as a keynote speaker (resource person) at numerous reputed international conferences held in India, Morocco, China, Belgium, and Bangladesh. He has served as a reviewer/editorial board member for several reputed international journals. He was previously an assistant professor at the HMR Institute of Technology and Management, New Delhi and a network engineer at HCL Infosystems Ltd., Noida. He has qualified GATE exams for successive years and gained the highest percentile of 98.48 in GATE 2013. He is also a member of numerous renowned bodies, including IEEE, IAENG, CSTA, SCIEI, IAE, and UACEE.

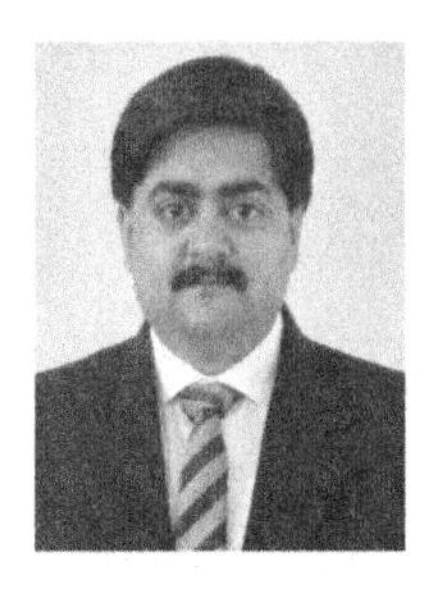

Nitin Rakesh is head of the Computer Science and Engineering Department for BTech/MTech (CSE/IT), BTech CSE-IBM Specializations, BTech CSE-I Nurture, BCA/MCA, BSc/MSc-CS at the School of Engineering and Technology, Sharda University, India. He earned a PhD in computer science and engineering with network coding as his specialization. He earned a master of technology degree in computer science and engineering and a bachelor of technology degree in information technology. Dr. Nitin has been instrumental in various industrial interfacing for academic and research at his previous assignments at various organizations (Amity University, Jaypee University, Galgotias, and others). He has 100+ research publications in reputed SCI or Scopus-indexed journals and international conferences. Currently, he is guiding eight PhD students at various universities and industries. He has also served as a reviewer for several prestigious international journals including *IEEE Transactions on Vehicular Technology* and *The Computer Journal*, Oxford Press. His research outlines emphasis on network coding, interconnection networks and architecture, and online phantom transactions. Dr. Nitin has accorded several other awards for best paper published, session chairs, highest cited author, best students thesis guided, and many others. He has also initiated an IoT and network lab at Sharda University, which will be a new technology initiative for graduate, postgraduate, and doctoral students. He is a recipient of the IBM Drona Award and Top 10 State Award Winner. He is an active member of professional societies such as IEEE (USA), ACM, SIAM (USA), Life Member of CSI, and other professional societies.

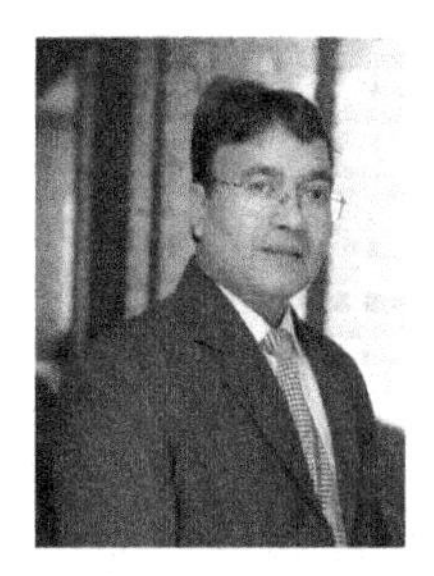

Parma Nand Astya is the dean of the School of Engineering Technology at Sharda University Greater Noida. He has over 26 years of teaching, industry, and research experience. He has expertise in wireless and sensor network, cryptography, algorithms, and computer graphics. He earned a PhD at IIT Roorkee and an MTech and a BTech in computer science and engineering at IIT Delhi. He has been head/member of many committees including board of studies, faculty and staff recruitment committee, academic council, advisory committee, monitoring and planning board, research advisory committee, accreditation committee, etc. He has been president of the National Engineers Organization. He is a senior member of IEEE (USA). He is a member of the Executive Council of IEEE UP section (R10), a member of the Executive Committee IEEE Computer and Signal Processing Society, a member of the Executive of India Council Computer Society, a member of the Executive Council Computer Society of India, Noida section, and has acted as an observer at many IEEE conferences. He also has active memberships in ACM, CSI, ACEEE, ISOC, IAENG, and IASCIT. He is a lifetime member of the Soft Computing Research Society (SCRS) and ISTE. He has delivered many invited/keynotes talks at international and national conferences/ workshops/seminars in India and abroad. He has published more than 85 papers in peer-reviewed international/national journals and conferences and has filed two patents. He is an active member of the advisory/technical program committees of reputed international/national conferences and a reviewer of a number of reputed journals, including Springer, Elsevier.

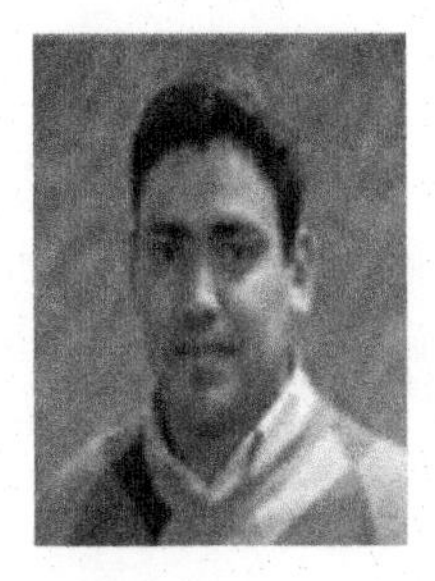

Yousef Farhaoui is a professor at Moulay Ismail University, Faculty of Sciences and Techniques, Morocco, and the local publishing and research coordinator, Cambridge International Academics in the United Kingdom. He earned a PhD in computer security at the Ibn Zohr University of Science. His research interests include learning, e-learning, computer security, big data analytics, and business intelligence. Dr. Farhaoui has authored three books in computer science. He is a coordinator and member of the organizing committee, a member of the scientific committee of several international congresses, and he is a member of various international associations. He has authored four books and many book chapters with reputed publishers such as Springer and IGI. He served as a reviewer for IEEE, IET, Springer, Inderscience, and Elsevier journals. He is also the guest editor of many journals with Wiley, Springer, Inderscience, etc. He has been the general chair, session chair, and panelist at several conferences. He is a senior member of IEEE, IET, ACM, and EAI Research Group.

Contributors

G. Abirami
Department of Computer Science
SRM Institute of Science and Technology (SRMIST) Kattankulathur
Kattankulathur, Tamil Nadu, India

Mustafa A. Al-Asadi
Department of Computer Engineering
Selçuk University, Konya
Konya, Turkey

Gufran Ahmad Ansari
B.S. Abdur Rahman Crescent Institute of Science and Technology
Vandalur, Tamil Nadu, India

Vincenzo Barrile
Università Mediterranea di Reggio Calabria
Reggio Calabria, Italy

Ernesto Bernardo
Università Mediterranea di Reggio Calabria
Reggio Calabria, Italy

Salliah Shafi Bhat
B.S. Abdur Rahman Crescent Institute of Science and Technology
Vandalur, Tamil Nadu, India

Biswajit R. Bhowmik
National Institute of Technology Karnataka
Mangalore, Karnataka, India

Giuliana Bilotta
Università Mediterranea di Reggio Calabria
Reggio Calabria, Italy

Gajanan K. Birajdar
Department of Electronics Engineering
Ramrao Adik Institute of Technology
Nerul, Navi Mumbai, India

Ankita Biswas
Department of Computer Engineering
University of Calcutta
Kolkata, West Bengal, India

Rafik Bouaziz
Department of Computer Science
University of Sfax
Sfax, Tunisia

Safa Brahmia
Department of Computer Science
University of Sfax
Sfax, Tunisia

Zouhaier Brahmia
Department of Computer Science
University of Sfax
Sfax, Tunisia

Kanyaka Chakraborty
Department of Computer Engineering
University of Calcutta
Kolkata, West Bengal, India

Anal Chatterjee
Department of Mathematics
Barrackpore Rastraguru Surendranath College
Kolkata, West Bengal, India

Shruti Dambhare
Galgotias University, Noida
Uttar Pradesh, India

Anindya Das
SRM Institute of Science and Technology (SRMIST), Kattankulathur
Kattankulathur, Tamil Nadu, India

Namrata Das
University of Calcutta
Kolkata, West Bengal, India

Ajitabh Dash
Birla Global University
Bhubaneswar, Odisha, India

Antonino Fotia
Università Mediterranea di Reggio Calabria
Reggio Calabria, Italy

Suchandra Ganguly
University College of Nursing
College of Medicine and J.N.M. Hospital
Kalyani, West Bengal, India

Ahona Ghosh
Department of Computer Science and Engineering
Maulana Abul Kalam Azad University of Technology
Kalyani, West Bengal, India

Ananya Ghosh
Department of Computer Engineering
University of Calcutta
Kolkata, West Bengal, India

Nikita Ghosh
University of Calcutta
Kolkata, West Bengal, India

R. Girija
Vellore Institute of Technology (VIT) Chennai
Chennai, Tamil Nadu, India

Fabio Grandi
University of Bologna
Bologna, Italy

Om Prakash Jena
Department of Computer Science
Ravenshaw University
Cuttack, Odisha, India

Sachin Kamley
Department of Computer Applications
Samrat Ashok Technological Institute
Vidisha, Madhya Pradesh, India

Bhakti Kaushal
Department of Electronics and Telecommunication Engineering
Ramrao Adik Institute of Technology
Nerul, Navi Mumbai, India

Ömer Köksal
Aselsan
Ankara, Turkey

Adarsh Kumar
National Institute of Technology Karnataka
Mangalore, Karnataka, India

Rahul Kumar
National Institute of Technology Karnataka
Mangalore, Karnataka, India

Sanjay Kumar
Galgotias University, Noida
Uttar Pradesh, India

Arion Mitra
University of Calcutta
Kolkata, West Bengal, India

Mukesh Patil
Department of Electronics and Telecommunication Engineering
Ramrao Adik Institute of Technology
Nerul, Navi Mumbai, India

Ebin Deni Raj
Indian Institute of Information Technology, Kottayam
Valavoor, Kerala, India

Smitha Raveendran
Department of Electronics Engineering
Ramrao Adik Institute of Technology
Nerul, Navi Mumbai, India

Barnali Sahu
Department of Computer Science and Engineering
Siksha 'O' Anusandhan University
Bhubaneswar, Odisha, India

Sitarashmi Sahu
Foundation for Technology and Business Incubation (FTBI)
National Institute of Technology Rourkela
Rourkela, Odisha, India

Navneeth Sreenivasan
SRM Institute of Science and Technology (SRMIST) Kattankulathur
Kattankulathur, Tamil Nadu, India

Sakir Tasdemİr
Department of Computer Engineering
Selçuk University, Konya
Konya, Turkey

Jeena Thomas
Indian Institute of Information Technology, Kottayam
Valavoor, Kerala, India

Shrinidhi Anil Varna
National Institute of Technology Karnataka
Mangalore, Karnataka, India

Abir Zekri
University of Sfax
Sfax, Tunisia

1 Machine Learning in Healthcare
An Introduction

Shruti Dambhare and Sanjay Kumar
Galgotias University, Noida, Uttar Pradesh, India

CONTENTS

1.1 INTRODUCTION

Technology and its continuous advancements have paved the way to exhilarating and effective innovations in various walks of human lives. Healthcare is one such key segment that is continuously witnessing the ripple effects of technological innovations via the new cutting-edge technologies like big data, Internet of things,

DOI: 10.1201/9781003189053-1

cloud computing and machine learning, etc. Over the past decade, the healthcare industry and its various segments have seen a radical shift in its way of functioning and if it is to be defined in a most simple way the answer would be that, it has become more "digital", "smart" and provides interoperability feature. Healthcare is a huge industry, and the amalgamation of machine learning in healthcare has resulted in the creation and development of life-altering applications. These applications, which were once only a part of science fiction and human imagination, are today's reality and ubiquitous to human lives.

With exponentially growing digitalization in all major sectors, the way "data" is seen and handled for example: data management, data sharing and data processing, is a task of high importance. When such data comes from the health and medical segment, it's even more important to utilize such data. At this point, such machine learning techniques and applications aids in providing valuable solutions to the ever-increasing medical needs. The healthcare industry, which has seen over 10 to 12 trillion dollars of global investments, is still crippled by the high operational cost, insufficient health workforce and poor infrastructure and many other shortcomings like transparency, no placement service delivery, changing health policies and laws.

To overcome such staggering challenges, machine learning can be effectively used. Ranging from simple chatbots that offer preliminary medical support to creation of predictive models to diagnose an onset of disease, prognosis to prevent the wider complications due to an underlying aliment to personalized medicine; machine learning has some promising solutions to offer. Machine learning also has added another dimension to myriad of possibilities to tackle even the mammoth issue like the pandemic and can provide solutions with other new and emerging technologies like IoT, big data, biometrics, cloud computing, deep learning, etc.

The remainder of the paper is organized as follows. Section 1.2 gives an in-depth idea about "machine learning" and its fundamental workings and usage for general applications. It covers the basic difference between artificial intelligence and machine learning. It describes the reason why machine learning is widely accepted and applied over general statistics and the various machine learning techniques are elaborated in section 1.4. Section 1.5 gives an insight to the various segments of the healthcare industry and provides a detailed overview of the wide spectrum of these different segment, which makes the entire healthcare industry. Section 1.6 highlights the various applications of machine learning in healthcare ranging from medical diagnosis, prognosis, electronic health records (EHR), medical image analysis, disease prediction and pandemic combatting solutions to pandemic outbreak prediction and control measures is covered. This section is followed by section 1.7, which states research trends and the conclusion.

1.2 MACHINE LEARNING AND ITS BASIC WORKINGS

Artificial intelligence has revolutionized many domains related to human existence. The past century has witnessed a key surge in the application of machine learning in such domains exhibiting state-of-the-art performances. Such an amalgamation of machine learning technology and application of machine learning algorithms in various walks of life has become a normal phenomenon. A U.S. visionary of computer games and artificial intelligence, Arthur Samuel (1901–1990) coined in 1959 the word 'machine learning.' He identified it as "a study field that allows computers to learn without having to be programmed explicitly" [1–3]. Machine learning since then went through a lot of systematic changes and with the ever-growing new research and applications of machine learning in various areas fuelled by the demands of humans, this led to a bloom of this field which found its separate path from its mother branch, artificial intelligence.

A basic question which set off the so-called machine learning revolution [4]: could a computer learn without being specifically instructed how? The field of artificial intelligence developed machine learning models by integrating mathematical information with the computer's ability to transfer vast quantities of data faster than anyone else could. These models may take raw data, identify a pattern influencing it, and adapt to new circumstances what they learned. Computers, in other words, may discover the hidden truths in the data by themselves. A machine learning model depicts the patterns hidden in data. Machine learning model can also be stated as mathematical representation which exhibits the pattern found within a set of data Figure 1.1 demonstrates this machine learning process. When the machine learning model is trained (or constructed or adapted) to the training data, some ruling function is observed within those. The ruling function is then transformed or stated into rules that can be used for predictions in novel environments [5–8].

As a point of conclusion, we may infer that unlike traditional programming where we input program and get results or rule; in machine learning (which is a

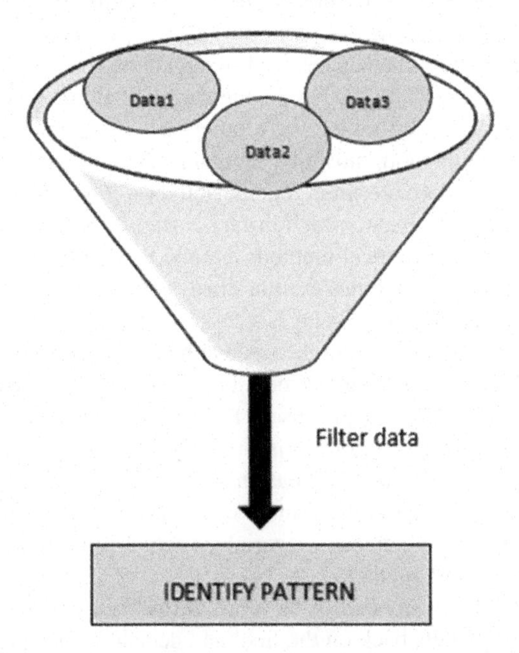

FIGURE 1.1 Machine learning process.

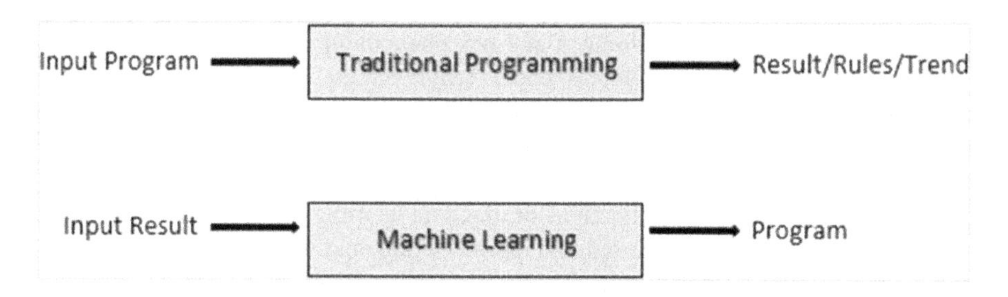

FIGURE 1.2 Traditional programming vs. machine learning.

sub-branch of artificial intelligence), the machine learns on its own rather than some prewritten algorithm which programs as shown in Figure 1.2. There are two key steps in this, one which is finding fresh interdependencies between two set of variables which are used as input and second is to predict new output with the known set of inter-dependability in the data variables.

1.3 WHY MACHINE LEARNING?

As per the definition given by Mitchell [9], machine learning is a branch of artificial intelligence that employs a variety of statistical, probabilistic and optimization tools to "learn" from past examples and to then use that prior training to classify new data, identify new patterns or predict novel trends.

Similar to statistics, machine learning used understand and examine data but the power of machine learning over statistics lies in the applicability of probabilistic methods, Boolean logic, conditional properties [10–12] as well as other systematic methods which help in training data sets and segregate patterns or relationships. The core strength of machine learning lies in the fact that it paves way to make inferences and decision making which were otherwise very difficult to make using conventional statistical method, most of which are based on multivariate regression or correlation analysis. If we consider general statistics, it usually loses its potential when relationships are nonlinear, which in fact is true for all biological systems in the natural settings [13]. Statistical methods assume that variables are independent.

Still, machine learning outcomes are not always correct and hence the practical applicability of machine learning being successful is not fixed. Undoubtedly with any method being used, clarity about the issue at hand and shortcomings of the data at disposal is mandatory. At the same time it is quite important to be aware of what-if scenario and issues with algorithm used. Probability of success increases manifold if the machine learning algorithm is properly designed and applied with the correct data set with efficient data validation process in hand [14]. In other words, refined and good quality data is the prime key to successful results. Also, another important parameter is the number of variables which must be appropriate with respect to the events to be predicted.

The statistical methods are said to be more efficient in comparison to machine learning, but it majorly falls back on the firsthand decisions made by the user about the inter dependability of data and data being non-linear. For handing this issue choosing an appropriate method for a required task is the key. Hence, it is extremely important to go for a best fit approach. Also machine learning is in every regard more efficient in find patterns in a set of data against human expert. An argument emphasizes that with more efforts and time even a human expert can correlate variables in a data set and define a trend however the key question is the time requirement for the same.

The mainstream use of machine learning is largely possible as a result of huge databases and significant progress in statistical and optimization techniques that help minimize over fitting. They are the two main guiding forces of machine learning's popularity today. This, along with the proliferation of interconnected machines or the Internet of Things (IoT) [15] has provided an enormous substrate on which to design predictive and intelligent systems. As the amount of health data available increases, machine learning becomes crucial. When more and more IoT-enabled systems are installed, a growing number of interconnected systems [16] would be needed to help sustain them.

1.4 MACHINE LEARNING TECHNIQUES

There are two common types of ML methods: supervised learning and unsupervised learning (Figure 1.3).

1.4.1 Supervised Learning

In supervised learning [17], a set of data called "labelled data" is used as training data. This set of labelled data is used by the model to find out the input data to the required output. Models use this labelled data to evaluate themselves during the training phase with an aim to improve the prediction functionality of a new test data. Supervised learning model focus on classification and regression algorithm.

Classification helps in tracing a function which aids in segregating the data set into classes based on different parameters. A computer program is trained on the training data set and based on that training, it categorizes the data into set of finite classes. In perspective of mapping, the use of a classification algorithm is to map any input "x" to output "y". In the field of healthcare, classification plays an

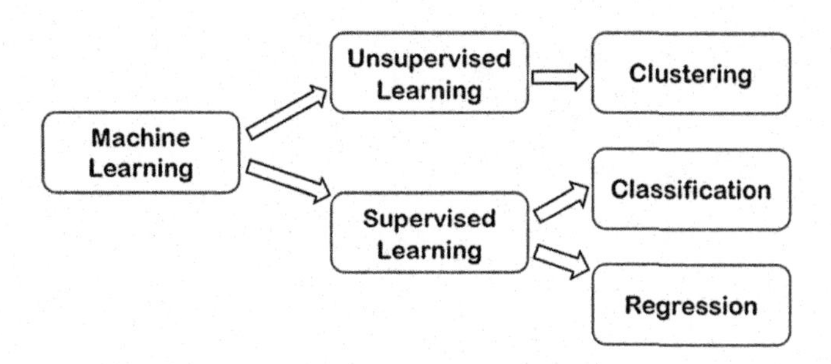

FIGURE 1.3 Machine learning techniques.

important rule that aids in evaluating the different set of data about patient health and diagnosing the disease or aliment. Classification has been widely adopted in other stages of prognosis and even patient treatment plan adoption [18].

The classification algorithms from the supervised learning group [18,19] are logistic regression, support vector machines (SVM), decision trees (DT), Naïve Bayes models, linear and random forest classification. And we can also train neural networks via supervised learning [20].

1.4.1.1 Workings of Support Vector Machine Algorithm

To understand the workings of SVM algorithm, the following instance can be taken into consideration. For instance, our data sets have two color tags, grey and black; and two sets of features x1 and y2 and we require a classifier that classifies the set x1 and x2 of coordinates in red or black. This is demonstrated in Figure 1.4, which shows tags black and grey.

We could easily separate the classes by a simple straight line, considering this is a two-dimensional space; however, we can have multiple straight lines that can segregate the two classes, as shown in Figure 1.5.

The objective of the SVM algorithm is to determine the best decision boundary, called "hyper plane", that can differentiate n-dimensional space into classes so that later we can easily put the new data point in the correct category. These extreme cases are called support vectors. This is also the reason why the algorithm is named a support vector machine. This is demonstrated in Figure 1.6.

Lately, SVMs are used extensively in the medical field majorly for disease prognosis and diagnosis [21,22] in a "Multi-disease prediction model using improved SVM-radial bias technique in healthcare monitoring system" accuracy of over 98 percent was achieved to predict chronic kidney disease, diabetes and heart disease [23]. In another, a proposed paper a novel IoT enabled Depth wise separable convolution neural network (DWS-CNN) with Deep support vector machine (DSVM) for COVID-19 diagnosis and classification [24].

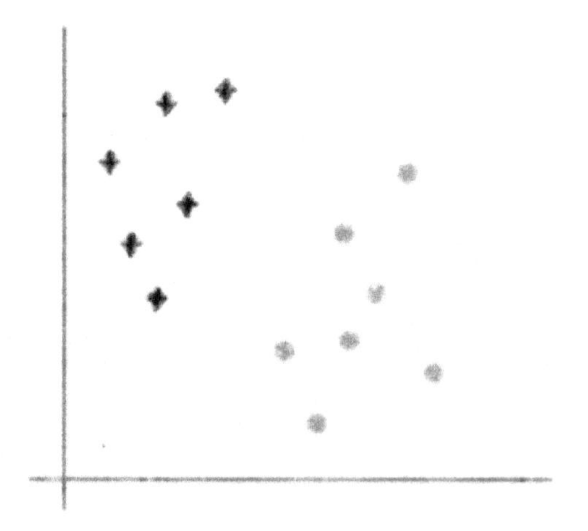

FIGURE 1.4 Tags (black and grey, x1 and x2).

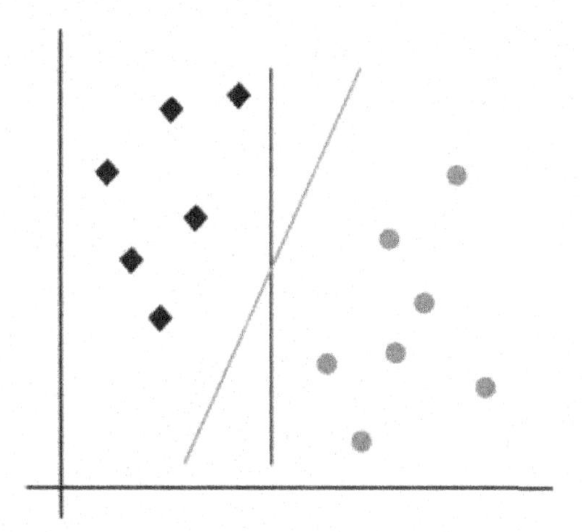

FIGURE 1.5 Separated classes by various lines.

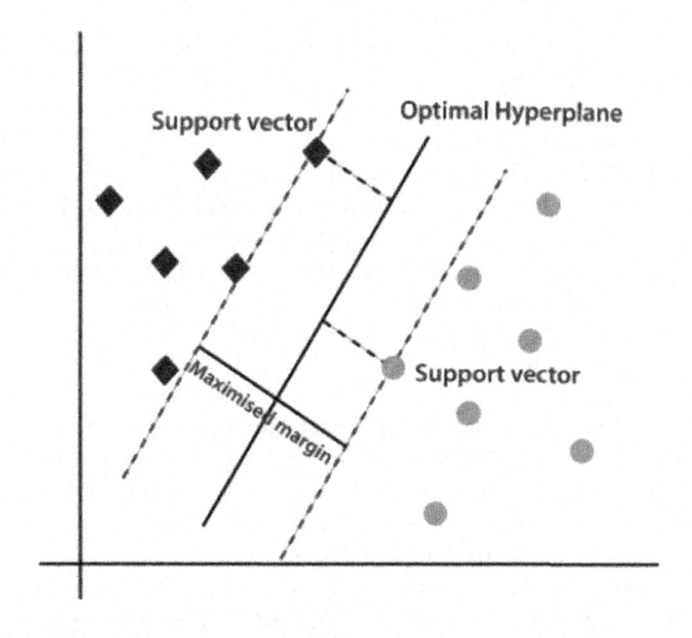

FIGURE 1.6 Linear support vector machine.

Logistic regression helps in determining a dependent variable from a set of independent variables. It states the output of discrete or categorical dependent variable logistic regression predicts the output of a categorical dependent variable [25,26]. Therefore, the outcome must be a categorical or discrete value. It states the probabilistic values between 0 and 1. Logistic regression is similar to linear regression except in how they are used. Linear regression is used for solving regression problems, whereas logistic regression is used for solving the classification problems.

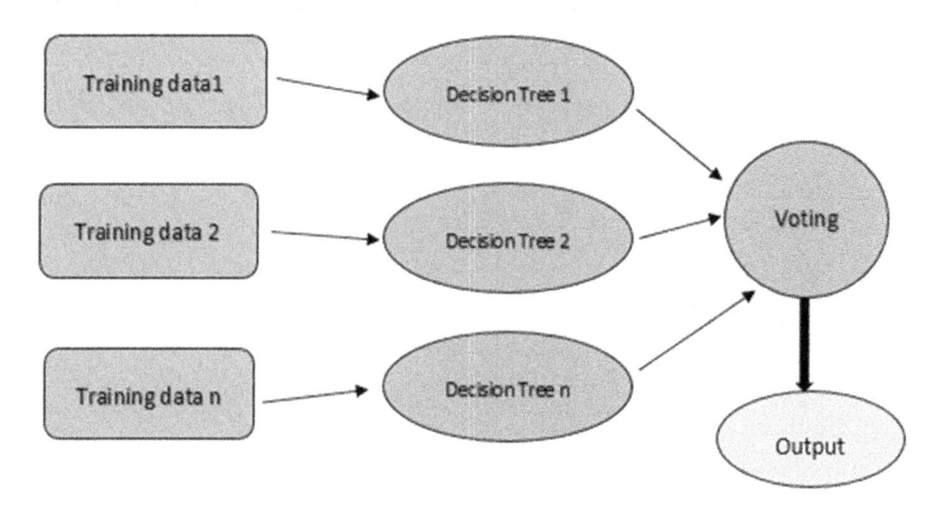

FIGURE 1.7 Random forest tree.

Based on the idea of ensemble learning, random forest is another supervised learning algorithm that is used for both classification and regression. It is a process of combining multiple classifiers to solve a complex problem and to improve the performance of the model [27–30].

To understand random forest, one must know the basics of decision trees [31]. As depicted in Figure 1.7, random forest takes into account the prediction from each tree and based on the voting makes a final prediction. Accuracy of this method of supervised learning is directly proportional to a number of decision trees. Gradient boosting is the process of enhancing any supervised algorithm.

1.4.2 Unsupervised Learning

In the unsupervised learning technique, models are not supervised [32]. They are not provided with any training data set. Alternatively, models itself identify the hidden patterns and trends from the given data. Unsupervised learning is particularly important because in the real world we have unlabeled or unstructured data and it's important to categorize this data to gain more insights.

In a theoretical framework we may say that human learning is very much similar to an unsupervised learning technique. The unsupervised learning algorithm can be further categorized into two types of problems, as shown in Figure 1.8.

Finding association means trying to find relationships between variables, particularly in huge and complex data sets, association mapping is very critical. Association rule method which is used for finding the relationships between variables in the large database [33]. Clustering is a method that clusters similar objects together by finding common elements between the different data and arrange them as group or batch. The presence or absence of common elements in the data object also helps in categorizing of data and creating clusters [34–36]. There are different types of clustering that is exclusive, agglomerative, overlapping and probabilistic.

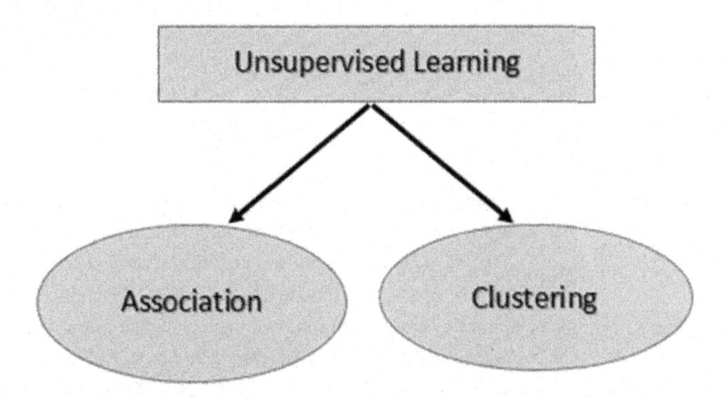

FIGURE 1.8 Unsupervised algorithm and its types.

1.4.2.1 Clustering Types

Under clustering, we have various clustering algorithms like KNN (k-nearest neighbors) [37], principle component analysis, hierarchal clustering and independent component analysis [38]. These are explained in Table 1.1.

1.5 UNDERSTANDING THE HEALTHCARE INDUSTRY

Machine learning has now found its place in almost all domains nowadays with the remarkable innovations seen over the past decade machine learning is well regarded as one of the most powerful tools that has the potential to change many prime areas and the way they function and one such fast-growing area is healthcare, which is a multi-faceted industry. The healthcare segment is estimated to reach $10 trillion by 2022 in terms of global investments. The healthcare sector [37], alternatively called the medical industry, which comprises of organizations that provide clinical services, diagnostic centers, disease prevention and outbreak control centers, drug discovery and manufacturing unit, pharmaceutical industry, medical equipment and medical toolkit providers, healthcare-related support services like care centers, rehabitation centers, along with patient centric provisions like medical insurance and personalized medicine and health plan [39,40].

The healthcare sector is a dynamic sector that is demonstrated in Figure 1.9 and shows how healthcare covers a wide spectrum of healthcare segments. These segments are prime areas ranging from primary-level healthcare to tertiary-level healthcare. Technology integration in each of these segment areas of healthcare stands as prime areas of potential transformation.

The driving force for such transformations is ongoing technological research and innovations, amalgamation of technology in medicine, need of more personalized medicine, need of fast and smart healthcare system and most importantly ever-growing population is a major driving force that places healthcare as a basic necessity for living. Such a digitized healthcare system will aim for improved diagnostic measures, better care and medical facilities, optimal operational cost and wider outreach to general public.

TABLE 1.1
Clustering Algorithms

Type	Detail
Hierarchical clustering	Clustering hierarchy is an algorithm which constructs a cluster hierarchy. It starts with all the data allocated to its own cluster. Two clusters will be in the same cluster here. This algorithm stops if only one cluster remains.
K-means clustering	K implies that it's an iterative algorithm that allows us to find the highest value for each iteration. The number of clusters you want are picked initially. You need to classify the data points into groups of k in this clustering process. A larger K is similar to smaller classes with greater granularity. A lower k refers to larger classes of less size. The algorithm output is a "label" category. It gives one of the k groups data point. Each group is identified by having a center for each group in k-means clustering. The centers are like the center of the cluster, where the nearest points are captured and added to it. K-means clustering further defines two subgroups: Agglomerative clustering and dendrogram.
K-NN (k nearest neighbors)	Also known as "lazy learner algorithm" It is one of the easiest supervised learning algorithms that does not learn from the training set. Rather, it stores the data set and afterwards, it assigns new data to categories that are almost the same. It basically works by identifying similarity and this non-parametric algorithm does not require any assumptions on the data. K-nearest neighbor can be used for regression problems, but it is mostly used for classification problems.
Principal component analysis	Principal computer analysis, or PCA, is a dimension-reduction technique that mostly reduces large data sets' dimensionality by turning a large number of variables into a smaller one with the most details still in the large range. In this a little compromise on accuracy is traded off in order to achieve simple data set.

1.6 APPLICATIONS OF ML IN HEALTHCARE

1.6.1 Machine Learning in Prognosis

Prognosis is a method of determining the expectancy of disease prior to its occurrence. Prognosis aids in identifying the symptoms and determining whether the symptoms are going to get better, stay mild or worse with respect to the disease progression. It adds to having clarity, whether the person affected will be able to cope up with respect to day-to-day activity. Prognosis stands as a prime factor in medical support, since it paves way for giving a serious attention towards the health aspects of person affected majorly because it gives risk assessment, prediction of complex issues that may arise, survival rate and relapse or reoccurrence of the disease.

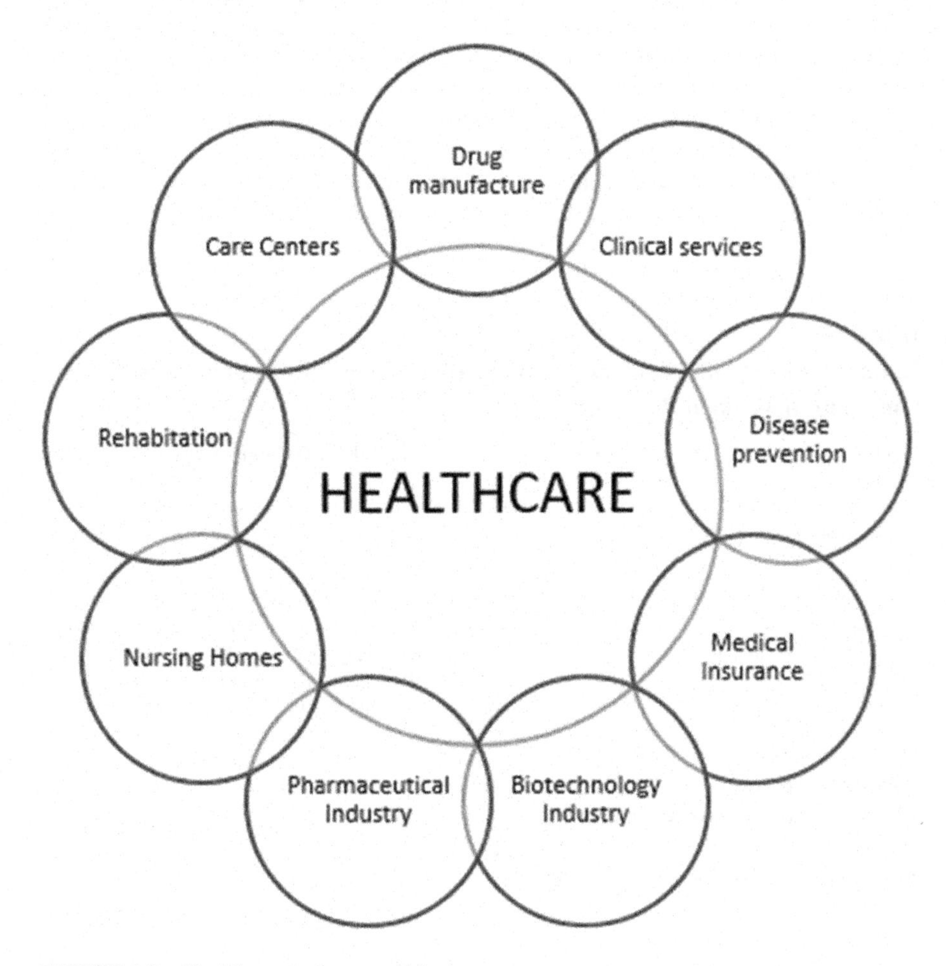

FIGURE 1.9 Healthcare industry and its segments.

For ease of understanding, the mentioned points can be stated as key parameters of prognosis:

1. Survival chances
2. Medical treatment sensitivity
3. Disease progression
4. Expected life/years prediction

In this regard, patient health data [41] plays a major role that can be used by the machine learning models in prognosis. Data collected for such modelling comes from various sources, like epidemiological, genomic (DNA sequencing, micro-arrays), histological, proteomic (protein chips, tissue arrays, immuno-histology), phenotypic, medical images (fMRI, PET, micro-CT), laboratory results or a combination of any of these, etc. Machine learning models such as artificial neural networks, fuzzy logic, genetic algorithm, support vector machine and other hybrid techniques have been largely used for one of the most deadly diseases, cancer, in which prognosis can be a lifesaving line of action (Table 1.2).

Many of these machine learning models are extensively deployed for determining and differentiating between various forms of cancers like lung, throat, melanoma skin, breast cancer, etc. [42–45]. Most of the research and application of machine learning methods work in three lines for cancer prognosis (Figure 1.10):

TABLE 1.2
Summary of Various Machine Learning Techniques and Applications Which Can Help in Medical Prognosis

Prognosis	Algorithms/Techniques Used
In cancer prognosis and prediction (lung, throat, oral, breast, skin)	Artificial neural networks (ANNs), Bayesian networks (BNs), support vector machines (SVMs) and decision trees (DTs)
Prognosis of the femoral neck fracture recovery	K-nearest neighbors algorithm, the semi-Naive Bayesian classifier, back propagation, linear regression, logistic regression, k-nearest neighbor (k-NN), support vector machine (SVM), random forest (RF), and natural language processing (NLP)
Prognosis in dermatology	
Prognosis of congenital heart disease	
Prognosis of type II diabetes	
Prognosis of Alzheimer's disease	
Severe dengue prognosis	
Prognosis of functional recovery in acute stroke	
Prognosis rate of kidney disease	

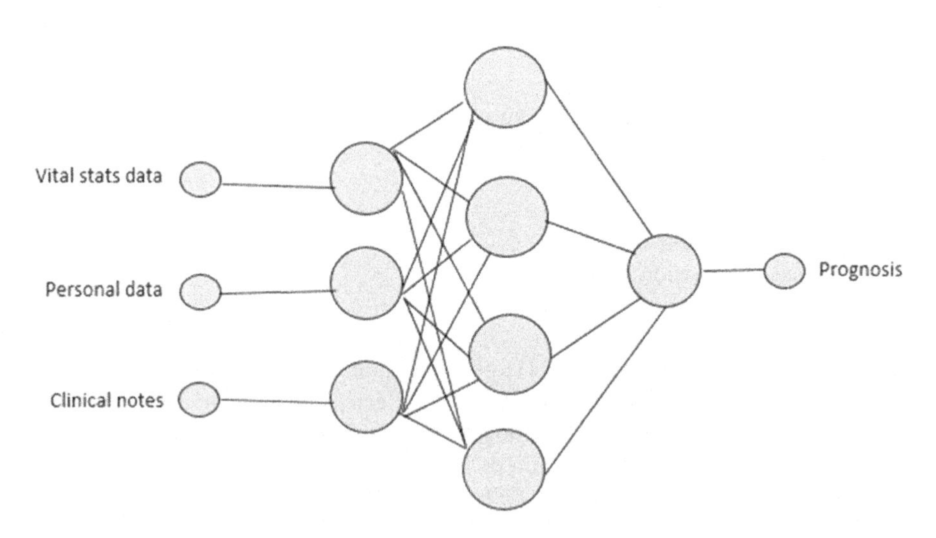

FIGURE 1.10 Medical prognosis using neural network.

1. Cancer prediction
2. Survival risk assessment
3. Cancer remission/reoccurrence

Below are the three basic steps that depict how to build and deploy a neural network for medical prognosis.

Step 1 is to generate a data set by accumulating all the data regarding all the major parameters related to the disease that may cover all the attributes like individual data, environmental data, health statistics and comorbidity data. Step 2 is to build a neural network that will help predict the outcome of new patients. The next graph illustrates a neural network for medical prognosis. Step 3 is to apply a training strategy to the neural network to find out the relationships between the variables or data set. With an aim to refine the prediction level of the model, we may also reiterate the model selection by selecting varied altered combinations of data, which is termed multi-modal data set. In the end, the model is tested and future full deployment of the model depends on the testing results, which finally helps in medical prognosis.

1.6.2 Machine Learning in Diagnosis

Diagnosis is a process that is a basic requirement for medical and clinical systems. It forms the very base of healthcare systems [46]. With correct and effective diagnosis, appropriate treatment can be planned, care and support functionalities can be provided and most importantly immediate treatment plan can be laid to curtail further damage. The additional enhancement and improved techniques in diagnostic testing and imaging has resulted in efficient diagnosis. However, the diagnosis based on knowledge by human scientific methods still stand remarkable and efficient over high-end technical expertise. Although a lot of human error in diagnosis have proved extremely dangerous and in some cases fatal in various incidences recorded worldwide. Such errors are a result of misjudged intuitive and to some extent it's caused due to gross mishandling of systems. Adjoining parameters like negligence in observatory span, involve misjudging the seriousness of given situation or medical complication, error in the considered hypothesis and general factors like wrong input, or miscalculations as well [47–49].

In such circumstances, machine learning stands out and outshines the conventional human expertise for diagnosis by providing what we call "intelligent data analysis". Today's healthcare facilities and clinics are having appropriate infrastructure and setups for data collection and surveillance compiled with large data management systems. This medical data set with diagnostic features is extremely valuable, since machine learning can utilize such massive data and predict trends and patterns and also analyses other correlated aliments. This data set of a patient's diagnosis can invariably be utilized in infinite ways for smart healthcare solutions. Figure 1.11 gives a brief pictorial representation of how clinical data can be used to produce a diagnostic model in the field of healthcare using machine learning techniques.

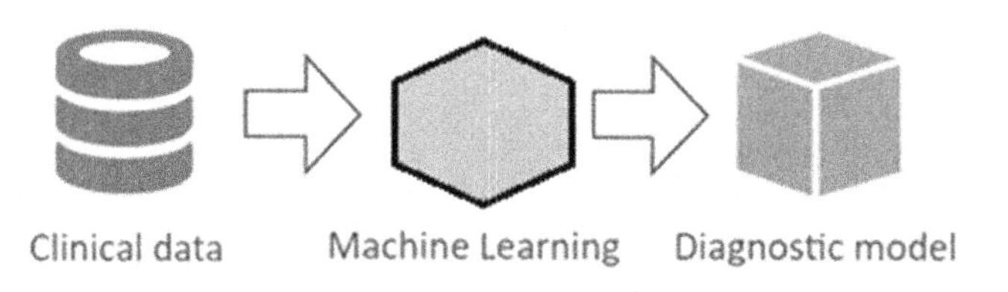

FIGURE 1.11 Machine learning for medical diagnosis.

Below are some of the various areas where machine learning techniques are used for diagnosis.

ONCOLOGY: The role of identifying a malignant tumor on time is critical in oncology. This is why, in this area, diagnostic accuracy and precision are critical. Oncologists can use machine learning to diagnose cancer in the early stages. Medical practitioners can reliably diagnose somatic mutations using techniques such as deep gene; in parallel to locating the tumor, machine learning can assess whether it is malignant or benign in milliseconds. While computer-based forecasts are not fault, recognition rate is remarkable at 88 percent.

CHRONIC HEALTH ISSUES: Chronic disease like certain skin conditions like psoriasis, rheumatoid arthritis, cardiovascular disease as heart attacks and brain stroke, diabetes and depression are diseases that affect the patient for a long time and requires lifelong treatment. Machine learning classification algorithms like random forest, decision trees and support vector machines have been widely used for diagnosis of these chronic diseases.

DERMATALOGY: Machine learning is used in dermatology to enhance clinical decision-making to ensure the skin condition assessments are accurate. Use of machine learning in this area will mitigate the needless biopsies that dermatologists must perform on patients. Machine learning can be used to further map the growth and improvements in skin moles, allowing for early detection of pathological conditions. Biomarkers for acne, nail fungus and seborrhea dermatitis and many other chronic skin conditions like psoriasis can also be identified using algorithms and also the growth and improvements in skin moles can also be traced, allowing for early detection of pathological conditions.

PATHALOGY: Given the global scarcity of pathologists, there is a strong case to be made for using machine learning to advance in this area. Pathology is therefore highly profitable for artificial intelligence deployment due to the need to process massive data sets. Here are some of the most promising applications of machine learning in medical diagnosis. Using automatic tissue and cell quantification to improve the accuracy of blood and culture analysis. On a diagnostic slide, mapping disease cells and highlighting areas is a concern with the creation of tumor management frameworks.We can increase the speed of profile scanning to improve the efficiency of healthcare professionals.

Psychological Issues/Illness: Psychological health issues are historically one of the most expensive diseases psychiatric illness if left untreated leads to severe consequences not only on individuals but on society at large. Machine learning offers a variety of solution for preliminary diagnosis of such disorders like bipolar disorder, and anxiety or other personality disorders. Machine learning offers

TABLE 1.3
Machine Learning Algorithms and Its Comparative Analysis for Diagnosis

Algorithm	Comparative Details
Support Vector Machine	SVMs are disease specific and needs alteration to be applicable for different diseases.
Decision Trees	Difficult to imply and takes a lot of time.
Naïve Bayes	Has shown excellent results with better accuracy.
Random Forest	RF has shown good results.
Back Propogation	Hidden units are already declared and time complexity is an issue.
Logistic Regression	Time consuming and recursive process.
Clustering	Accuracy is a problem for variety of disease.

chatbots and online counsellors or therapists and on a broad level help in prevention of mental illness through the creation of machine learning technologies that assist high-risk groups which showcase triggers like social alienation or suicidal history [50–52]. Table 1.3 given below gives a comparative details of the different machine learning algorithms used for diagnosis.

With the new age transformations in the medical treatment and flexible medical plans and services such wrong diagnosis can be identified and the better treatment possible for curable to incurable diseases and health issues [53]. Such errors can be reduced and cut down sharply with machine learning techniques and aid in better and efficient medical support and clinical interventions. Machine learning can provide better health analytics and can utilize clinical data in the most superlative order that paves the way to better medical support.

Machine learning has crafted a path and made the once seemingly impossible task like "creation of systems which learn and grown on their own" possible. Such techniques along with the 21st century cutting-edge technological advancements in the emerging fields like Internet of Things (IoT) [54,55], big data, biometrics [56], deep learning [57], block chain [58–60], etc. have given rise to trade services that cash in on such data and create products that are re-defining the healthcare and medical industry. One such unit of smart healthcare is electronic health records (EHRs).

1.6.3 Electronic Health Records

According to the National Coordinator for Health Information Technology (ONC) "Electronic health record (EHR) is a real-time, patient-centered record that makes information available instantly and securely to authorized users". An EHR comprises health-related data as well as medical history of the patient, and in other words can be visualized as a digital format of patient health card. The various elements of an EHR is shown in Figure 1.12. As non-eccentric as it may seem, EHR encapsulates a broader spectrum of data about patients that come from pharmacy, insurer, care provider data, vital signs and data from the patient's past history along

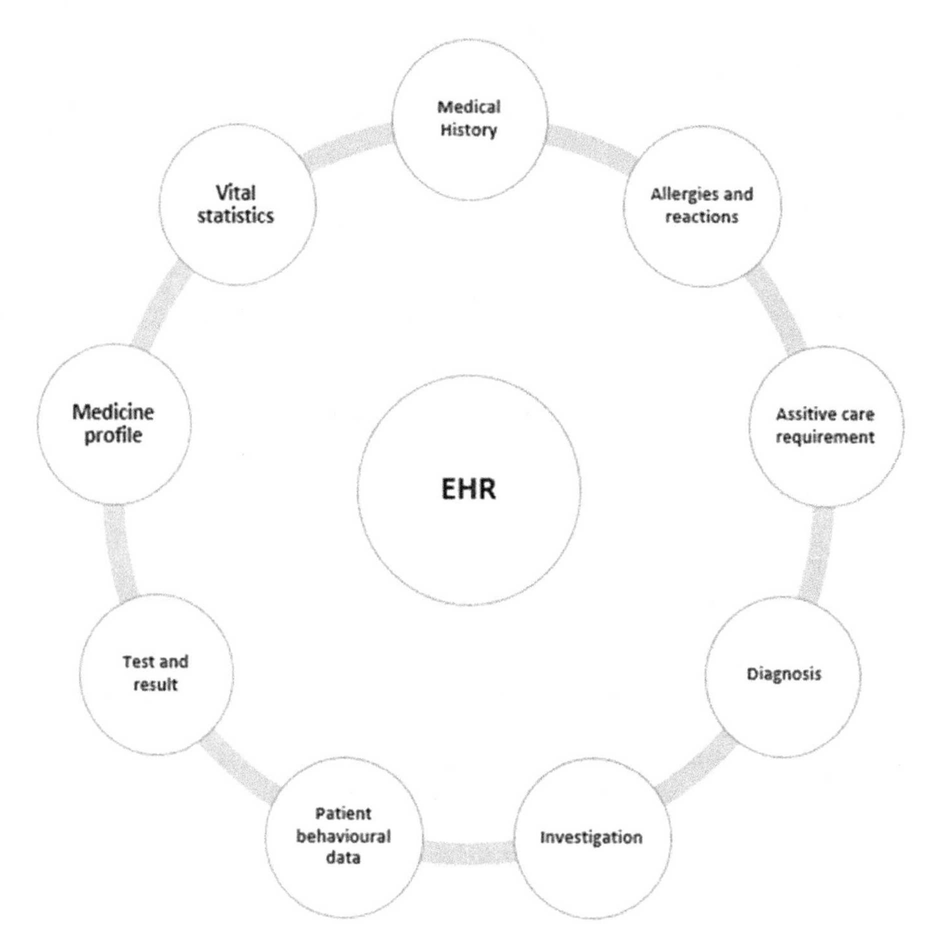

FIGURE 1.12 Electronic health record data.

with clinical data about test and diagnosis, drug dosage, treatment plans, radiological images, and variety of health insights [61–64].

Around the globe, the usage and maintenance of electronic health records (EHRs) is growing majorly because of the IT Act and government reformative policies and laws. Complete health records of patients are maintained by many medical centers and hospitals and such as huge databases create the electronic health records (EHRs) on a regular basis. Such a database consists of raw as well as refined data. Many developed and developing countries like the United States of America (USA), Canada, United Kingdom, and gulf countries like United Arab Emirates, etc. have invested to a great extent in digitization of healthcare units in their country. The law enforcement and many other fiscal medical policies have made maintaining electronic health records a customary thing. The core objective of such law enforcement is to act as a catalyst to the adoption of digital methods to hold, share and communicate as well as reuse this electronic medical data of patients and proliferate it further in using it for many different medical objectives.

The Indian government has also strongly advocated the adoption of electronic health records and it came up with the Electronic Health Record Standards of India (EHRSI) that emphasizes the creation and maintenance of uniform EHRs across India.

Such detailed EHRs also prove to be an excellent tool for one stop point for information about a patient and aid primarily in the decision-making process to medical practitioners and physicians towards the course of treatment. This adds extensively to relax the decision-making process with respect to the amount of critical care procedures to be taken into consideration that also means a personalized approach is touched upon due to the very existence of EHRs.

EHRs also make it easy for the care providers and medical experts to align the treatment that is to be time tracked and makes it easier to set key alarms and safeguard the treatment strategy to yield better results with the help of the 24 into 7 reminders provision. Such reminders certainly help further in subsiding the human error chances and aid in systematic interventions. Another facet of EHRs is the interoperability between second-party caregivers like pharmaceuticals, insurers and assistive healthcare staff.

Such a wide range of data provided by EHRs not only improve the healthcare efficiency but also have found its place in numerous clinical data applications such as disease tracking, feature extraction and disease projection evaluation.

1.6.3.1 Electronic Health Records and Machine Learning

Since EHRs encompass massive amounts of data, they can be used to train models and identify patterns and generate new parameters that may help in decision making and prediction. Machine learning algorithms like supervised, semi-supervised and unsupervised are used with EHR data. Support vector machine (SVM) algorithms are used for various bifurcation requirements based on clinical data of patients such as identifying smoking status and predicting further answers related to life quality in the future. EHR data was used to identify which patients are most at risk for post-hospitalization veno-thromboembolism (VTE) [65] [66]. In this study, which was conducted on a set of patients, their medical health history data was extracted from EHRs and machine learning methods were used to get a classification of patients as per a different level of risk like high risk, low risk and susceptible. In the field of radiation oncology, the machine learning model has been used to predict recurrence patterns after intensity modulated radiotherapy (IMRT) for nasopharyngeal cancer. Prediction of diabetes using EHR data has been done [67]. ML has been used to predict which patients are more prone to chronic diseases like psoriasis [68] and other autoimmune diseases.

1.6.4 Applications of ML in Medical Image Analysis

A systematic process in many of the medical interventions for a variety of disease and aliments calls for taking in consideration the help and utilization of medical imaging. Various internal organs that might be deeply affected due to an underlying health issue needs to be examined and this is where medical imaging becomes such a remarkable gamechanger. It totally eliminates the requirement of open surgery and complex procedures and saves so much time and effort to help in prognosis, diagnosis and several other clinical interventions. It indirectly reduces a lot of risk that comes along with any simple or complex surgery that ranges from risk of infection, heart failure or even paralytic stroke.

However, it also brings in a lot of need for physicians, radiologists and pathologists and other diagnostic experts to be well trained. Many cases of human error, negligence and careless interpretations of medical image data have resulted in wrong diagnosis and also to a great extent affected the prognosis process. Not only the manual analysis of medical images and interpretations is costly, takes time and is prone to be incorrect but it hinders the purpose of quality healthcare with repeated errors.

In the healthcare sector, medical images come from a variety of sources such as positron emission tomography (PET), imaging (MRI), computed tomography (CT), images from ultrasound and X-rays, etc. These sets of different medical image sources provide valuable and extremely important data about patient and its various organs and body parts that is affected due to an ailing disease. Such medical images are very important and careful and in-depth analysis of them may open a doorway to various sets of data that can further aid in disease management and control. Most importantly for both prognosis and diagnosis, medical image analysis is a critical process in a majority of health issues.

Medical image analysis [69] is a stream in itself which in amalgamation of advanced computational techniques is crafting its way towards automated and intelligent medical image processing and diagnosis system. The most prominent tasks in medical image analysis include image identification, image detection, classification, segmentation, retrieval, reconstruction and image registration, as shown in Figure 1.13.

Image enhancement and identification is the process in which medical images are studied carefully to find out the pattern and abnormality that was mostly manually examined by physicians; however, such examination may majorly have false identifications due to image error or in other case minute abnormality or changes in pattern may go unnoticed even by expert physicians. In such a scenario, machine learning may add an extra edge to identify patterns easily with a trained model. Image segmentation is the process in which the digital or gray-scale image is segmented into different units or image objects. This way the segmented image objects are created, which are easier and more meaningful to analyses. Feature extraction [70] in medical imaging is a process that works for dimensionality reduction, which has the prime objective to take out maximum information from an image and represent it in a small dimensionality. Image classification helps in categorizing the images as per the given set of unstructured data finding commonality between them.

Machine learning techniques like deep learning (DL) and artificial neural networks (ANNs) are used for classifying medical image data. Medical images often are prone to degradation that are due to noise or environmental disturbances that get added during the manual recording process of them. Such noisy and outlier data if taken into consideration for medical analysis is prone to give incorrect prognosis or

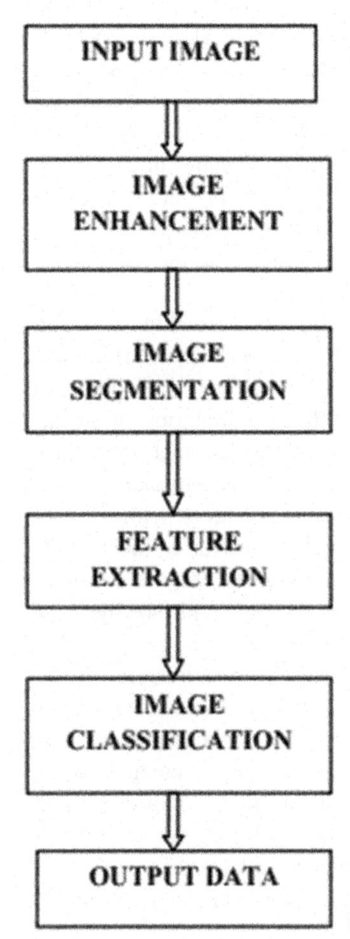

FIGURE 1.13 Medical image processing.

diagnosis, which may ruin the overall purpose of proving medical support in the first place. Hence, enhancing the images and removing the noise is extremely important. Many machine learning and deep learning methods are often used for removing the noise and upgrade the images such as convolutional denoising auto encoders.

1.6.5 Machine Learning in Natural Language Processing of Medical Documents and Literature

As discussed in the previous section about electronic health records, one key findings of some of the recent research is that we do have mandates and laws to maintain electronic health records but we are failing big time in setting up the infrastructure to maintain the ever-growing number of records, which are due to the huge volumes of data generated each day in the healthcare units and increasing number of patients.

Getting these huge volumes of data streamlined and using it to align the medical efficiency and meet the demand requirement of health is the need of the hour. However, the currently existing physical set of documents that are non-digitized prove to be a bottleneck in ensuring quality outcomes. Implementation of methods or human personnel to transfer these physical data into digital format can take many hours and will be a cumbersome process. Machine learning can play a vital role to eliminate these issues by the application of natural language processing (NLP), which is a sub-branch of artificial intelligence that is concerned with the computer's ability to understand text and spoken words.

By scanning EHR documents, and extracting readable data from the text and applying image processing techniques to spot key words can help in churning out very important data that can be added to the database. Similarly, all the medial data recorded in terms of clinical notes and patient past history in terms of health symptoms, doctor's findings or notes can be annotated. However, such extraction of data can be difficult if the data has not been articulated appropriately or has misspelt words that may lose their essence. Hence, a formal document with written-on details may be helpful to maintain the required documents instead of loose notes or handwritten rough data. NLP along with machine learning techniques can help in curating a patient-centric clinical decision support system with the help of preexisting records.

In a recent study an NLP-based algorithm efficiently helped in determining and finding the severity of aortic stenosis from semi-structured and unstructured echocardiogram reports taken from electronic health records' data. The study further supports the potential value of NLP to enhance quality improvement and research efforts for this condition. In another application of NLP, a paper claimed accurate mapping of the onset of psychosis in youth based on the recorded interview conducted with them, over a span of 2.5 years. Similarly, NLPs have been successfully identified at the onset of cancer from the clinical notes and history of a patient extracted from electronic health records.

Doctors' notes and annotated medical documents have become immensely important as a way of communicating complex information and insights for patient's healthcare and their database. Analysis of such data is complex because of the variability and incompleteness of knowledge retrieval at higher levels of generality. Machine learning is starting to produce important effects in conducting these dynamic analyses [71].

These natural language processing (NLP) techniques possess the potential to transform the unstructured data, unstructured healthcare information, evaluate the grammatical aspect, find out the meaning and reuse this important extracted information in the medical record. Such techniques aid in reducing not only the time to refine data but also increase the efficiency of healthcare systems.

1.6.6 Machine Learning and Pandemic Combatting

Pandemics [72] are known to have existed right from 430 BC and the current century that is still witnessing the crippling effect of one such deadly pandemic, COVID-19, which has already affected over 270 million people worldwide.

In the past, pandemics such as Middle East Respiratory Syndrome (MERS), Swine flu, ZIKA, EBOLA, SARS (severe acute respiratory syndrome), etc. have caused severe impact on economy, infrastructure, failure or overburdening of healthcare, partial and total shutdown or lockdown of regions affecting people and general way of living [73]. The existence and such pandemic over the years outlines the importance that science and technology have to gear up for preparing against the outbreak of such infectious disease and a strong public health surveillance system should be set up to combat against all the major ill effects that come due to the onset of such pandemics. Scientists and researchers are progressively applying and exploring the potential of artificial intelligence (AI), natural language processing (NLP) and machine learning for understanding the onset, spread and ways to contain such infectious disease.

At the hindsight, the healthcare sector is well aware of where the answers lie; it lies in 'data' that is central and is most important to come up with viable technological solutions to combat pandemics [74]. Also before the occurrence and rapid spread of an epidemic into global pandemic, various measures are needed to be put in place for counter-control of such sporadic spread. This also places a lot of importance on understanding the effect and control process of pandemic. The flow diagram showcases the key states that occur once the outbreak of any pandemic happens (Figure 1.14).

From the pandemic outbreak control model given in Figure 1.13, it can be understood that we need two most concrete solutions when it comes to a pandemic:

1. Pandemic detection/prediction model (pre-pandemic)
2. Pandemic control model (after pandemic)

1.6.7 Applications of ML in Pandemic Predictions

The electronic health records of the mass public can be examined for finding changes in the structure or detect abnormality. In most of the infectious diseases and past pandemic, changes in computed tomography (CT) scan and X-ray images [75] were noted. These data can aid in early detection and help in alarming the public surveillance systems about a possible outbreak. Thus, the machine learning algorithm coupled with medical image analysis can help in identifying the underlying risk [76,77].

An interesting path-breaking link to emergence of infectious diseases is the changes in the global temperatures recorded in recent years. Such climatic abruptions resulting from elevated temperatures and precipitation have been linked to the spread of infectious disease. It has been found that the disease-carrying vectors that play a key role in disease transmission and from animal chain to human have been affected [78]. This, along with rising population and enhanced mobility by humans, have contributed adversely to the rise and spread of infectious diseases [79].

Another effective way for aiding in setting out early warning signs to the general public of a possible outbreak is by analyzing the massive amounts of open-source data available over the internet, social media feeds and news, which

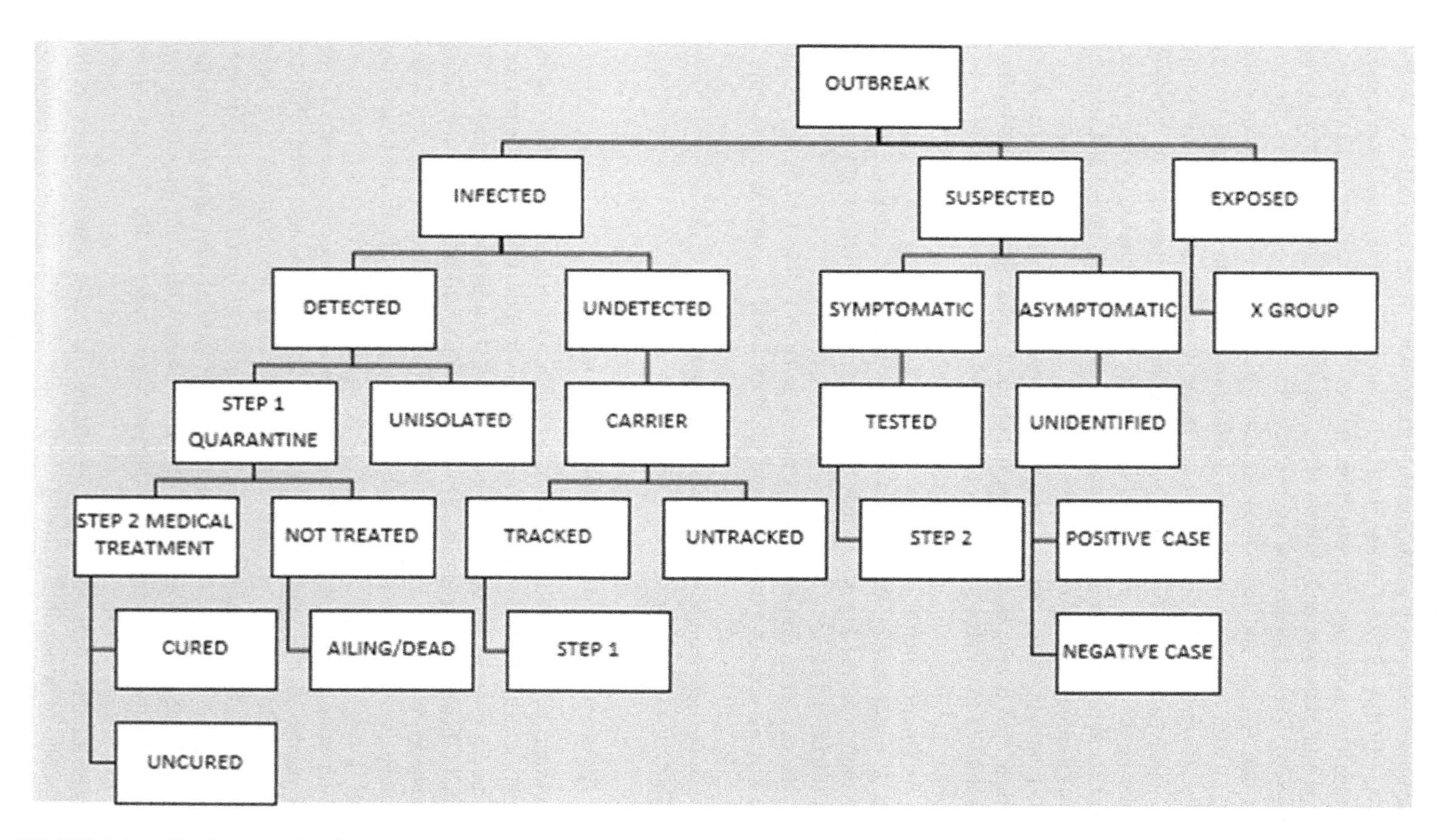

FIGURE 1.14 Pandemic outbreak control model depicting various stages.

tends to be unstructured. This is termed an event-based surveillance system (EBS) [80]. Machine learning algorithms, along with natural language processors, can be used to analyze this exuberant amount of unstructured data and classify them to generate a data model. Further using systematic algorithms can identify set triggers that in turn can help to predict the outbreak.

Over the years, conventional machine learning algorithms like auto-regressive integrated moving average model (ARIMA) and generalized autoregressive conditional heteroscedasticity (GARCH) [81] have been deployed to project the time of a pandemic outbreak; however, new and efficient algorithms such as long short term memory (LSTM) have been clearly outcasted in terms of efficiency of the generic approach.

1.6.8 Applications of ML in Pandemic Controls

After the spread and outbreak of the pandemic, machine learning can aid in a wide range of control applications like tracking affected individuals, aiding in the quarantine process by contact tracing, identifying the high-risk patients and aiding in medical treatment of affected and suspected untracked individuals. It may also help in identifying the people who need immediate medical support and further contribute in allocating medical resources to those who are in acute need. This can majorly relieve the burden from healthcare and medical support sector and add on to streamline the services. Machine learning applications for drug discovery is also a prime area for pandemic management and control. Also, contact tracing of affected individuals and identification of areas with a surge in the number of positive cases is important.

In the current scenario, the PCR-polymerase chain reaction test is the most widely used for identifying the presence of the COVID strain. Apart from being expensive and time consuming, the PCR tests are increasingly stated to have given false positive and negative results, as per the surge in recorded cases of faulty diagnosis via PCR. This is majorly due to the insufficient measure via sample collection, sample handling and low-quality measures that have given rise to the need of alternative approaches for such mass testing. Machine learning techniques that are used over X-ray and CT scans are widely being explored. Recently, a convolutional neural network model was devised by using CT scan images to differentiate between COVID and pneumonia. A wide range of machine learning models that have shown upscale performances for diagnosis of infection have been practically applied in various research. These models are SVM, CNN, RNN, transfer learning, XGBoost and others [82–84].

In spite of the upscale results, the general applicability of these models is still a big issue owing to low precision and limited applicability. Machine learning techniques are especially useful because they provide a range of tools to enhance the process of drug discovery and development for specific contexts, using accurate and high-quality information. As result, a considerable attempt has been made to implement pharmacological AI/ML solutions. Similar machine learning techniques are applied to find out the mortality risk in patients who are affected by the pandemic.

1.7 CONCLUSION

Machine learning in healthcare has a very key role to play and has promising and exciting innovations and trend generation potential for the future. From disease prognosis, outbreak prediction and diagnosis to drafting medical plans, machine learning has an answer for all aspects of healthcare issues provided accurate machine learning models are generated and that depends on a lot of data and its accuracy. Emerging technological advances like the Internet of Things (IoT), big data, data science, data mining and other technical aspects from the streams of biology and computer science have created room for providing power to boost more research and accelerate the scientific studies rate. Such complex and interoperable intelligent systems with a massive wealth of data sets are pioneers to bring in change in the healthcare sector. Precision medicine and individualized medical plans are paving the way to precision medicine. As much as machine learning aids in creating and envisioning smart and intelligent healthcare system [85], there do lie many ethical and other important considerations to make it a practical, viable system. Predictive modelling on electronic health records and using this data for further medical care and treatment will also be helpful to avoid human errors and such steps will also aid in saving finances and valuable time.

Medical image analysis has already uprooted the need of performing surgeries and convenient evaluation of the internal bod parts is now possible. Machine learning has now been effectively used for pandemic combatting and its general ability to detect patterns remains open to be applicable in variety of provisions like chat bots, drug discovery for pandemic prevention, tracking and monitoring of ailing patients, ensuring quarantine facility. The application of natural language processing (NLP) [86] has also brought the possibility of retrieving data from medical EHRs and other audio or text bases data to be processed into valuable information. The healthcare sector is already experiencing a revolutionary change [87] in all segments and machine learning has proved its mettle to be a gamechanger.

However, with all the upsurge in research and application of machine learning in the healthcare sector, many concerns like reliability of the developed applications and their practical use in clinical settings is still a major bottleneck. The data set used for training the models, which is highly unstructured and non-linear, pose another concern. Also, a major question also comprises the accuracy and results but also on the legal, technical and ethical concerns with respect to the data used in various machine learning applications in the first place [88,89].

REFERENCES

[1] Witten Ian and Frank Eibe. Data mining: practical machine learning tools and techniques Morgan Kaufmann (2005).

[2] Bishop Christopher M. *Pattern recognition and machine learning*. Springer, New York, (2006).

[3] Mitchell Tom M. The discipline of machine learning: Carnegie Mellon University. Carnegie Mellon University, School of Computer Science, Machine Learning Department (2006).

[4] Dean Jeff, Patterson David, and Young Cliff. "A new golden age in computer architecture: Empowering the machine-learning revolution." *IEEE Micro* 38, no. 2 (2018): 21–29.

[5] Murdoch W. James, Singh Chandan, Kumbier Karl, Abbasi-Asl Reza, and Yu Bin. "Definitions, methods, and applications in interpretable machine learning." *Proceedings of the National Academy of Sciences* 116, no. 44 (2019): 22071–22080.

[6] Carleo, Giuseppe, Cirac Ignacio, Cranmer Kyle, Daudet Laurent, Schuld Maria, Tishby Naftali, Vogt-Maranto Leslie, and Zdeborová Lenka. "Machine learning and the physical sciences." *Reviews of Modern Physics* 91, no. 4 (2019): 045002.

[7] Simeone, Osvaldo. "A very brief introduction to machine learning with applications to communication systems." *IEEE Transactions on Cognitive Communications and Networking* 4, no. 4 (2018): 648–664.

[8] Alpaydin, Ethem. *Introduction to machine learning*. MIT press, (2020).

[9] Kersting, Kristian. "Machine learning and artificial intelligence: two fellow travelers on the quest for intelligent behavior in machines." *Frontiers in big data* 1 (2018): 6.

[10] Bzdok, Danilo, Altman Naomi, and Krzywinski Martin. "Points of significance: statistics versus machine learning." (2018): 233–234. https://doi.org/10.1038/nmeth.4642

[11] Van Calster, Ben. "Statistics versus machine learning: definitions are interesting (but understanding, methodology, and reporting are more important)." *Journal of Clinical Epidemiology* 116 (2019): 137.

[12] Sra, Suvrit. "Directional statistics in machine learning: A brief review." *Applied Directional Statistics: Modern Methods and Case Studies* 225 (2018): 1–12.

[13] Dangeti, Pratap. *Statistics for machine learning*. Packt Publishing Ltd, 2017.

[14] Qin, S. Joe, and Chiang Leo H. "Advances and opportunities in machine learning for process data analytics." *Computers & Chemical Engineering* 126 (2019): 465–473.

[15] Zeadally, Sherali, and Tsikerdekis Michail. "Securing Internet of Things (IoT) with machine learning." *International Journal of Communication Systems* 33, no. 1 (2020): e4169.

[16] Grassia, Marco, De Domenico Manlio, and Mangioni Giuseppe. "Machine learning dismantling and early-warning signals of disintegration in complex systems." arXiv preprint arXiv: 2101.02453 (2021).

[17] Verma, Rajat, Nagar Vishal, and Mahapatra Satyasundara. "Introduction to supervised learning." *Data Analytics in Bioinformatics: A Machine Learning Perspective* 1, (2021): 1–34.

[18] Mali, Barasha, Yadav Chandrasekhar, and Kumar Santosh. "Supervised Learning-Based Classifiers in Healthcare Decision-Making." In Proceedings of International Conference on Computational Intelligence and Data Engineering, pp. 83–91. Springer, Singapore, 2021.

[19] Sen, Pratap Chandra, Hajra Mahimarnab, and Ghosh Mitadru. "Supervised classification algorithms in machine learning: A survey and review." In Emerging technology in modelling and graphics, pp. 99–111. Springer, Singapore, 2020.

[20] Osisanwo, F. Y., Akinsola J. E. T., Awodele O., Hinmikaiye J. O., Olakanmi O., and Akinjobi J. "Supervised machine learning algorithms: Classification and comparison." *International Journal of Computer Trends and Technology (IJCTT)* 48, no. 3 (2017): 128–138.

[21] Cicchetti, Domenic V. "Neural networks and diagnosis in the clinical laboratory: State of the art." *Clinical Chemistry* 38, no. 1 (1 January 1992): 9–10

[22] Huang, Shujun, Cai Nianguang, Pacheco Pedro Penzuti, Narrandes Shavira, Wang Yang, and Xu Wayne. "Applications of support vector machine (SVM) learning in cancer genomics." *Cancer Genomics-Proteomics* 15, no. 1 (2018): 41–51.

[23] Harimoorthy, Karthikeyan, and Thangavelu Menakadevi. "Multi-disease prediction model using improved SVM-radial bias technique in healthcare monitoring system." *Journal of Ambient Intelligence and Humanized Computing* 12, no. 3 (2021): 3715–3723.
[24] Manju, Bala, Athira V., and Rajendran Athul. "Efficient multi-level lung cancer prediction model using support vector machine classifier." In IOP Conference Series: Materials Science and Engineering, vol. 1012, no. 1, p. 012034. IOP Publishing, 2021.
[25] Menard, Scott. *Logistic regression: From introductory to advanced concepts and applications*. Sage, 2010.
[26] Pampel, Fred C. *Logistic regression: A primer*. Vol. 132. Sage publications, 2020.
[27] Biau, Gérard, and Scornet Erwan. "A random forest guided tour." *Test* 25, no. 2 (2016): 197–227.
[28] Ren, Shaoqing, Cao Xudong, Wei Yichen, and Sun Jian. "Global refinement of random forest." In Proceedings of the IEEE Conference on Computer Vision and Pattern Recognition, pp. 723–730. 2015.
[29] Qi, Yanjun. "Random forest for bioinformatics." In *Ensemble machine learning*, pp. 307–323. Springer, Boston, MA, 2012.
[30] Nicodemus, Kristin K., Malley James D., Strobl Carolin, and Ziegler Andreas. "The behaviour of random forest permutation-based variable importance measures under predictor correlation." *BMC Bioinformatics* 11, no. 1 (2010): 1–13.
[31] Song, Yan-Yan, and Ying Lu. "Decision tree methods: applications for classification and prediction." *Shanghai Archives of Psychiatry* 27, no. 2 (2015): 130.
[32] Sutskever, Ilya, Jozefowicz Rafal, Gregor Karol, Rezende Danilo, Lillicrap Tim, and Vinyals Oriol. "Towards principled unsupervised learning." arXiv preprint arXiv: 1511.06440 (2015).
[33] Koh Yun Sing, and Ravana Sri Devi. "Unsupervised rare pattern mining: A survey." *ACM Transactions on Knowledge Discovery from Data (TKDD)* 10, no. 4 (2016): 1–29.
[34] Hu, Wenjian, Singh Rajiv, R.P., and Scalettar Richard T. "Discovering phases, phase transitions, and crossovers through unsupervised machine learning: A critical examination." *Physical Review E* 95, no. 6 (2017): 062122.
[35] Sato, Yuki, Izui Kazuhiro, Yamada Takayuki, and Nishiwaki Shinji. "Data mining based on clustering and association rule analysis for knowledge discovery in multiobjective topology optimization." *Expert Systems with Applications* 119 (2019): 247–261.
[36] Venkatkumar, Iyer Aurobind, and Kondhol Shardaben Sanatkumar Jayantibhai. "Comparative study of data mining clustering algorithms." In 2016 International Conference on Data Science and Engineering (ICDSE), pp. 1–7. IEEE, 2016.
[37] Du, Mingjing, Ding Shifei, and Jia Hongjie. "Study on density peaks clustering based on k-nearest neighbors and principal component analysis." *Knowledge-Based Systems* 99 (2016): 135–145.
[38] Nordhausen, Klaus, and Oja Hannu. "Independent component analysis: A statistical perspective." *Wiley Interdisciplinary Reviews: Computational Statistics* 10, no. 5 (2018): e1440.
[39] Budrionis, Andrius, and Bellika Johan Gustav. "The learning healthcare system: where are we now? A systematic review." *Journal of Biomedical Informatics* 64 (2016): 87–92.
[40] Panch, Trishan, Szolovits Peter, and Atun Rifat. "Artificial intelligence, machine learning and health systems." *Journal of Global Health* 8, no. 2 (2018).
[41] Injadat, Mohammad Noor, Moubayed Abdallah, Nassif Ali Bou, and Shami Abdallah. "Machine learning towards intelligent systems: applications, challenges, and opportunities." *Artificial Intelligence Review* (2021): 1–50.

[42] Monaghan, Timothy, Manski-Nankervis Jo-Anne, and Canaway Rachel. "Big data or big risk: general practitioner, practice nurse and practice manager attitudes to providing de-identified patient health data from electronic medical records to researchers." *Australian Journal of Primary Health* 26, no. 6 (2021): 466–471.
[43] Ray, Susmita. "A survey on application of machine learning algorithms in cancer prediction and prognosis." In *Data Management, Analytics and Innovation*, pp. 349–361. Springer, Singapore, 2021.
[44] Lee, Changhee, Light Alexander, Alaa Ahmed, Thurtle David, van der Schaar Mihaela, and Gnanapragasam Vincent J. "Application of a novel machine learning framework for predicting non-metastatic prostate cancer-specific mortality in men using the Surveillance, Epidemiology, and End Results (SEER) database." *The Lancet Digital Health* 3, no. 3 (2021): e158–e165.
[45] Zhu, Wan, Xie Longxiang, Han Jianye, and Guo Xiangqian. "The application of deep learning in cancer prognosis prediction." *Cancers* 12, no. 3 (2020): 603.
[46] Balakumar, Ayshwarya, and Senthil S. "Machine learning is the future for lung cancer prognosis and prediction." In *Applications of Deep Learning and Big IoT on Personalized Healthcare Services*, pp. 176–196. IGI Global, Hershey, Pennsylvania, 2020.
[47] Saritas, Ismail, Ozkan Ilker Ali, and Sert Ibrahim Unal. "Prognosis of prostate cancer by artificial neural networks." *Expert Systems with Applications* 37, no. 9 (2010): 6646–6650.
[48] Chang, Siow-Wee, Abdul-Kareem Sameem, Merican Amir Feisal, and Zain Rosnah Binti. "Oral cancer prognosis based on clinicopathologic and genomic markers using a hybrid of feature selection and machine learning methods." *BMC Bioinformatics* 14, no. 1 (2013): 1–15.
[49] Richens, Jonathan G., Lee Ciarán M., and Johri Saurabh. "Improving the accuracy of medical diagnosis with causal machine learning." *Nature Communications* 11, no. 1 (2020): 1–9.
[50] Heinrichs, Bert, and Eickhoff Simon B. "Your evidence? Machine learning algorithms for medical diagnosis and prediction." *Human Brain Mapping* 41, no. 6 (2020): 1435–1444.
[51] Raval, Dhaval, Bhatt Dvijesh, Kumhar Malaram K., Parikh Vishal, and Vyas Daiwat. "Medical diagnosis system using machine learning." *International Journal of Computer Science & Communication* 7, no. 1 (2016): 177–182.
[52] Khamparia, Aditya, Singh Prakash Kumar, Rani Poonam, Samanta Debabrata, Khanna Ashish, and Bhushan Bharat. "An internet of health things-driven deep learning framework for detection and classification of skin cancer using transfer learning." *Transactions on Emerging Telecommunications Technologies* 32, (2020): e3963.
[53] Jussupow, Ekaterina, Spohrer Kai, Heinzl Armin, and Gawlitza Joshua. "Augmenting medical diagnosis decisions? An investigation into physicians' decision-making process with artificial intelligence." *Information Systems Research* (2021): 35–48.
[54] Goyal, Sukriti, Sharma Nikhil, Bhushan Bharat, Shankar Achyut, and Sagayam Martin. "Iot enabled technology in secured healthcare: applications, challenges and future directions." In *Cognitive Internet of Medical Things for Smart Healthcare*, pp. 25–48. Springer, Cham, 2021.
[55] Jindal, Mansi, Gupta Jatin, and Bhushan Bharat. "Machine learning methods for IoT and their Future Applications." In 2019 International Conference on Computing, Communication, and Intelligent Systems (ICCCIS), pp. 430–434. IEEE, Greater Noida, India, 2019.

[56] Sharma, Nikhil, Kaushik Ila, Bhushan Bharat, Gautam Siddharth, and Khamparia Aditya. "Applicability of WSN and biometric models in the field of healthcare." in *Deep Learning Strategies for Security Enhancement in Wireless Sensor Networks.* (Sagayam K. Martin, Bhushan Bharat, Diana Andrushia A., and Hugo Victor de Albuquerque C., eds.), 304–329. Hershey, PA: IGI Global, 2020. 10.4018/978-1-7998-5068-7.ch016

[57] Kumar S., Bhusan B., Singh D. and Choubey D. K., "Classification of diabetes using deep learning," 2020 International Conference on Communication and Signal Processing (ICCSP), 2020, pp. 0651–0655, 10.1109/ICCSP48568.2020.9182293.

[58] Patra, Sudhansu Shekhar, Jena Om Praksah, Kumar Gaurav, Pramanik Sreyashi, Misra Chinmaya, and Singh Kamakhya Narain. "Random forest algorithm in imbalance genomics classification." *Data Analytics in Bioinformatics: A Machine Learning Perspective* 1 (2021): 173–190.

[59] Panigrahi, Niranjan, Ayus Ishan, and Jena Om Prakash. "An expert system-based clinical decision support system for Hepatitis-B prediction & diagnosis." *Machine Learning for Healthcare Applications* 1 (2021): 57–75.

[60] Paramesha, K., H. L. Gururaj, and Om Prakash Jena. "Applications of machine learning in biomedical text processing and food industry." *Machine Learning for Healthcare Applications* 1 (2021): 151–167.

[61] Wong, Jenna, Horwitz Mara Murray, Zhou Li, and Toh Sengwee. "Using machine learning to identify health outcomes from electronic health record data." *Current Epidemiology Reports* 5, no. 4 (2018): 331–342.

[62] Adkins, Daniel E. "Machine learning and electronic health records: A paradigm shift." *The American Journal of Psychiatry* 174, no. 2 (2017): 93.

[63] Luz, Christian F., Vollmer Marcus, Decruyenaere Johan, Nijsten Maarten W., Glasner Corinna, and Sinha Bhanu. "Machine learning in infection management using routine electronic health records: tools, techniques, and reporting of future technologies." *Clinical Microbiology and Infection* 26, no. 10 (2020): 1291–1299. ISSN 1198-743X, https://doi.org/10.1016/j.cmi.2020.02.003

[64] Gianfrancesco, Milena A., Tamang Suzanne, Yazdany Jinoos, and Schmajuk Gabriela. "Potential biases in machine learning algorithms using electronic health record data." *JAMA Internal Medicine* 178, no. 11 (2018): 1544–1547.

[65] Khanna, Raman, and Auerbach Andrew D. "Automating venous thromboembolism risk calculation using electronic health record data upon hospital admission: the automated Padua Prediction Score." *Journal of Hospital Medicine* 12, no. 4 (2017).

[66] Tritschler, Tobias, Kraaijpoel Noémie, Le Gal Grégoire, and Wells Philip S. "Venous thromboembolism: Advances in diagnosis and treatment." *JAMA* 320, no. 15 (2018): 1583–1594.

[67] Li, Lin, Lee Chuang-Chung, Zhou Fang Liz, Molony Cliona, Doder Zoran, Zalmover Evgeny, Sharma Kristen, Juhaeri Juhaeri, and Wu Chuntao. "Performance assessment of different machine learning approaches in predicting diabetic ketoacidosis in adults with type 1 diabetes using electronic health records data." *Pharmacoepidemiology and Drug Safety* 30 (2021): 610–618.

[68] Eder, Lihi, Li Quan, Jerome Dana, Farrer Chandra, Yeung Jensen, and Rahman Proton. "The efficacy of genetic testing for early detection of psoriatic arthritis in patients with Psoriasis." (2021). 10.21203/rs.3.rs-147804/v1

[69] Shen, Dinggang, Wu Guorong, and Suk Heung-Il. "Deep learning in medical image analysis." *Annual Review of Biomedical Engineering* 19 (2017): 221–248.

[70] Nixon, Mark, and Aguado Alberto. *Feature extraction and image processing for computer vision.* Academic press, 2019.

[71] Morens, David M., Daszak Peter, Markel Howard, and Taubenberger Jeffery K. "Pandemic COVID-19 joins history's pandemic legion." *Mbio* 11, no. 3 (2020): e00812-20. 10.1128/mBio.00812-20

[72] Qiu, Wuqi, Rutherford Shannon, Mao A., and Chu Cordia. "The pandemic and its impacts." *Health, Culture and Society* 9 (2017): 1–11.

[73] Afshar, Parnian, Heidarian Shahin, Enshaei Nastaran, Naderkhani Farnoosh, Rafiee Moezedin Javad, Oikonomou Anastasia, Faranak Babaki Fard, Samimi Kaveh, Plataniotis Konstantinos N., and Mohammadi Arash. "COVID-CT-MD: COVID-19 Computed Tomography (CT) scan data set applicable in machine learning and deep learning." arXiv preprint arXiv: 2009.14623 (2020).

[74] Al-Karawi, Dhurgham, Al-Zaidi Shakir, Polus Nisreen, and Jassim Sabah. "Machine learning analysis of chest ct scan images as a complementary digital test of coronavirus (covid-19) patients." medRxiv (2020).

[75] Kadry, Seifedine, Rajinikanth Venkatesan, Rho Seungmin, Raja Nadaradjane Sri Madhava, Rao Vaddi Seshagiri, and Thanaraj Krishnan Palani. "Development of a machine-learning system to classify lung CT scan images into normal/covid-19 class." arXiv preprint arXiv: 2004.13122 (2020).

[76] Akhtar, Naveed, Nawaz Naveed, BiBi Sadaf, and Ahmad Muhammad. "Impact of climatic factors on viability of SARS-CoV-2 and transmission prospective of COVID-19: An overview." *Microbes and Infectious Diseases* 1, no. 3 (2020): 118–125.

[77] Carteni, Armando, Di Francesco Luigi, and Martino Maria. "How mobility habits influenced the spread of the COVID-19 pandemic: Results from the Italian case study." *Science of the Total Environment* 741 (2020): 140489.

[78] Balajee, S. Arunmozhi, Salyer Stephanie J., Greene-Cramer Blanche, Sadek Mahmoud, and Mounts Anthony W. "The practice of event-based surveillance: concept and methods." *Global Security: Health, Science and Policy* 6, no. 1 (2021): 1–9.

[79] Zhu, Wenbohao, Li Xiaofeng, and Sun Bo. "Research and Prediction on China's Novel Coronavirus (2019-nCoV/COVID-19) Epidemic—Based on Time Series ARIMA Model." *International Conference on Education, Management, Computer and Society (EMCS2020)*, pp 310–316.

[80] Barstugan, Mucahid, Ozkaya Umut, and Ozturk Saban. "Coronavirus (covid-19) classification using ct images by machine learning methods." arXiv preprint arXiv: 2003.09424 (2020).

[81] Aslan, Muhammet Fatih, Unlersen Muhammed Fahri, Sabanci Kadir, and Durdu Akif. "CNN-based transfer learning–BiLSTM network: A novel approach for COVID-19 infection detection." *Applied Soft Computing* 98 (2021): 106912.

[82] Islam, Md Milon, Islam Md Zabirul, Asraf Amanullah, and Ding Weiping. "Diagnosis of COVID-19 from X-rays using combined CNN-RNN architecture with transfer learning." medRxiv (2020).

[83] Suzuki, Yoshiro, and Suzuki Ayaka. "Machine learning model estimating number of COVID-19 infection cases over coming 24 days in every province of South Korea (XGBoost and MultiOutputRegressor)." medRxiv (2020).

[84] Baker, Stephanie B., Xiang Wei, and Atkinson Ian. "Internet of things for smart healthcare: Technologies, challenges, and opportunities." *IEEE Access* 5 (2017): 26521–26544.

[85] Yuvaraj, D., Ayoobkhan Mohamed Uvaze Ahamed, and Sivaram M. "A study on the role of natural language processing in the healthcare sector." *Materials Today: Proceedings* (2021). 10.1016/j.matpr.2021.02.080

[86] Ghosh, Ananya. "Artificial intelligence in bringing about a revolution in the healthcare industry." *BODHI International Journal of Research in Humanities, Arts and Science* 5, no. 1: 98.

[87] Zaouiat, C. E. Ait, and Latif A. "Internet of things and machine learning convergence: The e-healthcare revolution." In Proceedings of the 2nd International Conference on Computing and Wireless Communication Systems, pp. 1–5. (2017).
[88] Chen, Irene Y., Pierson Emma, Rose Sherri, Joshi Shalmali, Ferryman Kadija, and Ghassemi Marzyeh. "Ethical machine learning in health care." arXiv e-prints (2020): arXiv-2009.
[89] Char, Danton S., Shah Nigam H., and Magnus David. "Implementing machine learning in health care—addressing ethical challenges." *The New England Journal of Medicine* 378, no. 11 (2018): 981.

2 A Machine Learning Approach to Identify Personality Traits from Social Media

Arion Mitra, Ankita Biswas, Kanyaka Chakraborty, Ananya Ghosh, Namrata Das, and Nikita Ghosh
Department of Computer Science and Engineering, University of Calcutta, Kolkata, India

Ahona Ghosh
Department of Computer Science and Engineering, Maulana Abul Kalam Azad University of Technology, Kalyani, West Bengal, India

CONTENTS

DOI: 10.1201/9781003189053-2

2.1 INTRODUCTION

Social media plays an important role in the modern world. It is an online platform where people share contents such as images, videos, songs, logs, reviews, and so on. Social media over time has seen an exponential growth in the user base with almost everyone using some form of social media platform or the other. Through social media, people can easily express themselves to the whole world, which is impossible physically [1,2]. They enjoy the circumstances in which they can interact with other people without meeting the person physically [3], i.e., without seeing them, or specifically completely obscuring their feelings. It is convenient for them to hide their true emotions, and make a statement to the outside world [4]. It is usually observed that the posts shared by users on social media have a direct correlation with their ideologies and personalities [5]. It might not be possible to understand the traits by judging one or two posts shared by him/her, but by observing the posts for a limited period, some patterns can be identified through which the personality of the person can be predicted. For instance, a preliminary classification can be made based on the gender of the person. Statistically, it is observed that women are more prone to post selfies, group pictures, and other media than men [2,6]. Among women, depending upon their social circles, the posts may differ quite a bit. For example, if someone has a bigger social circle and is outspoken, they usually post about various events in their lives, most of which are various social interactions with her circle [4]. Whereas someone with limited social interaction does not have a lot to post about his/her daily life [7,8]. In a similar context, someone who is shy is not usually observed to be very active in social media platforms, [9,10] whereas someone who is bold is usually much more active. Based on this trend, it can be predicted that the person is introverted or extroverted depending on their posts and their activity on social media platforms [3] which include how often they are online, or, frequency at which they post, etc. [11]. Analysing these patterns, their perspectives, opinions, sensitivity, and judgement can be predicted. Posts that are related to a specific topic which can be in agreement, disagreement or general to the topic, can talk about the likes and dislikes of that person [12]. Similarly, individuals with anxiety or depression can also be reflected through their social activities sometimes [13].

For predicting such behaviors, high agreeableness and neuroticism are the two most important predictors [14,15]. High agreeableness refers to the sympathetic trait of a person towards others and neuroticism is the trait representing the degree to which a person experiences stress, self-doubt, and other negative feelings. The three properties, such as extraversion, agreeableness, and neuroticism are connected with the likelihood of expressing one's true image. Among these three properties, neuroticism is important for the expression of hidden thoughts [3]. So, it is clearly visible that online social networking, broadly known as OSN, plays a vital role in identifying the behavioural traits [16,17]. The attitude of taking someone's own selfie while discarding the other people of a group depicts some form of narcissism [18]. Similarly, in a group picture, removing others or cropping or editing others' faces or presence and only focusing upon himself/herself presents a valuable point in personality analysis [19,20]. Analysing the posts from various online sites like Twitter, Facebook, and Instagram may state that people with different mentality opt for different platforms [21,22]. For instance, people with narcissistic traits, who love to put their own photos, or photos that are directly related to themselves often in social media, are most likely to use Instagram [7]. On the other hand, those who love to put writings or posts, not directly related to themselves, and maintain anonymity, are more active in Reddit [23]. Similarly, people who want social media as an informative platform mostly use Twitter [24]. Those who regularly post their daily life, pictures and videos alike, along with writings, are found to use Facebook extensively [25,26]. Thus, depending upon their likes, dislikes, and behaviour patterns, the choice of social media also differs. Since personality analysis is possible by observing public posts on various social media, therefore, we can generate a personality profile based on the usage patterns and the content [17].

The following section will discuss existing works and analyse their different benefits and loopholes/disadvantages. The gaps found in existing literature motivated us to consider the domain for further research to overcome them. Section 2.3 will describe our proposed methodology and Section 2.4 will present the experimental result and evaluate its performance using performance metrics like accuracy, validation loss, etc. Section 2.5 discusses results and compares the various models, Section 2.6 provides the future scope of the work, and Section 2.7 concludes the paper.

2.2 RELATED WORKS

The contributions of machine learning in healthcare can be classified broadly in two fields; one is physical health [27–31] and the other mental health. For the counseling of a person, it is very important to know more about his/her personality. The MBTI is considered to be one of the reliable and popular methods to predict personality. Recently in 2020, Mohammad Hossein Amirhosseini and Hassan Kazemian [32] used neuro-linguistic programming (NLP) to predict the personality of an individual based on the Myers-Briggs test. They compared the accuracy and reliability of the study with other existing methods. The performance of the study was better in comparison to the others. They established a new machine learning algorithm based on the MBTI indicators for automating the process of program and personality prediction. The gradient boosting library tools they used for implementing the process were the natural language processing toolkit (NLTK) and XGBoost for implementing the machine algorithms for the gradient boosting framework. The methodology proposed had better accuracy than the most successful existing model that used Kaggle's Myers–Briggs personality type data set.

One of the primitive studies on personality prediction was done by Golbeck et al. [5]. They presented a procedure to predict the personality of the user from the information available in his or her Twitter profile. They collected publicly accessible data from the user profile from the Twitter API and found small correlations in them. The two structural features of the profile that they considered were network density and their number of friends. They used this data to train two machine learning algorithms Gaussian processes and ZeroR. In 2011, Michael Komisin and Guinn [33] collected the MBTI and in-class writing samples from 40 graduate students. They used the support vector machine (SVM) and Naïve-Bayes technique to predict the personality from the choice of words that are made. They analysed the performance of both the methods and concluded that Naïve-Bayes works better on their data set than the SVM technique. Other than the Myers-Briggs personality model, the Big Five personality model is also a popular model to predict personality. Unlike MBTI, the Big Five personality system predicts the measurable features in an individual's life, like marital status, income, etc [34]. In 2013, Wan et al. [35] tried to predict the Big Five personality types of users from the texts they collected from a Chinese social networking site, Weibo, using machine learning techniques. They were successful in their work. In another study, Li, Wan, and Wang [36] used three different models namely the multi-tasking model, the multi-regression model, and the grey prediction model to predict the personality of individuals based on the Big Five personality model. They concluded that the grey prediction model is more efficient than the other two models. In 2017, Hernandez and Knight [37] tried to build a classifier that will be capable of assorting people into their Myers-Briggs Type Index (MBTI) personality type depending on text samples collected from their social media posts. The main motivation of their work was extensive use of social media will provide them with a huge amount of data to execute the personality test permitting more people to receive access to their MBTI test and their classifier could work as a verifier for the initial tests to allow people to have confidence in the result obtained. They used various models like GRU, simple RNN, LSTM, and bi-directional LSTM to build the classifier. The overall accuracy of their model was 0.028.

Another study in 2017, by Tandera et al. [38], used some deep learning architectures to predict the personality of users based on their Facebook posts using the Big Five personality model. They made a comparison between their model and older machine learning algorithms used to do the same. Their accuracy was 74.17%, which was better than the previous results. In 2007, Chung and Pennebaker [39], introduced and applied a new method of using commonly used adjectives from self-descriptive essays and analyzing them to find a psychological factor behind using them. Mihai Gavrilescu [40], in his work, used a neural-network-three-layer architecture to determine the personality type by using the correlation between MBTI personality traits and handwriting features. In 2013, Andrew Schwartz [41] analysed 700 million words, topic instances, and phrases collected from volunteers and used LIWC features and open-vocabulary DLA (differential language analysis) to guess the personality of Facebook users based on their status and posts. In a study by Brandon Cui and Calvin Qi [42], in conjunction with machine learning, various NLP techniques are used to predict the personality of an individual based on the Myers-Briggs model using their social media posts. They used baseline Naïve-Bayes and SVM models for performing their work.

In a study on the relation between mental health and personality of the individuals and associated workers by Pujol [43], he stated that the mental health of an individual is not only related to his personality traits but also his co-workers' personality characteristics. This context proves the importance of the personality test in today's world. In a similar study, Husin and Zaidi [44] discussed the correlation between the employees' personality and their job satisfaction. In 2010, Sitaram Asur and Bernard A. Huberman [45] in their study demonstrated how to predict the real-world outcomes from the social media contents. They showed that a model based on the rate at which the tweets are created about any topic can give better accuracy than the market-based predictors. The table shows the summarisation of the implementation-based related works; additionally, some scholarly articles published over the recent three to four years in the domain of personality prediction with the help of machine learning methods have also been listed in Table 2.1.

Along with the food industry [52], the contribution of machine learning in healthcare is remarkable in every aspect [53,54]. Usually, personality tests are based on filling a questionnaire, but the idea of using social media posts is much more practical and easier to carry out. We, therefore, focus on using social media posts to predict the personality traits of people. The following sections will present the methodology used, and the experimental results and the inference drawn.

2.3 PROPOSED METHODOLOGY

From the social media posts, the stop words are removed, word embedding is generated and the entire post is tokenised. Then based on MBTI four classes of personality are considered for prediction. Then the tokenised posts are classified into four categories. The description of the classifiers used is discussed below.

2.3.1 Classification Using Random Forest

Among several machine learning algorithms, random forest is a diverse, flexible, stable, and quite accurate mechanism that runs on large data sets efficiently to produce optimal outcomes. This method can be applied to regression or classification, both types of problems, solvable by the construction of multiple decision trees. All these decision trees are then united to predict a stable solution accurately. This is a very well-known supervised learning algorithm that uses a bagging approach [55], where the original input data subsets of equal size are extracted with replacement, and then the model is executed on them; later they assemble together. In decision trees feature importance is one of the main processes to identify the features of the data points. It is calculated by taking the node probability of a node for a tree to reach the node. The more the probability, the more important the feature is. The importance of features is calculated using equation (2.1).

$$\mathrm{fi}_{\mathrm{i}} = \frac{\sum_{j:node\ j\ splits\ on\ feature\ i} ni_j}{\sum_{k \in all\ nodes} ni_k} \tag{2.1}$$

TABLE 2.1
Comparative Study of Related Works

Ref. No.	Objective	Methods Used	Result	Benefits	Loopholes
[33]	Using document classification methods, identification of different personalities.	MBTI personality model. Naïve-Bayes and SVM classifier based on text analysis tool Linguistic Inquiry and Word Count (LIWC) and word choice of a personality.	Evaluation of SVM and Naïve-Bayes classifiers using leave-one-out cross-validation.For SVM, both word-based and LIWC performed poorly compared to Naïve-Bayes.	In the word-based Naïve-Bayes trials, S-N and T-F perform better. Removal of lower clarity scored authors improved S-N, T-F, and J-P in precision and recall to >73%, which is considered as better performance than LIWC based features.	Less than 70% accuracy yielded by LIWC-based features in all dichotomies because of the study context. Feature space is not large enough and the sample size is small. Poor results for E-I and J-P.
[5]	Predicting personalities of users of Twitter	Big Five Personality Model ZeroR and Gaussian Process with 10-fold cross-validation, each executed 10 epochs.	Pearson correlation values between personality scores and feature scores. Regression analysis in Weka for score prediction of a personality feature. Normalised mean absolute error for Big Five personality traits individually, fitted using Gaussian process and ZeroR.	For every personality trait prediction, the maximum deviation of 11–18% was observed from their actual values. For openness and agreeableness, this value is restricted below 11% where extraversion, neuroticism, and conscientiousness yielded worse results up to 18%.	Personality scores between friends or connected personalities on social media are overlooked. Absence of large samples of data.

(*Continued*)

[35]	Prediction personality based on all characters of users' social media information.	Big Five Personality Model Logistic regression and Naïve-Bayes algorithm, each with 10-fold cross-validation with 10 iterations. The Linguistic Inquiry and Word Count (LIWC) dictionary is used for analyzing the content of Weibo content.	Pearson correlation coefficient reveals the relationship between a user's personality and all types of information. It is used as the standard to select features based on dependency matrices theory. Logistic regression and Naïve-Bayes to compute the personality result of the test set. Both the algorithms have similar performance in terms of recall.	Naïve-Bayes gives more accuracy in terms of Precision. The mean precision of the two algorithms was 0.707.	Absence of large data sets. Less number of participants. The relation between the user's personality and their close friends is not revealed.
[40]	Determining the Myers-Briggs personality type based on the individual's handwriting.	MBTI personality predictor model. A three-layer neural network	Personality recognition results are based on the handwriting samples and subjects built upon the proposed neural network, along with its accuracy score for each trait category.	86.7% accuracy for predefined handwriting samples and 78.8% when applied on random handwritten texts, with best accuracies for E-I and T-F classes. The computation time of the system <1 minute, hence, better than a questionnaire and practical use. Robust system.	Absence of large no. of subjects for each personality category in the data set. Higher error rates for prediction of S-I and J-P.
[36]	Personality prediction of social network users.	MBTI Personality Model Big Five Personality Model Multitask Regression Model, Gray Prediction Model, and Multiple Regression Model	A relation is found between the personality and the behavioral characteristics of a user by comparative analysis of the prediction models.	The traditional multiple regression model is simple and easy to implement. Gray prediction has an excellent ability to fit in nonlinear regression, due to its generalisation ability. Gray gives a good result even if the state of social data is not good.	The results predicted by the traditional multiple regression model are not ideal. The non-linear predictions are not satisfactory most of the time.

(*Continued*)

TABLE 2.1 (Continued)
Comparative Study of Related Works

Ref. No.	Objective	Methods Used	Result	Benefits	Loopholes
[42]	Personality prediction by NLP using ML algorithms.	MBTI Personality prediction. Naïve-Bayes, regularised SVM, deep learning model	Comparison of various deep learning hyperparameters and analysis of dev and test accuracies. Performance comparison of different methods for MBTI personality predictions, with the best train and test accuracy of 40% and 38%, respectively using deep learning.	On individual personality types, regularised SVM is more accurate than Softmax and Naïve-Bayes. Moreover, deep learning models give better results than SVM. Overall final accuracy may not be satisfactory, but individual categorical results came better.	Limited data set without any metadata for posts. Absence of well-known word embeddings and attention mechanism on top of the current framework.
[46]	To observe if personality traits vary due to culture and language.	Deep learning algorithms, Poisson regression, ordinal regression, etc.	Two models were built on two different Twitter data sets: Turkish and Korean. The model which was trained on the Turkish data set was used to predict the personality of Korean users, and vice versa.	Other features(No. of hashtags, no. of retweets, etc.) along with the posts were also considered. Common top words from both cultures were listed for noting down similarities between the cultures.	The methodology is only proposed and not implemented. Good accuracy is not guaranteed.
[38]	Predicting personalities of users of Facebook.	Big Five Personality Prediction by myPersonality and manual gathered data set. Traditional ML algorithms like Naïve-Bayes, SVM, gradient boosting are compared to CNN, LSTM i.e., deep learning algorithms.	Comprehensive accuracy analysis of traditional ML classification algorithms and deep learning models.	Average accuracy: 74.17%, better than traditional methods. Best Accuracy: (myPersonality data set) MLP and (manual gathered data set) LSTM+CNN 1D.	Results are obtained for only two data sets, larger data sets are not used. XGBoost is not used among traditional ML models.

(Continued)

[47]	Predicting personalities of users of Facebook.	Big Five Personality Model Logistic regression, SVM, gradient boosting, and XGBoost on feature sets SNA, LIWC, and SPLICE, individually and then combined.	Comparative performance analysis of the models predicted with individual sets of features on the four different machine learning algorithms and then combined set of features on the same four ML methods for each personality trait separately and altogether as well.	Social network features are better than linguistic features. By the use of separate SNA sets of features on XGboost, extraversion was predicted most accurately, i.e., 78.6% accurately, whereas the combined set is 74.2% accurate. Individual sets of features, neuroticism, and agreeableness performed better than combined ones.	Absence of a larger data set that may allow a diverse range of features for performance optimisation
[48]	Classifying Borderline Personality Disorder (BPD) and Bipolar Disorder using a signature-based model.	Regression using random forest.	The signature feature set was extracted from self-reported mood data and analyzed using random forest. The BPD group was distinct among the others.	Second-order signature gave higher accuracy.	Medical changes of the patients during the study were not considered. Self-reported data can't be fully trusted.
[49]	Optimising Automatic Personality Prediction model trained on Bahasa Twitter data set.	Gradient boosting, stochastic gradient descent, stacking.	Improvement of machine learning algorithms was done by feature selection, tuning of hyperparameters, sampling, reducing noise.	The highest ROC AUC score of 1.0 was achieved.	Possibility of biased results due to small data set size.

(Continued)

TABLE 2.1 (Continued)
Comparative Study of Related Works

Ref. No.	Objective	Methods Used	Result	Benefits	Loopholes
[50]	Machine learning algorithms for advancement of personality analysis.	Construct validation perspective on assessment of personality.	Undiscovered insights into personality structure, development, processes. For a more robust analysis of personalities, nine specific recommended approaches of ML techniques.	Among the three steps of construct validation, traditional MLPA focused on one aspect of external validity, here, some other aspects are explored and particularly nine recommendations of MLPA are proposed.	Myers-Briggs Type Indicator not taken into account, some more aspects of construct validation could have been explored.
[51]	Applications of machine learning for research and assessment of different personalities.	Survey of past implementations of ML algorithms in personality psychology.	Methodological challenges dealt with by application of machine learning and considering potential loopholes.	Evaluation of personality scales derived using machine learning methods.	Construct validation perspective on assessment of personality is ignored here.
[32]	MBTI personality prediction using machine learning approach.	Extreme gradient boosting	Type indicators of MBTI were trained individually. Accuracy of Introversion-Extroversion and Intuition-Sensing improved upon configuration; however, the other two type indicators did not show any significant changes.	Accuracy improved in comparison to the RNN model that uses classification methodology.	The accuracy of the Feeling-Thinking type indicator in gradient boosting was less than that of the RNN model.

where fi_i is the importance of feature i and ni_j is the importance of node j. The values obtained are then normalised between 0 and 1 using equation (2.2).

$$normfi_i = \frac{fi_i}{\sum_{j \in all\ features} fi_j} \tag{2.2}$$

The final features that are to be taken into consideration are calculated using equation (2.3).

$$RFfi_i = \frac{\sum_{j \in all\ trees} normfi_{ij}}{T} \tag{2.3}$$

where $RFfi_i$ is the importance of features i calculated from all trees in the random forest model, $normfi_{ij}$ is the normalised feature importance for i in tree j, and T is the total number of trees.

Random forest performs two forms of randomisations to create trees. The first is bootstrap sampling, where for estimation of a population parameter, bagging is done. For the second randomisation, for the construction of the trees, a finite number of independent variables are selected.

2.3.2 KNN or K-Nearest Neighbour

KNN algorithm, also regarded as the k-nearest neighbour mechanism, is a supervised machine learning algorithm that is very basic and convenient for dealing with both classification and regression problems. This algorithm does not make any assumption on fundamental data so it is called a non-parameterised algorithm. The KNN algorithm stores the training data set first and then performs its actions. This is why it is also known as the lazy-learner algorithm. During the training phase of the KNN algorithm [56], the data set is only stored for future use. Later, when the new data set arrives, the training data set is classified in a similar category as the new data set. The KNN algorithm stands upon the concept that similar data points can be classified together. The similarity of these data points is more often than not is calculated using the general Euclidean distance shown in equation 2.4.

$$d(p, q) = d(q, p) = \sqrt{(q_1 - p_1)^2 + (q_2 - p_2)^2 + \ldots + (q_n - p_n)^2} \tag{2.4}$$

where p, q are data points and d(p, q) is the distance between them.

The KNN algorithm judges the similarity among all the available data and classifies a new data point. So, by using the KNN algorithm, a new data point can be easily classified into a category that suits it.

2.3.3 SVM or Support Vector Machine

One of the algorithms that work smoothly for both classification and regression problems is SVM, or support vector machine. SVMs are efficient in high-dimensional spaces. A SVM is quite efficient for saving memory space since it works with support vectors which are a decision function's subset of training points. The three main concepts in a SVM are support vectors, hyperplane, and margin [33]. The support vectors are the hyperplane's nearest data points. With the help of these data points, the separating lines are defined. A hyperplane is the decision space or plane that classifies the different classes separately. The gap between the separating lines is the margin. The perpendicular distance from the support vectors to the line is measured to calculate margin. Wider margins are called good margins, whereas narrow margins are bad margins. We can understand hyperplanes by taking a two-dimensional example. The linearly separable data in a 2-D space can be separated by a line. The equation of a line is $y = ax + b$. Let us take x as x_1 and y as x_2. Therefore, we get $ax_1 - x_2 + b = 0$. If we take x as (x_1, x_2) and w as $(a, -1)$ then the equation is:

$$w. x + b = 0 \tag{2.5}$$

This is the equation of the hyperplane and can be extended to any number of dimensions.

A SVM aims to divide the data set in a fashion such that the maximum marginal hyperplane is achieved between the classes. Two steps are needed for doing this. At first, hyperplanes are generated iteratively by a SVM that separates the classes in the finest approach. Finally, a SVM will choose the hyperplane that detaches the classes efficiently. The classifier in a SVM works with the following logic:

$$h(x_i) = \begin{cases} +1, & if\ w.x + b \geq 0 \\ -1, & if\ w.x + b < 0 \end{cases} \tag{2.6}$$

Therefore, the points above the hyperplane are classified as class +1 and the points below as class −1.

2.3.4 Naïve-Bayes

The probabilistic Bayes's theorem constructs a classification problem which is known as the Naïve-Bayes method. Naïve-Bayes can be considered as a probabilistic machine learning algorithm. It makes a strict assumption against feature dependency. It uses a decision rule to classify unknown texts, using the word frequencies for each class's bag-of-words, which is known as the maximum apriori (MAP) [33]. Given enough data, Naïve-Bayes can also handle single-label multinomial decisions. It has no complicated iterative parameter estimation. This algorithm performs quite well in many cases even though it is a simple one to implement. It even performs better than many sophisticated classification methods at times.

The way to calculate posterior probability P(d|y), from class prior probability P (d), predictor prior probability P(y), and the likelihood P(y|d) is provided by the Bayes's theorem [25]. Class conditional independence is assumed by the Naïve-Bayes classifier, i.e., the effect of y (the predictor value) on d (given class) is independent of the other values of y.

$$P(d|y) = \frac{p(y|d)P(d)}{p(y)} \tag{2.7}$$

$$P(d\,|Y) = P(y_1|d) \times P(y_2|d) \times \ldots \times P(y_n|d) \times P(d) \tag{2.8}$$

2.3.5 Long Short Term Memory or LSTM

Long short term memory (LSTM) network is a modified form of recurrent neural network or RNN. RNNs have feedback loops that help them to remember sequential information over time; however, for much longer sequences, this creates a problem. With time the gradient of loss function decays exponentially, causing the vanishing gradient problem. LSTM structure improves upon the RNN structure by including a memory cell that can store information for a comparatively long time period. There are gates that control the flow of information through the cells. A LSTM network is made of a cell, an input gate, an output gate, and a forget gate. LSTM networks are well suited to classifying problems consisting of longer sequences of data such as a very long article in our article. The dependencies of the words are stored and analysed over a time period that would not have been possible in the RNN structure. This is why LSTM networks are quite common for natural language processing problems, which contain a lot of textual data. In Figure 2.1, an example of a LSTM network is shown.

2.3.6 Convolutional Neural Networks or CNN

A convolutional neural network is generally used for the processing of images. It is a special multi-layered neural network algorithm that is used to detect and analyse objects present in an image or any input data. CNN is a deep learning model

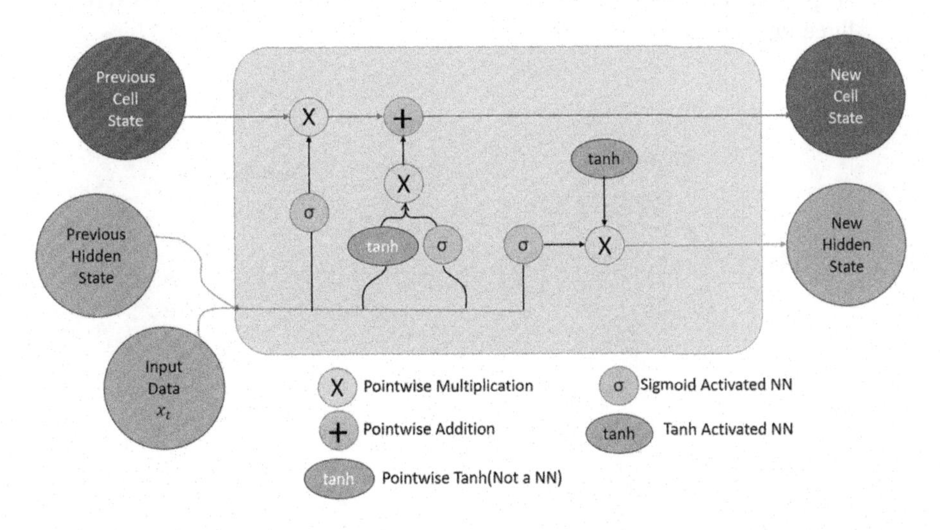

FIGURE 2.1 LSTM network.

designed specially to work with two-dimensional image data. ConvNet requires much less pre-processing compared to other classification algorithms. Figure 2.2 shows a CNN model with six convolution layers and three output layers. For our proposed model, we have implemented CNN to identify the key features in the input data, i.e., the posts of users from the data set. CNN consists of two major parts:

A. Convolutional Layer – This layer scans the input and finds patterns in the data.
B. Down-Sampling Layer – This layer is used to decrease the feature map dimensionality which helps in much faster computations, thus increasing the performance of the model. This layer is also known as pooling.

For our data, the posts are quite lengthy, and therefore identifying key features from the posts is quite important. This is why CNN is beneficial for this task. Figure 2.2 shows the structure and workings of a CNN model.

2.4 EXPERIMENTAL RESULT AND PERFORMANCE EVALUATION

This section includes the data set description and visualisation method followed by the pre-processing technique and the description of the classifiers used here.

2.4.1 Data Set Preparation

An open-source data set [57] containing over 8,600 rows of data has been used here, where each row presents a person's:

- Type (The person's four-letter MBTI code/type)
- A specific portion of each of their last 50 posts (Every record delimited by three pipe characters, i.e., "|||")

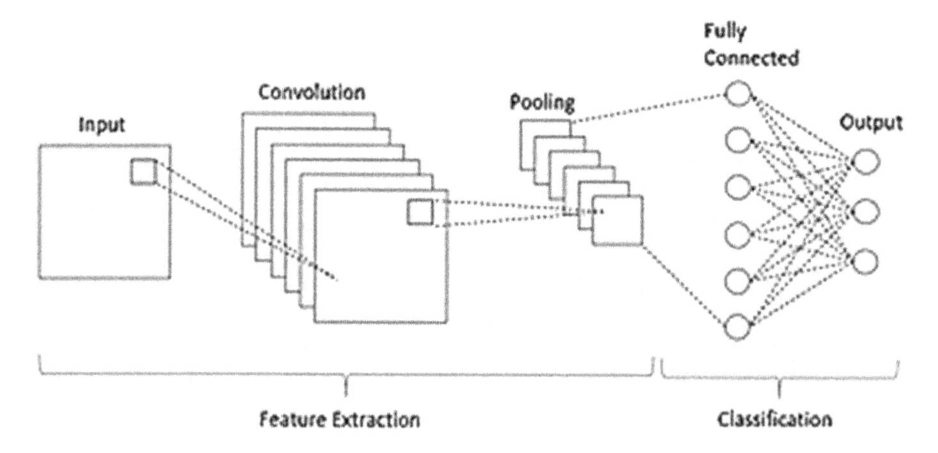

FIGURE 2.2 Structure of CNN.

A person's personality is determined by the four-letter codes (E/I), (N/S), (T/F), (J/P). In our data set, there is a single column containing this four-letter code corresponding to each user's post. From these four letters, there are 16 possibilities possible; hence, we have used binary representation to understand the encoding. We have taken four columns where each column represents one of the traits. For example, for the first column, a binary value of 1 represents Extrovert (E) and 0 represents Introvert (I), and so on.

2.4.1.1 Data Set Visualisation

The original data set containing the posts and the corresponding personality types is shown in Figure 2.3.

The modified data set containing the binary representation of the personality types is shown in Figure 2.4.

2.4.2 Pre-processing of Data

Pre-processing is a necessary step for any textual data which cleans unnecessary items from the text, resulting in better training of the model and thus better prediction of results. There are a lot of pre-processing methods that are followed, the most common among them is tokenisation, stemming, lemmatisation, stop word removal, lowercasing, etc. We have used cleaning of text by removing the lowercasing, punctuations, numbers, single characters, and multiple spaces and stopword removal while using the Keras word embeddings. Figure 2.5 shows a glimpse of the process of how the pre-processing is done.

2.4.3 Classification

MBTI, or the Myers-Briggs Type Indicator, is a method of classification into 16 distinct personality types for each person depending on their traits:

	type	posts
0	INFJ	'http://www.youtube.com/watch?v=qsXHcwe3krw|||...
1	ENTP	'I'm finding the lack of me in these posts ver...
2	INTP	'Good one _____ https://www.youtube.com/wat...
3	INTJ	'Dear INTP, I enjoyed our conversation the o...
4	ENTJ	'You're fired.|||That's another silly misconce...

FIGURE 2.3 Original data set.

	posts	E-I	S-N	T-F	J-P
0	'http://www.youtube.com/watch?v=qsXHcwe3krw|||...	0	0	0	1
1	'I'm finding the lack of me in these posts ver...	1	0	1	0
2	'Good one _____ https://www.youtube.com/wat...	0	0	1	0
3	'Dear INTP, I enjoyed our conversation the o...	0	0	1	1
4	'You're fired.|||That's another silly misconce...	1	0	1	1

FIGURE 2.4 Modified data set.

```
In [1]: import re
        def preprocess_text(sen):
            # Remove punctuations and numbers
            sentence = re.sub('[^a-zA-Z]', ' ', sen)
            # Single character removal
            sentence = re.sub(r"\s+[a-zA-Z]\s+", ' ', sentence)
            # Removing multiple spaces
            sentence = re.sub(r'\s+', ' ', sentence)
            return sentence

In [2]: sentence=" Hello 123, this is    a noisy sample.....Let's clean it!"
        print(sentence)
        print(preprocess_text(sentence))

         Hello 123, this is    a noisy sample.....Let's clean it!
         Hello this is noisy sample Let clean it

In [13]: string = "Hello, This is a sample text from which all the stopwords will be removed"
         stop_words = ['the', 'a', 'and', 'is', 'be', 'will', 'This', 'from', 'be']
         string = ' '.join([word for word in string.split() if word not in stop_words])
         print(string)

         Hello, sample text which all stopwords removed
```

FIGURE 2.5 Pre-processing of data.

- Extroversion (E) – Introversion (I)
- Sensing (S) – Intuition (N)
- Thinking (T) – Feeling (F)
- Judging (J) – Perceiving (P)

As an instance, if somebody goes after extroversion, sensing, feeling, and judging, they should be considered as an ESFJ for MBTI.

2.4.3.1 Random Forest

An ensemble classifier, RandomForestClassifier, is imported from the scikit-learn package and fitted on the data set [57], by setting the no. of trees (n_estimators) parameter to 400 and keeping the value of the other parameters to their defaults. The model is trained as a multi-label classifier but we have considered its performance based on the individual accuracy of each predicted label, i.e., the four categories. As we know, random forest deals with the overfitting problem quite well; hence, only the testing accuracy of the model is shown in Figure 2.6.

2.4.3.2 K-Nearest Neighbour

KNeighborsClassifier is also imported from the scikit-learn package and fitted on the data set [57] by setting the no. of neighbors (n_neighbors) parameter to 400. This model also has been trained as a multi-label classifier, but we have considered its performance based on the individual accuracy of each predicted label, i.e., the four categories of MBTI. Both the training and testing accuracy of the model are shown in Figure 2.7.

2.4.3.3 Support Vector Machine

To implement SVM also, the help of the scikit-learn package was essential and we created a pipeline to standardise the data first, followed by the SVC classifier itself.

	Introvert - Extrovert	Intuition - Sensing	Thinking - Feeling	Judging - Percieiving
test	0.777949	0.861698	0.533999	0.590088

FIGURE 2.6 Testing accuracy for each of the four categories using random forest.

	Introvert - Extrovert	Intuition - Sensing	Thinking - Feeling	Judging - Percieiving
train	0.765936	0.862131	0.541262	0.610114
test	0.777949	0.861698	0.540530	0.590088

FIGURE 2.7 Training and testing accuracy for each of the four categories using KNN.

	Introvert - Extrovert	Intuition - Sensing	Thinking - Feeling	Judging - Percieiving
train	0.800362	0.873826	0.860484	0.759842
test	0.777949	0.861698	0.525163	0.589320

FIGURE 2.8 Testing and training accuracy for each of the four categories using SVM.

All the parameters of the SVC function are kept to their default values. For larger data sets, SGDClassifier or Linear SVC could have been used to get better values, but for our data set, SVC seems to be a fine model itself. Unlike the previous two methods, here, we have not used SVC as a multilabel classifier; instead, each column is predicted in isolation and their accuracies are also calculated separately. This has been possible as the four categories are independent of each other and one does not affect other labels' predictions. Both training and testing accuracies are visualised in Figure 2.8 for each category.

2.4.3.4 Naïve-Bayes

For the Naïve-Bayes approach, the classifier is imported from nltk (natural language toolkit) package along with the utility function to predict MBTI personality traits. Similar to SVM, here also the model is not used as a multilabel classifier; instead, each column is predicted separately and accuracies are also calculated accordingly. This has been possible as the four categories are independent of each other and one does not affect other labels' predictions. Both training and testing accuracies are depicted in Figure 2.9 for each category, but as the result shows, the overfitting problem seems to be a problem for each category prediction for this algorithm.

	Introvert - Extrovert	Intuition - Sensing	Thinking - Feeling	Judging - Percieiving
train	0.811244	0.701452	0.800346	0.797934
test	0.582047	0.544626	0.594132	0.544055

FIGURE 2.9 Training and testing accuracy for each of the four categories using Naïve-Bayes.

2.4.3.5 Convolutional Neural Network

For the analysis of a text followed by feature extraction from it, we have used the CNN model. The CNN model comprises an embedding layer that takes in the input vector. This passes through a convolutional layer followed by a pooling layer. SpatialDropout1D lowers the correlation between the feature maps and increases the effective learning rate. The value of SpatialDropout1D was varied and when the value was set to 0.9, it was experimentally observed that the CNN algorithm gave the best accuracy.

In the dense layer, we have used the activation function ReLU or rectified linear unit to solve vanishing gradient problems. ReLU handles the problem of non-linearity by returning 0 for negative values and the actual value for positive values. So, the output value is never negative, and as a result, the value doesn't diminish while moving through the layers. The optimal epoch value was found to be 13 experimentally. It was observed that if we increased the epoch further, the training accuracy increased and testing accuracy decreased, which indicated overfitting.

As we have considered only binary values in our problem, this falls under the category of binary classification, and thus the suitable loss function for this case was binary cross-entropy. The CNN model consists of nine layers. The full model architecture is given in Figure 2.10.

This model was trained on each column, and the results are shown. Figure 2.11 is the accuracy graph for the first column "Extrovert-Introvert" or "E-I".

Figure 2.12 is the loss graph for the first column "Extrovert-Introvert" or "E-I".

Figure 2.13 is the accuracy graph for the second column "Sensing-Intuition" or "S-N".

Figure 2.14 is the loss graph for the second column "Sensing-Intuition" or "S-N".

Figure 2.15 is the accuracy graph for the third column "Thinking-Feeling" or "T-F".

Figure 2.16 is the loss graph for the third column "Thinking-Feeling" or "T-F".

Figure 2.17 is the accuracy graph for the fourth column "Judging-Perceiving" or "J-P".

Figure 2.18 is the loss graph for the fourth column "Judging-Perceiving" or "J-P".

The training and testing accuracy of the CNN model is shown in Figure 2.19.

The training and testing loss of the CNN model is shown in Figure 2.20.

2.4.3.6 Long Short Term Memory

The LSTM model is implemented using a sequential layer containing an embedding layer to take the word embedding vector as input. We have used bidirectional LSTM layers so that context of a word can be analysed from both sides of the input sequence; this helps in better semantic context understanding. The training and testing accuracy of the LSTM model is shown in Figure 2.21.

The LSTM model's training and testing loss are shown in Figure 2.22.

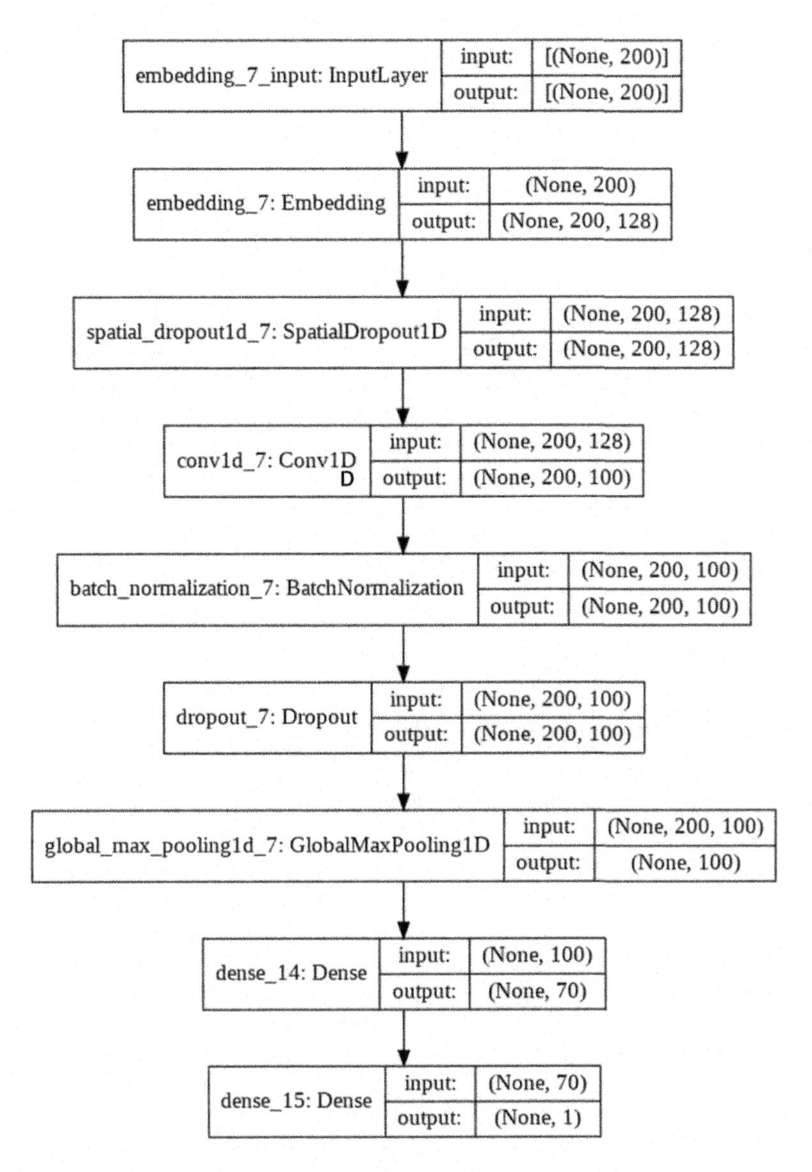

FIGURE 2.10 The CNN layers with their dimensions.

2.5 RESULTS

We approached the problem of predicting a person's Myers-Briggs personality from their social media post by taking into consideration the four type indicators: Introversion/Extroversion, Intuition/Sensing, Feeling/Thinking, Perceiving/Judging. Instead of trying to predict 1 of 16 possible personalities, we tried to predict each of these four type indicators corresponding to a certain social media post. This reduced the complexity of our problem. Further, for a particular model, we trained the data

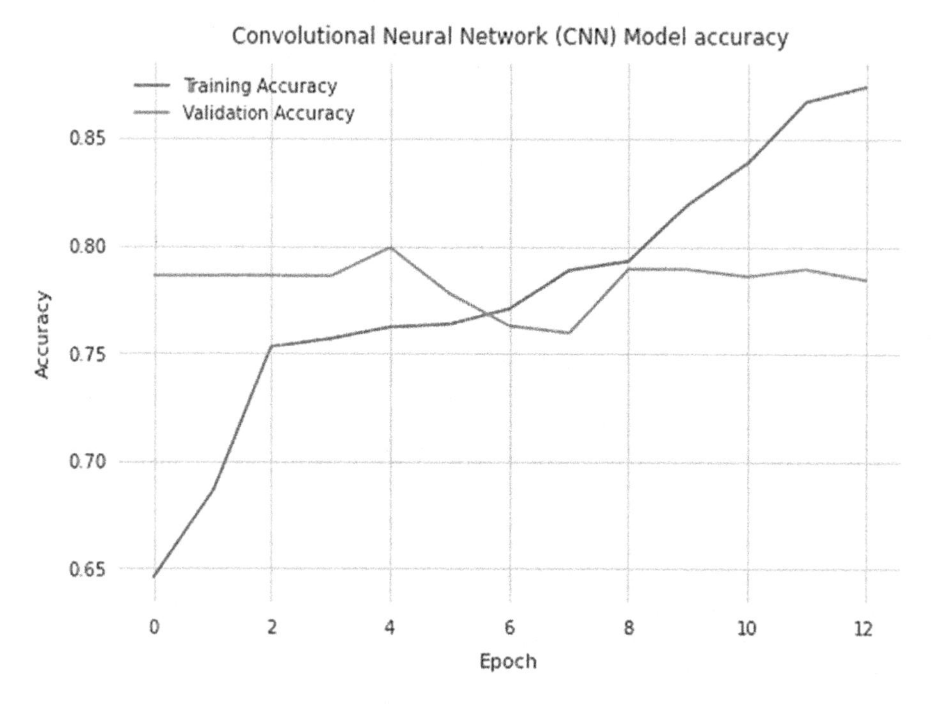

FIGURE 2.11 Accuracy graph for "E-I" column.

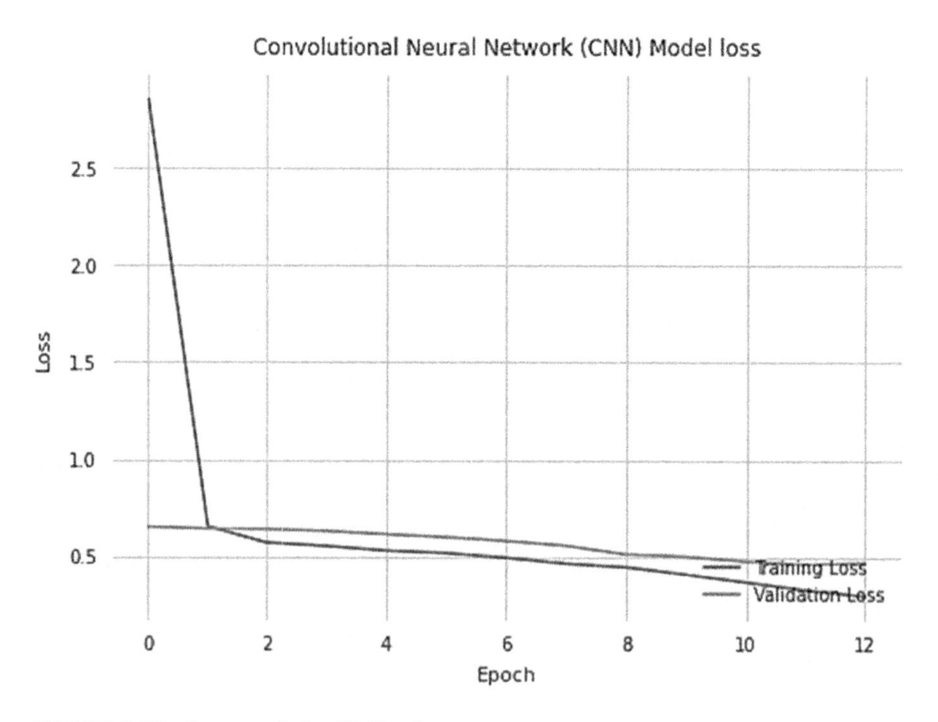

FIGURE 2.12 Loss graph for "E-I" column.

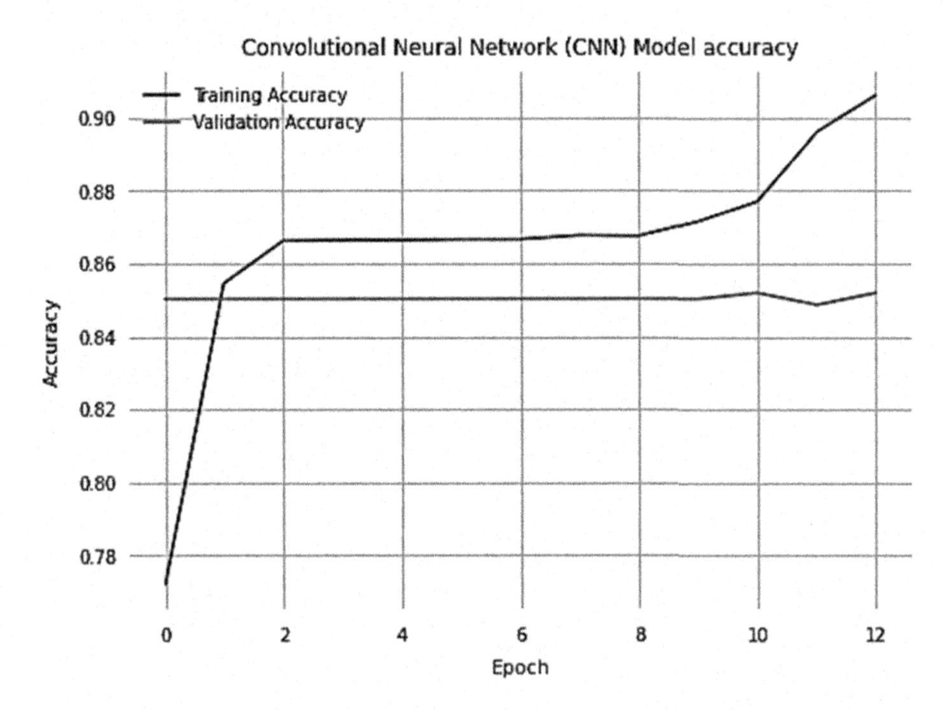

FIGURE 2.13 Accuracy graph for "S-N" column.

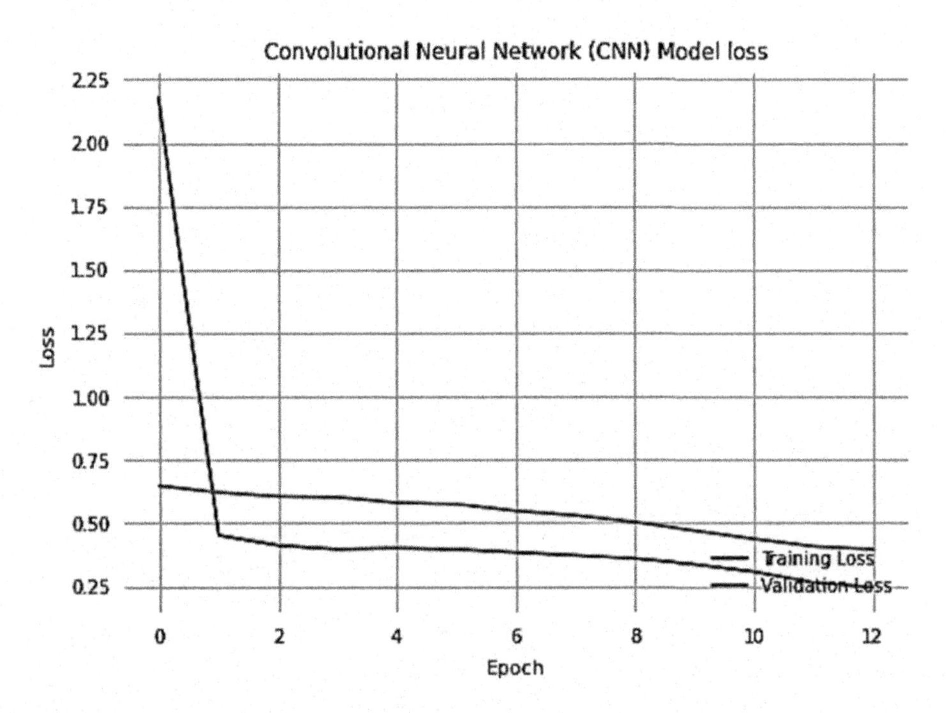

FIGURE 2.14 Loss graph for "S-N" column.

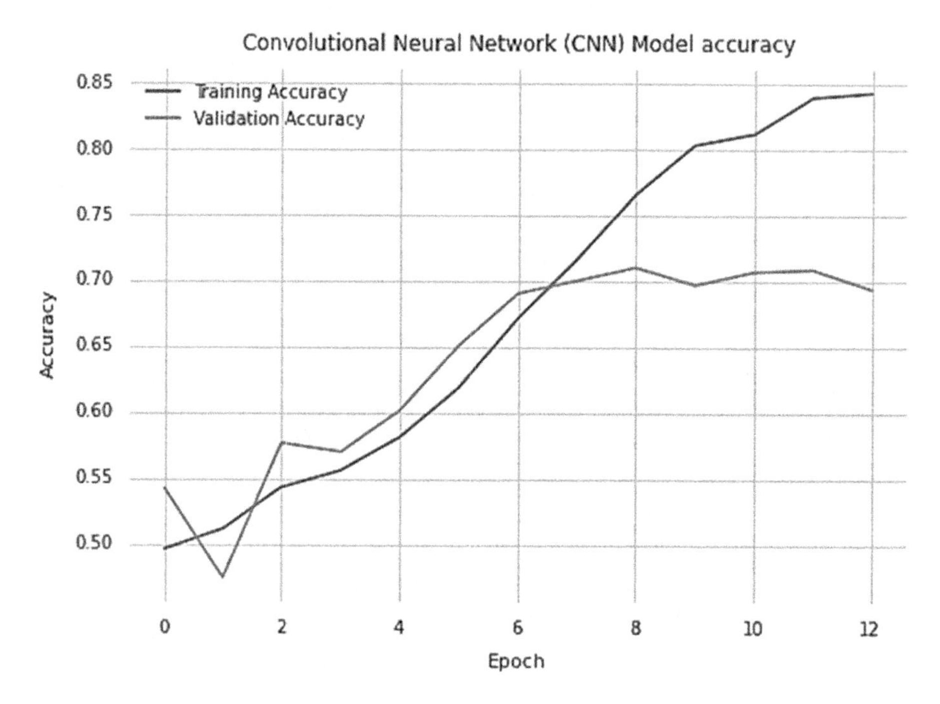

FIGURE 2.15 Accuracy graph for "T-F" column.

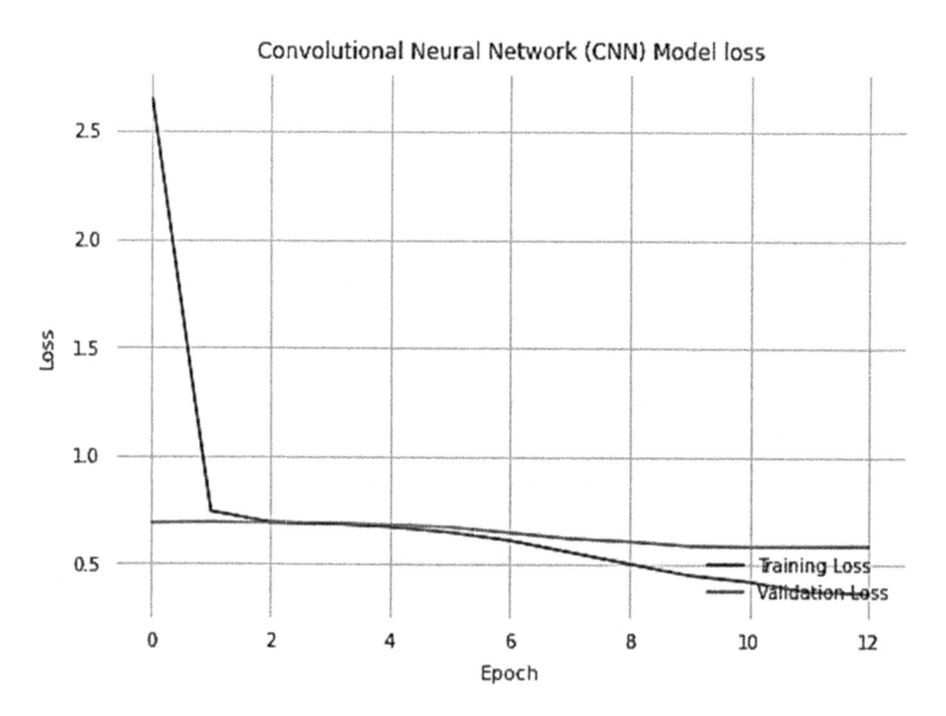

FIGURE 2.16 Loss graph for "T-F" column.

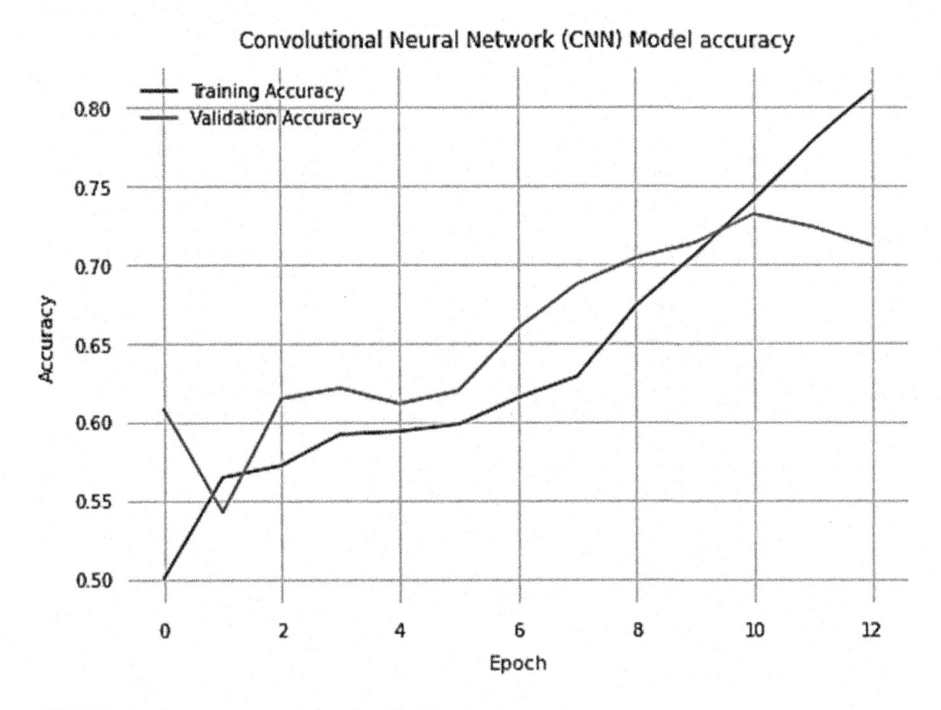

FIGURE 2.17 Accuracy graph for "J-P" column.

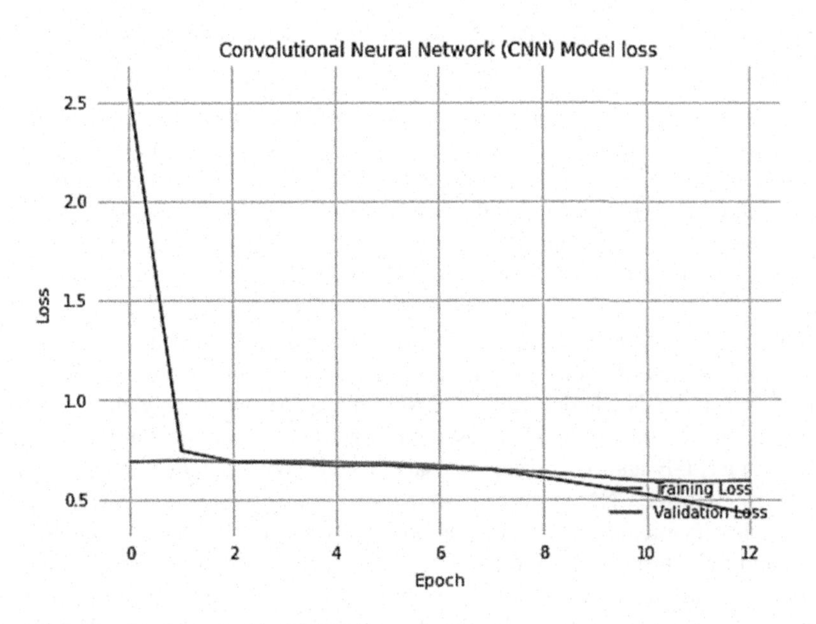

FIGURE 2.18 Loss graph for "J-P" column.

	Extrovert-Introvert	Sensing-Intuition	Thinking-Feeling	Judging-Perceiving
train	0.906785	0.922431	0.893939	0.869236
test	0.791779	0.855551	0.732232	0.700730

FIGURE 2.19 Training and testing accuracy for each of the four categories using CNN.

	Extrovert-Introvert	Sensing-Intuition	Thinking-Feeling	Judging-Perceiving
train	0.305477	0.237088	0.367782	0.433882
test	0.487538	0.386378	0.556300	0.592036

FIGURE 2.20 Training and testing loss for each of the four categories using CNN.

	Extrovert-Introvert	Sensing-Intuition	Thinking-Feeling	Judging-Perceiving
train	0.887352	0.927701	0.95504	0.878294
test	0.777948	0.850557	0.73761	0.696888

FIGURE 2.21 Training and testing accuracy for each of the four categories using LSTM.

	Extrovert-Introvert	Sensing-Intuition	Thinking-Feeling	Judging-Perceiving
train	0.350483	0.258757	0.234569	0.398891
test	0.484485	0.398717	0.527617	0.590183

FIGURE 2.22 Training and testing loss for each of the four categories using LSTM.

for each type indicator independently in isolation, rather than taking all of the four type indicators at once. We did so because we wanted to focus on increasing the accuracy of predicting each type indicator instead of the whole personality trait. Taking all four type indicators all at once resulted in poor accuracies of both training and testing. With this approach, we used deep learning models as well as some machine learning models to train the data and compared their performances in Table 2.2.

It is evident from Table 2.2 the performance of our deep neural network model CNN is the best among all, whereas if we consider column by column accuracy, then for E-I and S-N, random forest, KNN, and SVM, all three yielded the best accuracies but failed to capitalise as their performance for the third and fourth columns, i.e., T-F and J-P, were not satisfactory compared to our deep neural models. In contrast, CNN performed well for all four categories and even for the first two classifications, and predicted almost as well as the best performing models for E-I and SN. During the training phase, initially, a larger epoch value was set to observe the pattern of training the data. It was observed that when the training accuracy increased beyond a point, the testing accuracy started to fall. This indicated overfitting, i.e., the model started to learn unnecessary and random fluctuations in data and hence was making the function fit too closely for a limited set of

TABLE 2.2
MBTI Category-Wise Training and Testing Accuracy

Models	Training Accuracy				Testing Accuracy			
	E-I (%)	S-N (%)	T-F (%)	J-P (%)	E-I (%)	S-N (%)	T-F (%)	J-P (%)
Random Forest Classifier	98.6278	99.3612	94.2555	94.4321	77.7949	86.1698	53.3999	59.0088
K-Nearest Neighbour	76.5936	86.2131	54.1262	61.0114	77.7949	86.1698	54.0530	59.0088
Support Vector Machine	80.0362	87.3826	86.0484	75.9842	77.7949	86.1698	52.5163	58.9320
Naïve-Bayes	81.1244	70.1452	80.0346	79.7934	58.2047	54.4626	59.4132	54.4055
Convolutional Neural Network (CNN)	90.6785	92.2431	89.3939	86.9236	79.1779	85.5551	73.2232	70.0730
Long Short Term Memory (LSTM)	88.7352	92.7701	95.5040	87.8294	77.7948	85.0557	73.7610	69.6888

data points. The maximum testing accuracy was achieved at epoch 13, so the epoch was set to that value.

2.6 FUTURE SCOPE

The machine learning algorithms can be optimised by using techniques like random search, grid search, or Bayesian optimisation and by tuning the hyperparameters to improve performance. We can combine the machine learning models along with the neural network models to obtain better results for each trait. We have used the basic Keras word embedding. Some different and well-known word embedding approaches such as Glove, Google's Word2Vec, and FastText can be implemented to improve the accuracy of our model. While cleaning the data, instead of removing hyperlinks, we can extract some content from that link to find some possibly useful data and replace the hyperlink with that data.

2.7 CONCLUSION

The current chapter has attempted to detect the personality traits of users from their social media posts. The applicability of random forest, K-nearest neighbour, support vector machines, CNN, and LSTM has been evaluated to classify the four broader personality traits of Introversion/Extroversion, Intuition/Sensing, Feeling/Thinking, Perceiving/Judging. The accuracy of each model has been considered as the performance metric. The performance of each model has been compared with each other and in the future can be attempted to improve and more models can be tested further to have a future direction in this area of research.

REFERENCES

[1] Liu, Leqi, Preotiuc-Pietro Daniel, Samani Zahra Riahi, Moghaddam Mohsen E., and Ungar Lyle. "Analyzing personality through social media profile picture choice." In *Proceedings of the International AAAI Conference on Web and Social Media*, vol. 10, no. 1. 2016.

[2] Azucar, Danny, Marengo Davide, and Settanni Michele. "Predicting the Big 5 personality traits from digital footprints on social media: A meta-analysis." *Personality and Individual Differences* 124 (2018): 150–159.

[3] Jin, S. Venus, Muqaddam Aziz, and Ryu Ehri. "Instafamous and social media influencer marketing." *Marketing Intelligence & Planning* 37, no. 5 (2019). 10.1108/MIP-09-2018-0375

[4] Sorokowska, Agnieszka, Oleszkiewicz Anna, Frackowiak Tomasz, Pisanski Katarzyna, Chmiel Anna, and Sorokowski Piotr. "Selfies and personality: Who posts self-portrait photographs?." *Personality and Individual Differences* 90 (2016): 119–123.

[5] Golbeck, Jennifer, Robles Cristina, Edmondson Michon, and Turner Karen. "Predicting personality from twitter." In *2011 IEEE third international conference on privacy, security, risk and trust and 2011 IEEE third international conference on social computing*, pp. 149–156. IEEE, 2011.

[6] Guntuku, Sharath Chandra, Yaden David B., Kern. Margaret L, Ungar Lyle H, and Eichstaedt Johannes C. "Detecting depression and mental illness on social media: an integrative review." *Current Opinion in Behavioral Sciences* 18 (2017): 43–49.

[7] Walsh, Patrick, Clavio Galen, David Lovell M., and Blaszka Matthew. "Differences in event brand personality between social media users and non-users." *Sport Marketing Quarterly* 22, no. 4 (2013).

[8] Seidman, Gwendolyn. "Self-presentation and belonging on Facebook: How personality influences social media use and motivations." *Personality and Individual Differences* 54, no. 3 (2013): 402–407.

[9] Kavakci, Elif, and Kraeplin Camille R. "Religious beings in fashionable bodies: the online identity construction of hijabi social media personalities." *Media, Culture & Society* 39, no. 6 (2017): 850–868.

[10] Park, Gregory, Andrew Schwartz H., Eichstaedt Johannes C., Kern Margaret L., Kosinski Michal, Stillwell David J., Ungar Lyle H., and Seligman Martin E.P. "Automatic personality assessment through social media language." *Journal of Personality and Social Psychology* 108, no. 6 (2015): 934.

[11] Pratama, Bayu Yudha, and Sarno Riyanarto. "Personality classification based on Twitter text using Naïve-Bayes, KNN and SVM." In *2015 International Conference on Data and Software Engineering (ICoDSE)*, pp. 170–174. IEEE, 2015.

[12] Klassen, Karen Michelle, Borleis Emily S., Brennan Linda, Reid Mike, McCaffrey Tracy A., and Lim Megan S.C. "What people "like": Analysis of social media strategies used by food industry brands, lifestyle brands, and health promotion organizations on Facebook and Instagram." *Journal of Medical Internet Research* 20, no. 6 (2018): e10227.

[13] Conway, Mike, and O'Connor Daniel. "Social media, big data, and mental health: Current advances and ethical implications." *Current Opinion in Psychology* 9 (2016): 77–82.

[14] Coppersmith, Glen, Ngo Kim, Leary Ryan, and Wood Anthony. "Exploratory analysis of social media prior to a suicide attempt." In *Proceedings of the third workshop on computational linguistics and clinical psychology*, pp. 106–117. 2016.

[15] De Choudhury, Munmun, Gamon Michael, Counts Scott, and Horvitz Eric. "Predicting depression via social media." In *Proceedings of the International AAAI Conference on Web and Social Media*, vol. 7, no. 1. 2013.
[16] Kim, Ji Won, and Makana Chock T. "Personality traits and psychological motivations predicting selfie posting behaviors on social networking sites." *Telematics and Informatics* 34, no. 5 (2017): 560–571.
[17] Gaspar, Rui, Pedro Cláudia, Panagiotopoulos Panos, and Seibt Beate. "Beyond positive or negative: Qualitative sentiment analysis of social media reactions to unexpected stressful events." *Computers in Human Behavior* 56 (2016): 179–191.
[18] Kanuri, Vamsi K., Chen Yixing, and Sridhar Shrihari. "Scheduling content on social media: Theory, evidence, and application." *Journal of Marketing* 82, no. 6 (2018): 89–108.
[19] McCain, Jessica L., Borg Zachary G., Rothenberg Ariel H., Churillo Kristina M., Weiler Paul, and Keith Campbell W. "Personality and selfies: Narcissism and the Dark Triad." *Computers in Human Behavior* 64 (2016): 126–133.
[20] Shu, Kai, Sliva Amy, Wang Suhang, Tang Jiliang, and Liu Huan. "Fake news detection on social media: A data mining perspective." *ACM SIGKDD Explorations Newsletter* 19, no. 1 (2017): 22–36.
[21] Lou, Chen, and Yuan Shupei. "Influencer marketing: how message value and credibility affect consumer trust of branded content on social media." *Journal of Interactive Advertising* 19, no. 1 (2019): 58–73.
[22] Liu, Dong, and Baumeister Roy F. "Social networking online and personality of self-worth: A meta-analysis." *Journal of Research in Personality* 64 (2016): 79–89.
[23] Goodmon, Leilani B., Smith Patrick L., Ivancevich Danica, and Lundberg Sofie. "Actions speak louder than personality: Effects of Facebook content on personality perceptions." *North American Journal of Psychology* 16, no. 1 (2014).
[24] Wu, Tai-Yee, and Atkin, David. "Online news discussions: Exploring the role of user personality and motivations for posting comments on news." *Journalism & Mass Communication Quarterly* 94, no. 1 (2017): 61–80.
[25] Vembandasamy, K., Sasipriya R., and Deepa E. "Heart diseases detection using Naïve-Bayes algorithm." *International Journal of Innovative Science, Engineering & Technology* 2, no. 9 (2015): 441–444.
[26] Ehrenberg, Alexandra, Juckes Suzanna, White Katherine M., and Walsh Shari P. "Personality and self-esteem as predictors of young people's technology use." *Cyberpsychology & Behavior* 11, no. 6 (2008): 739–741.
[27] Khamparia, Aditya, Singh Prakash Kumar, Rani Poonam, Samanta Debabrata, Khanna Ashish, and Bhushan Bharat. "An internet of health things-driven deep learning framework for detection and classification of skin cancer using transfer learning." *Transactions on Emerging Telecommunications Technologies* 32, no. 7 (2020): e3963.
[28] Goyal, Sukriti, Sharma Nikhil, Bhushan Bharat, Shankar Achyut, and Sagayam Martin. "IoT enabled technology in secured healthcare: Applications, challenges and future directions." In *Cognitive Internet of Medical Things for Smart Healthcare*, pp. 25–48. Springer, Cham, 2020.
[29] Sharma, Nikhil, Kaushik Ila, Bhushan Bharat, Gautam Siddharth, and Khamparia Aditya. "Applicability of WSN and biometric models in the field of healthcare." In *Deep Learning Strategies for Security Enhancement in Wireless Sensor Networks*, pp. 304–329. IGI Global, Hershey, Pennsylvania, 2020.
[30] Jindal, Mansi, Gupta Jatin, and Bhushan Bharat. "Machine learning methods for IoT and their future applications." In 2019 International Conference on Computing, Communication, and Intelligent Systems (ICCCIS), pp. 430–434. IEEE, 2019.

[31] Kumar, Santosh, Bhusan Bharat, Singh Debabrata, and Choubey Dilip kumar. "Classification of diabetes using deep learning." In 2020 International Conference on Communication and Signal Processing (ICCSP), pp. 0651–0655. IEEE, 2020.

[32] Amirhosseini, Mohammad Hossein, and Kazemian Hassan. "Machine learning approach to personality type prediction based on the myers–briggs type indicator®." *Multimodal Technologies and Interaction* 4, no. 1 (2020): 9.

[33] Komisin, Michael C., and Guinn Curry. "Identifying personality types using document classification methods." PhD diss., University of North Carolina Wilmington, Wilmington, (2011).

[34] Hernandez, Rayne, and Ian Scott Knight. "Predicting Myers-Briggs type indicator with text." In *31st Conference on Neural Information Processing Systems (NIPS 2017)*. (2017).

[35] Wan, Danlin, Zhang Chuang, Wu Ming, and An Zhixiang. "Personality prediction based on all characters of user social media information." In *Chinese national conference on social media processing*, pp. 220–230. Springer, Berlin, Heidelberg, (2014).

[36] Li, Chaowei, Wan Jiale, and Wang Bo. "Personality prediction of social network users." In *2017 16th International Symposium on Distributed Computing and Applications to Business, Engineering and Science (DCABES)*, pp. 84–87. IEEE, (2017).

[37] Leung, Louis. "Generational differences in content generation in social media: The roles of the gratifications sought and of narcissism." *Computers in Human Behavior* 29, no. 3 (2013): 997–1006.

[38] Tandera, Tommy, Suhartono Derwin, Wongso Rini, and Prasetio Yen Lina. "Personality prediction system from Facebook users." *Procedia Computer Science* 116 (2017): 604–611.

[39] Chung, Cindy K., and Pennebaker James W. "Revealing dimensions of thinking in open-ended self-descriptions: An automated meaning extraction method for natural language." *Journal of Research in Personality* 42, no. 1 (2008): 96–132.

[40] Gavrilescu, Mihai. "Study on determining the Myers-Briggs personality type based on individual's handwriting." In *2015 E-Health and Bioengineering Conference (EHB)*, pp. 1–6. IEEE, 2015.

[41] Schwartz, H. Andrew, Eichstaedt Johannes C., Kern Margaret L., Dziurzynski Lukasz, Ramones Stephanie M., Agrawal Megha, Achal Shah et al. "Personality, gender, and age in the language of social media: The open-vocabulary approach." *PloS one* 8, no. 9 (2013): e73791.

[42] Cui, Brandon, and Qi Calvin. "Survey Analysis of Machine Learning Methods for Natural Language Processing for MBTI Personality Type Prediction." (2017).

[43] Pujol, Ramon Solves, Umemuro Hiroyuki, Murata Kensuke, Yano Kazuo, and Ara Koji. "Mental health assessment based on personality of individual and associated workers in workplace." In *2011 International Conference on Business, Engineering and Industrial Applications*, pp. 16–19. IEEE, 2011.

[44] Husin, Liatul Izian Binti Ali, and Zaidi Noor Ainn. "The correlation effects between big five personality traits and job satisfaction among support staff in an organization." In *2011 IEEE Colloquium on Humanities, Science and Engineering*, pp. 883–887. IEEE, 2011.

[45] Asur, Sitaram, and Huberman Bernardo A. "Predicting the future with social media." In *2010 IEEE/WIC/ACM international conference on web intelligence and intelligent agent technology*, vol. 1, pp. 492–499. IEEE, 2010.

[46] Catal, Cagatay, Song Min, Muratli Can, Kim Erin Hea-Jin, Tosuner Mestan Ali, and Kayikci Yusuf. "Cross-Cultural Personality Prediction based on Twitter Data." *JSW* 12, no. 11 (2017): 882–891.

[47] Tadesse, Michael M., Lin Hongfei, Xu Bo, and Yang Liang. "Personality predictions based on user behavior on the Facebook social media platform." *IEEE Access* 6 (2018): 61959–61969.
[48] Arribas, Imanol Perez, Goodwin Guy M., Geddes John R., Lyons Terry, and Saunders Kate E.A. "A signature-based machine learning model for distinguishing bipolar disorder and borderline personality disorder." *Translational Psychiatry* 8, no. 1 (2018): 1–7.
[49] Adi, Gabriel Yakub N.N., Tandio Michael Harley, Ong Veronica, and Suhartono Derwin. "Optimization for automatic personality recognition on Twitter in Bahasa Indonesia." *Procedia Computer Science* 135 (2018): 473–480.
[50] Bleidorn, Wiebke, and Hopwood Christopher James. "Using machine learning to advance personality assessment and theory." *Personality and Social Psychology Review* 23, no. 2 (2019): 190–203.
[51] Stachl, Clemens, Pargent Florian, Hilbert Sven, Harari Gabriella M., Schoedel Ramona, Vaid Sumer, Gosling Samuel D., and Bühner Markus. "Personality research and assessment in the era of machine learning." *European Journal of Personality* 34, no. 5 (2020): 613–631.
[52] Paramesha, K., Gururaj H. L., and Jena Om Prakash. "Applications of Machine Learning in Biomedical Text Processing and Food Industry." *Machine Learning for Healthcare Applications* (2021): 151–167. https://doi.org/10.1002/9781119792611.ch10
[53] Pattnayak, Parthasarathi, and Jena Om Prakash. "Innovation on Machine Learning in Healthcare Services—An Introduction." *Machine Learning for Healthcare Applications* (2021): 1–14. https://doi.org/10.1002/9781119792611.ch1
[54] Panigrahi, Niranjan, Ayus Ishan, and Jena Om Prakash. "An Expert System-Based Clinical Decision Support System for Hepatitis-B Prediction & Diagnosis." *Machine Learning for Healthcare Applications* (2021): 57–75. https://doi.org/10.1002/9781119792611.ch
[55] Sarica, Alessia, Cerasa Antonio, and Quattrone Aldo. "Random forest algorithm for the classification of neuroimaging data in Alzheimer's disease: a systematic review." *Frontiers in Aging Neuroscience* 9 (2017): 329.
[56] Moldagulova, Aiman, and Sulaiman Rosnafisah Bte. "Using KNN algorithm for classification of textual documents." In *2017 8th International Conference on Information Technology (ICIT)*, pp. 665–671. IEEE, Amman, Jordan, (2017).
[57] (MBTI) Myers-Briggs Personality Type Dataset https://www.kaggle.com/datasnaek/mbti-type (Date Last Accessed, March 27, 2021).

3 Influence of Content Strategies on Community Engagement over the Healthcare-Related Social Media Pages in India

Ajitabh Dash
Birla Global University, Bhubaneswar, Odisha, India

CONTENTS

3.1 INTRODUCTION

As per Korda and Itani [1], web-based social media incorporates an expansive range of online specialized devices and works through a few components. Social media can give a channel for social help and encourage a feeling of connectedness among people. They likewise notice that these online virtual communities let clients share data that is not only more user-centric but also generated and controlled by the users [2]. In general, social media has become solidly popular across all the socio-demographic segments in the community [2]. Recent advancements in technology

DOI: 10.1201/9781003189053-3

are fundamental to this development, as appropriation of personal digital devices associated with the Internet proceeds to develop across socio-demographic gatherings and geographic areas [3]. Social media gives a huge market to the healthcare industry with more than 3.6 billion social media clients worldwide that are projected to reach 4.46 billion by the end of 2025 [4]. In India, there are more than a 400 million active social media users [5] who spend about 2 hours and 36 minutes on average on the Internet [6]. These insights unmistakably portray the wide extent of social media and its wide reach in general wellbeing. Web-based social media can bring the entire healthcare industry readily available by systems administration with other industry pioneers and displaying potential clients their main goal and most noteworthy resources in a visual medium [3,7].

Interest in social media as an apparatus for healthcare-related communication has grown colossally in the previous decade [8]. Social media has become an amazing worldwide communication tool for health-related information, giving the community a wide scope of advanced healthcare facilities, and a medium for individuals to speak with each other also with the healthcare service providers and experts [9–,11]. Experts engaged in healthcare communication consistently look for new and proficient techniques for contacting individuals with different socio-demographic profile [12]. The utilization of innovative technology, all the more social media could be a critical system in assisting with addressing a portion of the difficulties looked at by those in the field of healthcare promotion. Intercessions joining web-based social media channels hold extensive potential for healthcare professionals and address a portion of the constraints seen by conventional healthcare promotion techniques by expanding the potential for better engagement through interaction and customization of content [13]. Ongoing studies in the field of social media marketing have additionally uncovered that organizations engaged in the healthcare sector have raised their social media spending and will continue to do so in the following five years. In India, even though Facebook, the most mainstream online media, with more than 6 million healthcare-related pages in India unfortunately has only a couple of them prevailing as far as online engagement is concerned [14]. This addresses that promoting via web-based social media has not yet arrived at the level of assumption for these healthcare service providers as they neglected to connect with their objective clients through their social media posts. Sharing, liking, and commenting on social posts are considered the indications of online engagement [15,16]. Thus, through this study, an attempt has been made to study how various kinds of content strategies such as vividness, novelty, and content type influence the online engagement on healthcare-related Facebook pages in India.

The outputs of this study will not only contribute to the existing literature of the social media content strategy but also will help the healthcare companies to craft their social media content strategy in the Indian context. Theoretically, the outcome of this research advocated a reliable operationalization for these content attributes that can too be used in future studies. With these improvements, this study proposed a robust model for explaining community engagement with better predictive power. Practically, the outcomes of this study also imply that healthcare service providers must emphasize sharing more informative content in comparison to entertaining and transactional content on their social media pages. They should also emphasize developing and disseminating novel content to garner a better rate of engagement.

In terms of structure, this paper follows the introduction section by concentrating on developing a set of hypotheses based on a thorough review of literature on the effect of social media content strategies on community engagement, especially in the healthcare sector. The third section of the paper focuses on the data analysis outcomes, with the fourth section focusing on the study's conclusions.

3.2 LITERATURE REVIEW

This section on literature review aimed to gain a comprehensive understanding of the use of social media and content strategies for community engagement in the healthcare industry. It served as the foundation for defining gaps, developing research hypotheses, and determining the directions for this study to contribute to the body of knowledge.

3.2.1 Social Media

Web-based social media is viewed as virtual communities that encourage a typical stage for individuals from assorted foundations to communicate and interact with each other [17]. As per Webster's dictionary [18], social media can be defined as a "system of online communication where users build virtual communities to disseminate ideas, information, and other audio-visual contents". The outcome of the past studies done concerning the availability of social media for interpersonal interaction shows that it is an ideal tool to reach the general public. Individuals can feel associated and experience a feeling of help without the requirement for up close and personal cooperation. Services of social media are accessible 24/7, making it conveniently available for everyone. It is an ideal method to impart because bustling individuals can exchange information quickly [14]. Web-based social media offers an option in contrast to conventional communication strategies for mass correspondence. An investigation by Buchholz [6] tracked down that a normal individual visits their social media account three times each day. As indicated by Keelery [5], social media incorporates a wide range of online specialized features and works through a few instruments. Online media can give a channel for social help and encourage a feeling of connectedness among people. Maybe generally significant, online media have become immovably settled across socio-segment gatherings. These highlights make web-based media appropriate and mainstream devices for promoting healthcare-related services [5].

3.2.2 Social Media and Healthcare

Healthcare promotion experts are not by any means the only experts receiving web-based social media as a way to arrive at people in general. Social networking sites have been received by certain specialists to disperse straightforward data to their patients, taking out holding uptime and an excursion to the center for some patients. As referred to by Cohen [19], Dr. J. James Rohack, leader of the American Medical

Association, was accounted to have said that correspondence with existing patients online can enhance the patient-doctor relationship [20,21]. Concurring to Korp [22], healthcare promotion interceded by the web has upgraded openings for patients to be all the more effectively occupied with their consideration since patients who utilize this structure of correspondence are more associated with adapting to their issues and in speaking with their primary care physician [23], thought about to the individuals who didn't utilize the web as a correspondence arbiter [20]. In an examination by Apenteng et al. [13], it was accounted for that, as of January 2020, about 90% of doctors were previously utilizing or were keen on utilizing doctors on the web networks, a sort of long-range interpersonal communication utilized distinctly for clinical purposes. Thus, medical care suppliers are ready to refresh patients in the important healthcare sector by straightforwardly conveying customized messages, updates, and cautions. Of course, carefulness should be utilized, because some data trade ought not to be overseen on the web. Even though it would be valuable for exercises like medicine tops-off and addressing basic wellbeing questions, online media would be improper and not practical for additional requesting demands like diagnostics and medicines, where face-to-face contact is required. In general, the social media presence of a healthcare service provider permits people to profit by simple admittance to preventive medication data [20,24]. Another significant utilization of social media is its capacity to empower people and associations to collaborate in all periods of crisis, relief, readiness, reaction, and recuperation [8]. Social media gives an exceptional chance to general society to lock in on basic general medical problems, like the COVID-19 pandemic, where sharing of data, cooperation, and intuitiveness are energized over social networking sites [25].

3.2.3 Engagement over Social Media

Community engagement in web-based social media is generally determined by the kind and nature of posts shared [13]. Community engagement is the sole purpose behind which organizations are utilizing social media as an instrument of advancement should plan those kinds of brand posts which can result in better client commitment and can build up a drawn-out relationship with them [17]. Engaging content not just speeds up the range of a brand post, it additionally cultivates their responsiveness towards the post [11]. Besides being a vital apparatus for estimating the presence of social media content, client commitment can improve the deals just as client reliability [16]. The greater part of the examinations on client commitment with brand posts is focussed on how the content system drives the clients' reaction regarding remarking, enjoying, or sharing the contents. Social media content strategy focuses on three significant components: novelty, distinctiveness, and content type [26].

Theoretically, vividness alludes to the capacity of the complete erotic capacities that a substance animates; what's more, the productivity of the insight that such inceptions make [13]. With regards to social media, any content utilizing only one image is nearly less engaging in contrast with content having a combination of the two or more images [27]. Subsequently, in a similar medium, various content can have an unusual level of vividness. Past investigations have affirmed a certifiable impact of vividness on community engagement concerning posts on different social networking sites [28]. Along these lines, the projected hypothesis is:

H_1: The greater vividness of content will result in better community engagement on the social media sites of different healthcare service providers.

The idea of novelty with regards to promoting correspondence with the prospective users can be applied to both the medium and the content [28]. Novelty indicates how much content is imaginative or unique among the others seen by the viewers [27]. The motivation behind novel content in the communication strategy measure is to catch the user's attention [26]. As social media users are exposed to a colossal amount of content in their newsfeed at a time, apprehending their consideration is the hardest test for promoters through their content [27] and, accordingly, the novelty in the content can help outstandingly in regards to this. Consequently, the projected hypothesis is:

H_2: Greater novelty of content will result in better community engagement on the social media sites of different healthcare service providers.

Organizations deliberately plan content for social media with informational, transactional, and entertaining qualities [16,17]. Content with entertaining ascribes encourage the users with fun and entertainment while content with informational qualities updates the user about the features of a product or service. At last, content with transactional traits potentially boosts the user with certain financial advantages [28]. With regards to the social media content of healthcare service providers, out of these three kinds of content, posts with the informational property can lead to a higher community engagement [13].

Accordingly, the projected hypothesis is:

H_3: Informative content will result in better community engagement on the social media sites of different healthcare service providers.

3.3 METHOD

The selection of the sample company for this study has emerged as a major challenge for this study. To overcome this challenge, this study took the help of socialbakers.com to select social media pages of five top-performing healthcare service providers in India. Other than their amazing follower base, these healthcare service providers kept an active presence on social media, especially on Facebook. Their social media pages were continually updated and included a rich assortment of content. Along with a high subscriber base, the social media pages of these healthcare service providers have elicited a significant volume of community engagement.

For this study, the sample size of 362 posts published by 10 different healthcare-related Facebook pages was selected for a period between 1 April and 1 July 2020.

Poisson regression analysis was performed to evaluate the effect of these post characteristics on online engagement. These promoters have kept a remarkable presence over social networking sites especially Facebook as well as have a generous follower base with an impressive degree of interaction in terms of likes, comments, and shares from them. Each post of these healthcare services provides was investigated cautiously in Microsoft Excel and 'R-language Version 3.0.2' was used to investigate and acquire significant knowledge from the information.

3.3.1 Variables Operationalization

In line with the past literature, the operationalizations of the chosen social media content attributes were done and are introduced in Table 3.1. Similarly, following the comprehension from the past investigations, community engagement was operationalized, utilizing the number of likes, comments, and shares as these are the form of normal reactions expected by the promoters [29].

TABLE 3.1
Variables Operationalization

Variable	Variation	Description
Brand post vividness (IV)	High	Content encompassing videos
	Moderate	Content encompassing two or more images
	Low	Content encompassing a solitary image
Brand Post Novelty (IV) (New offering; nique product display; brand events/competition)	High	Content demonstrating all the sources of novelty
	Moderate	Posts displaying any two of the sources of novelty
	Low	Posts demonstrating none of the three sources of novelty
Content-type (IV)	Entertainment	Posts about events associated with the service
	Informational	Posts about benefits associated with the service
	Transactional	Posts about deals and short term incentives
Online engagement (DV)	Number of likes	
	Number of shares	
	Number of comments	
Fan Number (CV)	Total number of fans for the brand page	

Source: Author's own.

3.3.2 Model Specification

Poisson regression analysis was used to gauge the impact of content characteristics on community engagement. The Poisson regression depends on the notion of Poisson or the discrete distribution of a variable under study. The number of likes, comments, and shares are considered the dependent variable for this study. As these dependent variables follow discrete distribution, the Poisson regression is chosen as a reasonable method for investigation. In this manner, the research model proposed for this study is mentioned as under:

$$\log(y_j) = \alpha_j + \beta_1 X_1 + \beta_2 X_2 + \beta_3 X_3 + \beta_4 X_4 + \beta_5 X_5 + \beta_6 X_6 + e \ldots\ldots\ldots\ldots\ldots\ldots \quad (3.1)$$

where

$Log(y_j)$: $log(y_1)$, $log(y_2)$, and $log(y_3)$ represent the log of likes and comments and shares earned on the contents shared on the social media page of selected healthcare service providers, respectively.

α_j: is α_1, α_2, and α_3, constant terms concerning likes, comments, and shares
βs are the coefficients of the independent variables to be estimated in this study.
X_1: Dummy variable elucidating high level of vividness in the content
X_2: Dummy variable elucidating the moderate level of vividness in the content
X_3: Dummy variable elucidating high level of novelty in the content
X_4: Dummy variable elucidating the moderate level of novelty in the content
X_5: Dummy variable elucidating entertainment kind of content
X_6: Dummy variable elucidating the informational kind of content
e: Error term for $log(y_1)$ or $log(y_2)$ or $log(y_3)$.

3.4 RESULTS

Descriptive measurements relating to the selected content attributes alongside long stretches of posting; furthermore, the average number of preferences and offers per content are introduced in Tables 3.2 and 3.3, separately.

Data presented in Table 3.2 uncovered that majority of the content shared by the healthcare promoters i.e., 156 (43%) out of 362 have demonstrated a high level of vividness, followed by 110 (30%) have demonstrated a moderate level of vividness, and the rest 96 (27%) have shown lowest level of vividness. Correspondingly, novelty-wise analysis of the contents shared by the promoters of healthcare service uncovered that the majority i.e., 41% of the contents shared by them are highly novel, followed by 36% are moderately novel, and only 23% of the total 362 contents have demonstrated the lowest level of novelty. Finally, analysis of the content in terms of their kind uncovered that the promoters of healthcare service providers are mostly sharing informative content (54%) on their social media page. Followed by informative content, they also preferred to share transactional (30%) and entertainment kind of content (16%) through their social media sites.

TABLE 3.2
Descriptive Analysis of Content Attributes

Variable	Variation	Frequency	Percentage
Vividness (IV)	High	156	43%
	Moderate	110	30%
	Low	96	27%
Novelty (IV)	High	147	41%
	Moderate	132	36%
	Low	83	23%
Content Type (IV)	Entertainment	58	16%
	Informational	196	54%
	Transactional	108	30%

Source: Author's calculation.

TABLE 3.3
Statistics of Engagement

Mode of interaction	Mean	Maximum	Minimum
Number of Likes	536	712	25
Number of Shares	92	117	3
Number of Comments	142	189	12

Source: Author's calculation.

Data presented in Table 3.3 attempts to uncover the average engagement earned by the contents shared by the healthcare service providers in terms of likes, comments, and shares. From the descriptive statistical analysis, it was inferred that the contents shared by the selected healthcare service providers have assimilated 142 comments, 92 shares, and 536 likes on average from their followers. These insights are comparable with the statistics reported in the earlier studies conducted in this domain.

3.4.1 Results of Poisson Regression

While trying to test the proposed hypothesis, the Poisson regression was performed and results are assessed and introduced in Table 3.4. The existence of homoscedasticity and multicollinearity were tested to inspect the robustness of the proposed model. Scrutiny of residual established the non-appearance of homoscedasticity as the standardized residuals of the dependent variables were distributed randomly. Likewise, a small variance inflation factor established the non-appearance of multicollinearity amongst the independent variables considered for this study. Figures presented in

TABLE 3.4
Coefficients

Variable	Variation	Log(Likes) β(t-Values)	Log(Shares) β(t-Values)	Log(Shares) β(t-Values)
Brand Post Vividness (IV)	High	0.12(3.24)	0.19(2.66)	0.05(0.39)
	Moderate	0.07(2.17)	0.04(1.11)	0.27(3.54)
	Low (Baseline)			
Brand Post Novelty (IV)	High	0.27(3.54)	0.18(2.19)	0.07(1.54)
	Moderate	0.19(4.25)	0.23(2.36)	0.11(2.007)
	Low (Baseline)			
Content Type (IV)	Entertainment	0.017(0.932)	0.2(−2.74)	0.15(2.28)
	Informational	0.68(32.51)	0.48(−3.76)	0.34(3.69)
	Transactional (Baseline)			
Constant		4.71	0.4352	1.1513
R^2		0.54	0.62	0.61
Adjusted R^2		0.49	0.57	0.58

Source: Author's calculation.

Table 3.4 give the aftereffects of the Poisson regression utilizing the model portrayed in equation 3.1.

The value of squared correlation (R^2) computed concerning "likes" on content is 0.54, which indicates that the novelty, vividness, and content type are responsible for 54% variation in community engagement in terms of "liking" a content shared by the healthcare service providers on their social media handle. As per the value of t-statistics computed for the "shares" model, it can be concluded that both a high ($\beta = 0.12$, t-statistics = 3.24) and a moderate ($\beta = 0.07$, t-statistics = 2.17) level of content vividness had a statistically significant effect on the likes. Thus, hypothesis-1 proposed for this study to examine the effect of vividness on community engagement was accepted so far as the likeability of content is concerned. Consequently, both a high ($\beta = 0.27$, t-statistics = 3.54) and a moderate ($\beta = 0.19$, t-statistics = 4.25) level of content novelty has a positive and significant effect on community engagement in terms of "likes". Accordingly, hypothesis-2 proposed for this study to examine the effect of content novelty on community engagement was accepted so far as the likeability of content is concerned. Similarly, only informational content ($\beta = 0.68$, t-statistics = 32.51) shared by the promoters of the healthcare sector has an affirmative effect on community engagement in terms of "likes". Therefore, hypothesis-3 proposed for this study to examine the effect of informational content on community engagement was accepted so far as the likeability of content is concerned.

The value of squared correlation (R^2) computed concerning "shares" on content is 0.62, which indicates that the novelty, vividness, and content type are responsible for 62% variation in community engagement in terms of "sharing" content shared by the healthcare service providers on their social media handle. As per the value of t-statistics computed for the "shares" model, it can be concluded that only a high ($\beta = 0.19$, t-statistics $= 2.66$) level of content vividness has a statistically significant effect on the likes. Thus, hypothesis-1 proposed for this study to examine the effect of vividness on community engagement is accepted only concerning high post vividness. Consequently, both a high ($\beta = 0.18$, t-statistics $= 2.19$) and a moderate ($\beta = 0.23$, t-statistics $= 2.36$) level of content novelty has a positive and significant effect on community engagement in terms of "shares". Accordingly, hypothesis-2 proposed for this study to examine the effect of content novelty on community engagement was accepted so far as sharing of content is concerned.

Similarly, both entertainment ($\beta = 0.2$, t-statistics $= -2.74$) and informational content ($\beta = 0.48$, t-statistics $= -3.76$) shared by the promoters of the healthcare sector have an affirmative effect on community engagement in terms of "shares". Therefore, hypothesis-3 proposed for this study to examine the effect of informational content on community engagement in terms of sharing the content uploaded by healthcare service providers was accepted.

The value of squared correlation (R^2) computed concerning "comments" on content is 0.61, which indicates that the novelty, vividness, and content type are responsible for 61% variation in community engagement in terms of giving a "comment" on the content shared by the healthcare service providers on their social media handle. As per the value of t-statistics computed for the "shares" model, it can be concluded that only a moderate ($\beta = 0.27$, t-statistics $= 3.54$) level of content vividness has a statistically significant effect on the commenting behavior of the community. Thus, hypothesis-1 proposed for this study to examine the effect of vividness on community engagement was accepted so far as commenting on content is concerned. Consequently, only a moderate ($\beta = 0.11$, t-statistics $= 2.007$) level of content novelty has a positive and significant effect on community engagement in terms of "comments". Accordingly, hypothesis-2 proposed for this study to examine the effect of content novelty on community engagement was accepted so far as comments on content are concerned. Similarly, both entertainment ($\beta = 0.15$, t-statistics $= 2.28$) and informational content ($\beta = 0.34$, t-statistics $= 3.69$) shared by the promoters of the healthcare sector have an affirmative effect on community engagement in terms of "comments". Therefore, hypothesis-3 proposed for this study to examine the effect of informational content on community engagement in terms of commenting on the content uploaded by healthcare service providers was accepted.

3.5 CONCLUSION

The outcomes of the current study underscore the necessity for the promoters of healthcare service providers to develop a deliberate content strategy for their social media handles. Based on these outcomes, the study proposes a couple of measures for crafting the content strategy. Promoters of healthcare service providers are required to boost the vividness of their content by broadcasting audiovisual content on their social media platforms. They should also focus on producing novel content, as new and innovative content causes a higher level of community engagement.

Content type also has a significant effect on community engagement. The informative content is a little more engaging than transactional and entertaining content. Thus, promoters of healthcare service providers must broadcast informative content more regularly than others.

3.6 LIMITATIONS

The outcomes of this study add to the current state of literature as well as help the promoters of healthcare service providers to create their content strategies for web-based social media in the Indian setting. Nonetheless, this study moreover envelops certain limitations as it focuses just on the brand posts overseen by healthcare service providers in India. Besides, just three significant factors, like content type, novelty, and vividness, were thought of for this study. Future investigations could improve the model and discoveries by fusing additional factors and applying them in different enterprises.

REFERENCES

[1] Korda, H., and Itani Z. "Harnessing Social Media for Health Promotion and Behavior Change." *Health Promotion Practice* 14, no. 15 (2011): 14–23.

[2] Adzharuddin, N. A., and Ramly N. M. "Nourishing healthcare information over Facebook." *Procedia-Social and Behavioral Sciences*. Elsevier, Kuala Lumpur, 2015. 383–389.

[3] Gupta, A., Tyagi M., and Sharma D. "Use of social media marketing in healthcare." *Journal of Health Management* 15, no. 3 (2013): 293–302.

[4] Statista. *Social Media & User-Generated Content*. 28 January. Accessed March10, 2021. https://www.statista.com/statistics/278414/number-of-worldwide-social-network-users/#:~:text=In%202020%2C%20over%203.6%20billion,almost%204.41%20billion%20in%202025, (2021).

[5] Keelery, S. *Social Media & User-Generated Content*. 16 October. Accessed March10, 2021. https://www.statista.com/statistics/278407/number-of-social-network-users-in-india / (2020).

[6] Buchholz, K. *Where Do People Spend the Most Time on Social Media?* 17 November. Accessed March03, 2021. https://www.statista.com/chart/18983/time-spent-on-social-media/ (2020).

[7] Mehmet, M., Roberts R., and Nayeem T. "Using digital and social media for health promotion: A social marketing approach for addressing co-morbid physical and mental health." *Australian Journal of Rural Health* 28, no. 2 (2020): 149–158.

[8] Antheunis, M. L., Tates K., and Nieboer T. E. "Patients' and health professionals' use of social media in health care: motives, barriers and expectations." *Patient Education and Counseling* 92, no. 3 (2013): 426–431.

[9] Khamparia, A., Singh P. K., Rani P., Samanta D., Khanna A., and Bhushan B. "An internet of health things-driven deep learning framework for detection and classification of skin cancer using transfer learning." *Transactions on Emerging Telecommunications Technologies* 32, no. 7 (2020), p. e3963.

[10] Kotsenas, A. L., Arce M., Aase L., Timimi F. K., Young C., and Wald J. T. "The strategic imperative for the use of social media in health care." *Journal of the American College of Radiology* 15, no. 1 (2018): 155–161.

[11] Cain, J. "Social media in health care: the case for organizational policy and employee education." *American Journal of Health-System Pharmacy* 68, no. 11 (2011): 1036–1040.

[12] Ukoha, C., and Stranieri A. "The delicate balance of communicational interests: A Bakhtinian view of social media in health care." *Journal of Information, Communication and Ethics in Society* ahead-of-print (ahead-of-print) 19, no. 2 (2020): 236–248. https://doi.org/10.1108/JICES-06-2020-0071

[13] Apenteng, B. A., Ekpo I. B., Mutiso F. M., Akowuah E. A., and Opoku S. T. "Examining the relationship between social media engagement and hospital revenue." *Health Marketing Quarterly* 37, no. 1 (2020): 10–21.

[14] Kalra, V., and Ahire N. "Social media usage in Indian Hospitals-Current scenarios and way ahead." *Annals of Tropical Medicine and Health* 23, no. 1 (2020): 232–315.

[15] Rasool, A., Shah F. A., and Islam J. U. "Customer engagement in the digital age: a review and research agenda." *Current Opinion in Psychology* 36, no. 1 (2020): 96–100.

[16] Van Doorn, J., Lemon K., Mittal V., Nass S., Pick D., Pirner P., and Verhoef P. "Customer engagement behavior: Theoretical foundations and research directions." *Journal of Service Research* 13, no. 3 (2010): 253–266.

[17] Boyd, D., and Ellison N. "Social Network Sites: Definition, History and Scholarship." *Journal of Computer-Mediated Communication* 13, no. 1 (2007): 210–230.

[18] Merriam-Webster. *Definition of Social Media.* 1 January. Accessed March16, 2021. https://www.merriam-webster.com/dictionary/social%20media, (2004).

[19] Cohen, E. *Should you "friend" your doctor on Facebook.* 28 February. Accessed February28, 2021. http://www.cnn.com/2009/HEALTH/09/03/ (2009).

[20] Levac, J. J., and O'Sullivan T. "Social media and its use in health promotion." *Revue interdisciplinaire des sciences de la santé-Interdisciplinary Journal of Health Sciences* 1, no. 1, (2010): 47–53.

[21] Panigrahi, N., Ishan A., and Jena O. P. "An Expert System-Based Clinical Decision Support System for Hepatitis-B Prediction & Diagnosis." in *Machine Learning for Healthcare Applications*, by (S. N. Mohanty, G. Nalinipriya, O. P. Jena and A. Sarkar), 57–75. India: John Wiley and Sons, (2021).

[22] Korp, P. "Health on the Internet: implications for health promotion." *Health Education Research* 21, no. 1, (2006): 78–86.

[23] Goyal, S., Sharma N., Bhushan B., Shankar A., and Sagayam M. "IoT Enabled Technology in Secured Healthcare: Applications, Challenges and Future Directions." in *Cognitive Internet of Medical Things for Smart Healthcare. Studies in Systems, Decision and Control*, (Hassanien A. E., Khamparia A., Gupta D. and Shankar K. by), 8. Cham: Springer, (2021).

[24] Pattnayak, P., and Jena O. P. "Innovation on Machine Learning in Healthcare Services—An Introduction." In *Machine Learning for Healthcare Applications*, by (Mohanty S. N., Nalinipriya G. and Jena O. P.), 1. India: John Wiley and Sons, (2021).

[25] Chen, Q., Min C., Zhang W., Wang G., Ma X., and Evans R. "Unpacking the black box: How to promote citizen engagement through government social media during the COVID-19 crisis." *Computers in Human Behavior* 110, no. 2 (2020): 106380.

[26] Geissinger, A., and Laurell C. "User engagement in social media–an explorative study of Swedish fashion brands." *Journal of Fashion Marketing and Management* 20, no. 2 (2016): 177–190.

[27] Lee, D., Hosanagar K., and H. S. Nair. "Advertising content and consumer engagement on social media: Evidence from Facebook." *Management Science* 64, no. 11 (2018): 5105–5131.

[28] Chauhan, K., and Pillai A. "Role of content strategy in social media brand communities: a case of higher education institutes in India." *Journal of Product & Brand Management* 22, no. 1 (2013): 40–51.
[29] Lipsman, A., Mudd G., Rich M., and Bruich S. "The power of "like": How brands reach (and influence) fans through social-media marketing." *Journal of Advertising Research* 52, no. 1 (2012): 40–52.

4 The Impact of Social Media in Fighting Emerging Diseases

A Model-Based Study

Anal Chatterjee
Department of Mathematics, Barrackpore Rastraguru Surendranath College, Kolkata, India

Suchandra Ganguly
University College of Nursing, College of Medicine and J.N.M. Hospital, Kalyani, West Bengal, India

CONTENTS

DOI: 10.1201/9781003189053-4

4.1 INTRODUCTION

In the 21st century along with human advancement, we are also witnessing evolution among various microbes like viruses and bacteria resulting in emerging and reemerging diseases. Emerging diseases refer to the infections caused by pathogens that are novel or newly evolved in recent times (in the past 20 years). These diseases usually have high transmissibility and if they acquire the capability of human-to-human transmission, they can lead to outbreaks or epidemics and pandemics. Some of the recent outbreaks we have witnessed include Ebola, Zika, influenza (swine flu), Nipah, SARS-CoV2, etc.

One of the major threats these diseases possess is the limited information regarding them. As the infections are relatively new, little is known about their disease pathology, characteristics, spreading mechanisms, etc. Moreover, the change in strains further aggravates the challenge. A lot of scientific and medical research is continuously going on in these areas. As a result, we not only get new information but also the past information keeps evolving and changing.

Awareness, vaccination and treatment are being identified as the three major pillars for combatting these emerging diseases. Vaccination requires time to develop and treatment for a new disease also requires time to be standardized and then also we may not find the perfect solution soon enough and have to depend on symptomatic treatment. Thus, awareness and proper information regarding the disease among the public forms our first line of defence against them. In this context, social media is becoming an undisputed tool for sharing and disseminating information regarding these emerging diseases, their outbreaks, health information and guidelines, etc. [1].

This motivated us to formulate and analyze a five-compartment epidemiological model to study the effect of social media by spreading awareness on emerging infectious diseases, in a time varying population. In our model, we have assumed five classes: unaware susceptible, aware susceptible, infected, media and recovery. A fraction of susceptible classes becomes aware of the disease due to the influence of the social media. Thus, the susceptible class further divides into susceptible unaware and susceptible aware classes. The susceptible aware class makes effort to avoid exposure from the infected ones. So, the chances of them getting infected is reduced as compared to the susceptible unaware class. Further, we assume that the cumulative density of the social media directly depends on mortality due to diseases from the infective class.

Based on the above assumptions, a mathematical model is formulated and the equilibrium point and stability of the system is examined. The main contributions can be highlighted as

- To investigate the effect of awareness of social media on emerging infectious diseases.
- To establish that immigration is vital in stabilizing the system.
- To examine the role of treatment rate and also it's combined effect with awareness on the proposed system.

The remaining sections are organized in the following order: Section 4.2 focuses on literature review, which includes awareness by social media, emerging infectious diseases and implementation of deep learning (DL) in the medical field. Section 4.3 represents the construction of a mathematical model based on some assumptions. Analytical results based on the model are discussed in Section 4.4, highlighting the condition for disease-free equilibrium, endemic equilibrium, Hopf-bifurcation and basic reproduction number. Section 4.5 showcases the numerical simulation and its results. Here, the effect of awareness, immigration, contact rate, treatment rate, etc. are described. The paper ends with a discussion about the major findings of the paper and conclusion in Section 4.6 and Section 4.7, respectively.

4.2 LITERATURE REVIEW

In the 21st century, we have witnessed an upsurge in the use of social media. During an epidemic or pandemic, public often refers to both social as well as traditional media for information [2]. Public digest the information they receive and often their behaviour, awareness and precautions they adopt are shaped by the social media [3]. This has opened up a new area of research and the authors are keen on analyzing the social media's ability to control an outbreak of an emerging disease.

In the article [4], the authors analyzed the influence of media by a mathematical model and concluded that media helps in delaying the infection peak and also reduces the infected population.

The authors in [5] developed a model to control the spread of infectious diseases by media coverage. Two equilibria, i.e, disease-free and endemic were found. The study concluded that media coverage alone is not enough in controlling the spread of diseases but plays an important role in reducing the cases of infected when its coverage is high.

The investigators in [6] developed a three-dimensional model to study the effect of media on control of infectious diseases and found three positive equilibria. They established that $R_o > 1$ and high media impact results in multiple equilibria.

The authors in [7] stated that awareness can be amplified and more effective if the social network and the network through which people communicate overlap. Moreover, the role of awareness spread through media on disease epidemiology considering immigration as an factor have been discussed in [8–11].

Deep learning (DL) is a new research field that has immense capability in medical field applications and has the potential to be used for emerging infectious diseases. Recently, the authors in [12] classified diabetes using the DL algorithm. Various activation functions, e.g. ELU and SELU, were introduced which helped in finding the solution for the neural network problem.

The authors in [13] utilized deep learning for not only the detection but also the classification of skin lesions as benign and malignant. The framework adopted had a very accurate classification that further improved network efficiency.

The scientists in [14] illustrated the "Internet of Things" (IOT) and showcased the application of machine learning to IOT and challenges encountered by IOT.

In recent past, the authors in [15] illustrated the application of big data, cloud computing, etc. in the medical field and healthcare system. On the other hand, the researchers in [16] studied the application of WSN and biometric models for online healthcare data.

Recently, many researchers are focusing on application of artificial intelligence (AI) and machine learning (ML). The researchers in [17] expressed that machine learning will aid in early identification of disease, better and personalised treatment and better outcome. Further, the researchers in [18] explained the application of machine learning techniques in sentiment analysis (SA) for drug reviews as narrated by users and also in food technology. In [19], the authors showcased the use of clinical decision support system (CDSS) for the diagnosis of Hepatitis-B.

Based on the literature review, we formulated our epidemiological model with the aim of establishing the beneficial impact of public awareness against emerging infectious diseases.

4.3 THE MATHEMATICAL MODEL

Here we consider five compartments: susceptible unaware population (S_w), susceptible aware population (S_a), infected population (I), media density M and recovery class R at time t. The rate of immigration is denoted by A. The parameter d represents the natural death rate of each class. We assume that contact between susceptible and infected classes only lead to spread in diseases.

Let λ be the dissemination rate of awareness by social media among susceptible. This leads to a new susceptible aware class. λ_0 is the transfer rate from aware to unaware susceptible class due to lacunae or negligence. Further, we assume that $\frac{\lambda M}{1+\gamma M}$, γ and $\frac{\lambda}{\gamma}$ represent the effect, limit of the effect and the maximum effect of awareness through social media on unaware susceptible population, respectively. Here, β represents the contact rate of S_w and I and β_1 is a fraction of $\beta(0 \leq \beta_1 \leq 1)$. Let α denote the disease-induced death rate from the infective class. We assume that the awareness density rate by social media is directly proportional to disease-related death rate α. Here, k is assumed as the proportionality constant. We assume that μ_0 is the depletion rate of awareness by social media due to prolonged time, monotonous information, etc. The parameter m represents the density level of social media focusing on the disease from outside areas. We know when a disease outbreaks, initial treatment is slow due to unavailability of proper drugs and correct health guidelines. As time progresses, with the availability of effective drugs and proper health information and health technologies, the treatment gains pace. Thus, in order to maintain balance, saturated treatment rate represented by $T(I) = \frac{aI}{1+bI}$ where a and b are positive constant is adopted. It clearly indicates that $\frac{a}{b} = \lim_{I\to\infty} T(I)$ is the maximum supply of resources including drugs per unit time. Also, $\frac{1}{1+bI}$ represents the reverse effect of infected ones who are delayed for treatment. The overall working principle of the model can be illustrated in Figure 4.1.

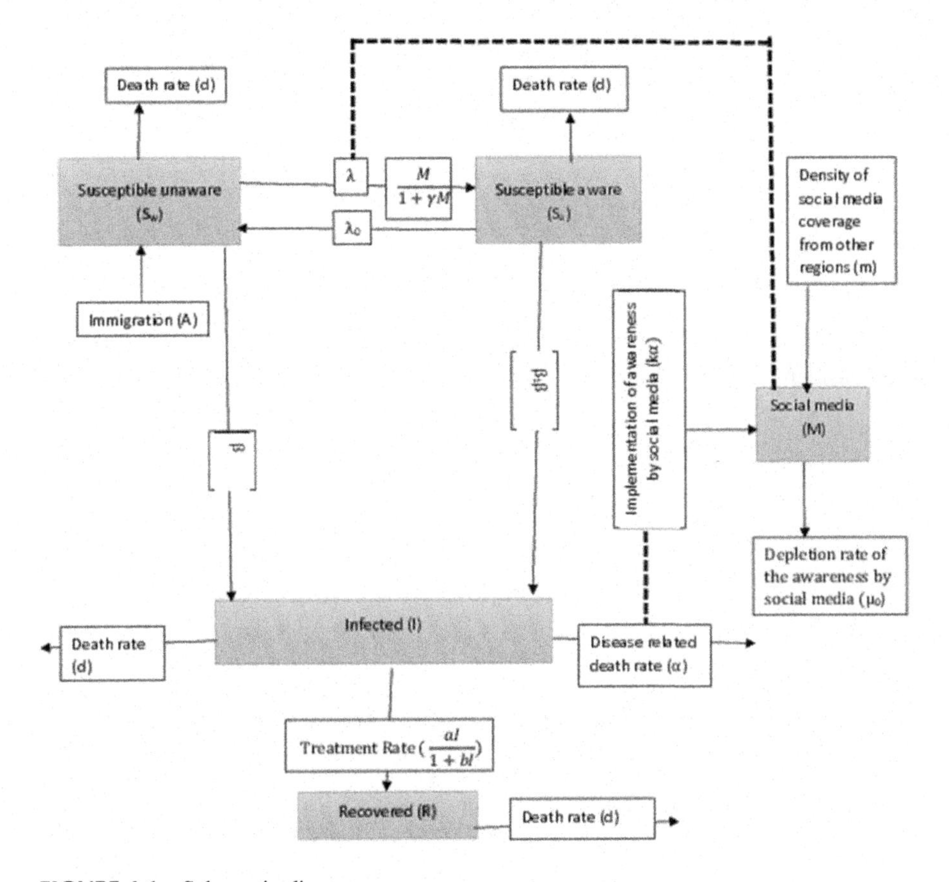

FIGURE 4.1 Schematic diagram.

With these above assumptions, our model system is:

$$
\left.
\begin{aligned}
\frac{dS_w}{dt} &= A - \beta S_w I - \frac{\lambda S_w M}{1+\gamma M} - dS_w + \lambda_0 S_a \\
\frac{dS_a}{dt} &= \frac{\lambda S_w M}{1+\gamma M} - \beta_1 \beta S_a I - dS_a - \lambda_0 S_a \\
\frac{dI}{dt} &= \beta S_w I + \beta_1 \beta S_a I - \alpha I - dI - \frac{aI}{1+bI} \\
\frac{dM}{dt} &= k\alpha I - \mu_0 M + m \\
\frac{dR}{dt} &= \frac{aI}{1+bI} - dR.
\end{aligned}
\right\}
\tag{4.1}
$$

We have carried out the analysis of the system (1) as per the initial conditions:

$$
S_w(0) > 0, \quad S_a(0) \geq 0, \quad I(0) \geq 0, \quad M(0) \geq 0, \quad R(0) \geq 0. \tag{4.2}
$$

From the above system (1) it is clearly indicates that S_w, S_a, I and M are independent from R as we assume that the recovered individuals gain immunity from the disease and is not further infected. Therefore, we consider the following subsystem rather than the previous system.

$$\left.\begin{aligned} \frac{dS_w}{dt} &= A - \beta S_w I - \frac{\lambda S_w M}{1+\gamma M} - dS_w + \lambda_0 S_a \\ \frac{dS_a}{dt} &= \frac{\lambda S_w M}{1+\gamma M} - \beta_1 \beta S_a I - dS_a - \lambda_0 S_a \\ \frac{dI}{dt} &= \beta S_w I + \beta_1 \beta S_a I - \alpha I - dI - \frac{aI}{1+bI} \\ \frac{dM}{dt} &= k\alpha I - \mu_0 M + m. \end{aligned}\right\} \tag{4.3}$$

We consider

$$N = S_w + S_a + I, \tag{4.4}$$

the system (3) transform to the following system:

$$\left.\begin{aligned} \frac{dN}{dt} &= A - dN - \alpha I - \frac{aI}{1+bI} \equiv G_1(N, S_a, I, M) \\ \frac{dS_a}{dt} &= \frac{\lambda(N - S_a - I)M}{1+\gamma M} - \beta_1 \beta S_a I - dS_a - \lambda_0 S_a \equiv G_2(N, S_a, I, M) \\ \frac{dI}{dt} &= \beta(N - (1-\beta_1)S_a - I)I - \left(\alpha + d + \frac{a}{1+bI}\right)I \equiv G_3(N, S_a, I, M) \\ \frac{dM}{dt} &= k\alpha I - \mu_0 M + m \equiv G_4(N, S_a, I, M). \end{aligned}\right\} \tag{4.5}$$

So, we choose to analyse system (5) instead of system (3). Here, the region of attraction is defined by $\Gamma = \left\{(N, S_a, I, M) \in R_+^4 : 0 \le S_w, I \le N \le \frac{A}{d}, 0 \le M \le \frac{k\alpha\left(\frac{A}{d}\right)+m}{\mu_0}\right\}$. As per the existence and uniqueness theorem, the trajectories are unable to approach the unfeasible domain from positive octant, which means that the solution will be in positive octant. This results in the system being well defined.

Explicitly, the jacobian matrix at $\bar{E} = (\bar{N}, \overline{S_a}, \bar{I}, \bar{M})$ is represented by

$$\bar{V} = \begin{bmatrix} -d & 0 & -\alpha - \frac{a}{(1+b\bar{I})^2} & 0 \\ \frac{\lambda\bar{M}}{1+\gamma\bar{M}} & -\left(\frac{\lambda\bar{M}}{1+\gamma\bar{M}} + \beta_1\beta\bar{I} + d + \lambda_0\right) & -\frac{\lambda\bar{M}}{1+\gamma\bar{M}} - \beta_1\beta\overline{S_a} & \frac{\lambda(\bar{N} - \overline{S_a} - \bar{I})}{1+\gamma\bar{M}} \\ \beta\bar{I} & -\beta(1-\beta_1)\bar{I} & \begin{array}{c}\beta\bar{N} - \beta(1-\beta_1)\overline{S_a} - 2\beta\bar{I} \\ -\left(\frac{a}{(1+b\bar{I})^2} + \alpha + d\right)\end{array} & 0 \\ 0 & 0 & k\alpha & -\mu_0 \end{bmatrix} \tag{4.6}$$

4.4 SOME PRELIMINARY RESULTS

4.4.1 EQUILIBRIA

The system (5) exhibits two equilibria like the disease-free equilibrium (DFE) $E_0 = \left(\frac{A}{d}, \frac{\lambda m A}{d[\lambda m + (d+\lambda_0)(\mu_0 + \lambda m)]}, 0, \frac{m}{\mu_0}\right)$ and endemic equilibrium $E^* = (N^*, S_a^*, I^*, M^*)$.

4.4.1.1 Disease-Free Equilibrium

E_0 is always feasible. The eigenvalues evaluated from (6) at E_0 are $-d < 0$, $-\frac{\lambda m}{\mu_0 + \gamma m} - d - \lambda_0 < 0$, $-\mu_0$ and $-\frac{\beta\lambda m A(1-\beta_1)}{d[\lambda m + (d+\lambda_0)(\mu_0 + \lambda m)]} + \frac{\beta A}{d}\left[\frac{(d+\lambda+a)d}{A\beta} - 1\right]$. Thus, it clearly indicates that E_0 is asymptotically stable if

$$R_0 = \frac{\beta A}{d(a + \alpha + d)} < 1 \tag{4.7}$$

hold. Here, the basic reproduction number is defined by R_0. Clearly, E^* exists for $R_0 > 1$.

4.4.1.2 Endemic Equilibrium

The endemic equilibrium at $E^* = (N^*, S_a^*, I^*, M^*)$ are $N^* = I^* + (1 - \beta_1)S_a + \frac{(d+\alpha+a)+b(d+\alpha)I^*}{\beta(1+bI^*)}$, $S_a^* = \frac{[(d+\alpha+a)+b(d+\alpha)I^*(k\alpha\lambda I^* + m\lambda)]}{\beta(1+bI^*)[\lambda(k\alpha I + m) + (d+\lambda_0+\beta_1\beta I^* - \lambda(1-\beta_1))](\mu_0 + k\alpha\gamma + m\gamma)}$, $M^* = \frac{k\alpha I^* + m}{\mu_0}$, while I^* is ensured by putting the value of N^* and S_a in the first equation of system (5). It is hard to find the positive root of I^* analytically. Therefore, we get the positive root of I^* with the help of numerical analysis.

At E^*, the jacobian matrix of system (5) can be written as

$$V^* = \begin{bmatrix} n_{11} & 0 & n_{13} & 0 \\ n_{21} & n_{22} & n_{23} & n_{24} \\ n_{31} & n_{32} & n_{33} & 0 \\ 0 & 0 & n_{43} & n_{44} \end{bmatrix}, \tag{4.8}$$

where

$$\theta_{11} = -d < 0,\ \theta_{13} = -\alpha - \frac{a}{(1+bI^*)^2} < 0,\ \theta_{21} = \frac{\lambda M^*}{1+\gamma M^*} > 0,$$
$$\theta_{22} = -\frac{\lambda M^*}{1+\gamma M^*} - \beta\beta_1 I^* - d - \lambda_0 < 0,\ \theta_{23} = -\frac{\lambda M^*}{1+\gamma M^*} - \beta_1\beta S_a < 0,$$
$$\theta_{24} = \frac{\lambda(N^* - S_a^* - I^*)}{1+\gamma M^*} > 0,\ \theta_{31} = \beta I^* > 0,\ \theta_{32} = -\beta(1-\beta_1)I^* < 0,\ \theta_{33} = -\beta I^* + \frac{abI^*}{(1+bI^*)^2}$$
$$\in R,\ \theta_{43} = k\alpha > 0,\ \theta_{44} = -\mu_0 < 0.$$

Now the corresponding characteristic equation is

$$\omega^4 + Q_1\omega^3 + Q_2\omega^2 + Q_3\omega + Q_4 = 0, \tag{4.9}$$

where the coefficients Q_I, $I = 1, 2, 3, 4$ are

$$\left.\begin{array}{l} Q_1 = -(\theta_{11} + \theta_{22} + \theta_{33} + \theta_{44}), \\ Q_2 = \theta_{11}\theta_{22} + \theta_{22}\theta_{33} + \theta_{33}\theta_{11} + \theta_{11}\theta_{44} + \theta_{22}\theta_{44} + \theta_{33}\theta_{44} - \theta_{23}\theta 32 - \theta_{13}\theta_{31}, \\ Q_3 = \theta_{13}\theta_{31}\theta_{44} + \theta_{23}\theta_{32}\theta_{44} + \theta_{11}\theta_{23}\theta_{32} + \theta_{13}\theta_{31}\theta_{22} - \theta_{11}\theta_{22}\theta_{44} - \theta_{11}\theta_{33}\theta_{44} \\ - \theta_{22}\theta_{33}\theta_{44} - \theta_{11}\theta_{22}\theta_{33} - \theta_{13}\theta_{21}\theta_{32} - \theta_{24}\theta_{32}\theta_{43}, \\ Q_4 = \theta_{11}\theta_{22}\theta_{33}\theta_{44} + \theta_{13}\theta_{21}\theta_{32}\theta_{44} + \theta_{11}\theta_{24}\theta_{32}\theta_{43} - \theta_{11}\theta_{44}\theta_{23}\theta_{32} - \theta_{13}\theta_{22}\theta_{31}\theta_{44}. \end{array}\right\} \tag{4.10}$$

Case 1: Clearly, $Q_1 > 0$ If $\theta_{33} < 0$.

Now, $Q_2 > 0$ if $\theta_{23}\theta_{32} > (\theta_{11}\theta_{22} + \theta_{11}\theta_{33} + \theta_{22}\theta_{33} + \theta_{11}\theta_{44} + \theta_{22}\theta_{44} + \theta_{33}\theta_{44} - \theta_{13}\theta_{31}$.
Also, $Q_3 > 0$ if $(\theta_{13}\theta_{31}\theta_{44} + \theta_{13}\theta_{31}\theta_{22} - \theta_{11}\theta_{22}\theta_{44} - \theta_{11}\theta_{33}\theta_{44} - \theta_{22}\theta_{33}\theta_{44} - \theta_{11}\theta_{22}\theta_{33} - \theta_{24}\theta_{32}\theta_{43}) > \theta_{13}\theta_{21}\theta_{32} - \theta_{11}\theta_{23}\theta_{32} - \theta_{23}\theta_{32}\theta_{44}$.
Here, $Q_4 > 0$ if $\theta_{11}\theta_{22}\theta_{33}\theta_{44} + \theta_{11}\theta_{24}\theta_{32}\theta_{43} - \theta_{13}\theta_{22}\theta_{31}\theta_{44} > \theta_{11}\theta_{22}\theta_{23}\theta_{44} - \theta_{13}\theta_{21}\theta_{32}\theta_{44}$.

Case 2: If $\theta_{33} > 0$ then $Q_1 > 0$ if $-(\theta_{11} + \theta_{22} + \theta_{44}) > \theta_{33}$.

Also, $Q_2 > 0$ if $\theta_{23}\theta_{32} - \theta_{11}\theta_{33} - \theta_{33}\theta_{44} > \theta_{11}\theta_{22} + \theta_{22}\theta_{33} + \theta_{11}\theta_{44} + \theta_{22}\theta_{44} - \theta_{13}\theta_{31})$. Also, $Q_3 > 0$ if $\theta_{13}\theta_{31}\theta_{44} + \theta_{13}\theta_{31}\theta_{22} - \theta_{11}\theta_{22}\theta_{44} - \theta_{24}\theta_{32}\theta_{43} > \theta_{11}\theta_{33}\theta_{44} + \theta_{22}\theta_{33}\theta_{44} + \theta_{11}\theta_{22}\theta_{33} + \theta_{13}\theta_{21}\theta_{32} - \theta_{11}\theta_{23}\theta_{32} - \theta_{23}\theta_{32}\theta_{44}$.
Here, $Q_4 > 0$ if $\theta_{11}\theta_{24}\theta_{32}\theta_{43} - \theta_{13}\theta_{22}\theta_{31}\theta_{44} > \theta_{11}\theta_{44}\theta_{23}\theta_{22} - \theta_{13}\theta_{21}\theta_{32}\theta_{44} - \theta_{11}\theta_{22}\theta_{33}\theta_{44}$.
Then, $Q_1Q_2 - Q_3 > 0$ if $Q_1Q_2 > Q_3$ as well as $Q_3(Q_1Q_2 - Q_3) - Q_1^2Q_4 > 0$ if $Q_3(Q_1Q_2 - Q_3) > Q_1^2Q_4$. As per the Routh-Hurwitz criterion, endemic equilibrium i.e., E^* is locally asymptotically stable which depends upon system parameters.

Remark 4.1: By fulfilling the following two conditions, the system may show Hopf-bifurcation at the endemic equilibrium.

$$Q_1(k_c)Q_2(k_c) - Q_3(k_c) = 0, \quad Q_1,(k_c)Q_2(k_c) + Q_1(k_c)Q_2,(k_c) - Q_3,(k_c) \neq 0. \tag{4.11}$$

4.4.2 Hopf Bifurcation at Coexistence

Theorem. (Hopf-Bifurcation)

If $\psi_1(k) > 0$, endemic equilibrium of (5) is locally asymptotically stable. For fulfilling the following conditions $\psi_1(k_c) = 0$ and $\left(\frac{d\psi_1}{dk}\right)|_{k_c} \neq 0$, and as k crosses $k_c \in R$, the system undergoes Hopf-bifurcation at E^* [20,21].

At E^*, we can write the characteristic equation in simplified form

$$\omega^4 + Q_1\omega^3 + Q_2\omega^2 + Q_3\omega + Q_4 = 0. \tag{4.12}$$

Let us define

$$\psi_1(k) = Q_1(k)Q_2(k)Q_3(k) - Q_3^2(k) - Q_1^2(k)Q_4(k). \tag{4.13}$$

Let the above characteristic equation have four roots $\omega_i (i = 1, 2, 3, 4)$.

Then we get

$$\left.\begin{aligned} &\omega_1 + \omega_2 + \omega_3 + \omega_4 = -Q_1, \\ &\omega_1\omega_2 + \omega_1\omega_3 + \omega_1\omega_4 + \omega_2\omega_3 + \omega_2\omega_4 + \omega_3\omega_4 = Q_2, \\ &\omega_1\omega_2\omega_3 + \omega_1\omega_3\omega_4 + \omega_2\omega_3\omega_4 + \omega_1\omega_2\omega_4 = -Q_3, \\ &\omega_1\omega_2\omega_3\omega_4 = Q_4. \end{aligned}\right\} \tag{4.14}$$

The Routh-Hurwitz criterion indicates that a minimum of one root will have a characteristic equation, say ω_1, with zero real parts if there exists $k_c \in R$ such that $\psi_1(k_c) = 0$. The fourth condition of (14) reveals that $Im\ \omega_1 = \omega_0 \neq 0$. Therefore, ω_2, then another root can be defined as $\omega_2 = \bar{\omega}_1$, since $\psi_1(k)$ represents a continuous function where ω_1 and ω_2 are complex conjugate roots in which k_c stay in an open interval of k. Thus, equation (4.14) can be derived in the following form at k_c:

$$\left.\begin{aligned} &\omega_3 + \omega_4 = -Q_1, \\ &\omega_0^2 + \omega_3\omega_4 = Q_2, \\ &\omega_0^2(\omega_3 + \omega_4) = -Q_3, \\ &\omega_0^2\omega_3\omega_4 = Q_4. \end{aligned}\right\} \tag{4.15}$$

First, equation of (14) follows that $2Re\ \omega_3 = -Q_1 < 0$ when ω_3 and ω_4 are complex conjugate. If ω_3 and ω_4 are real, evaluating first and fourth conditions of (15) indicates that $\omega_3 < 0$ and $\omega_4 < 0$. Also, after some calculations, it follows that

$$\frac{d}{dk} Re\,(\omega_1)_{k=k_c} = -\frac{Q_1}{2[Q_1^2 Q_4 + (Q_1Q_2 - 2Q_3)^2]}\frac{d\psi_1}{dk}\Big|_{k_c} \neq 0. \tag{4.16}$$

Hence, proof of the theorem.

4.5 NUMERICAL SIMULATIONS

Here we investigate the effects of the various parameters on the qualitative behaviour of the system by using MATLAB. We begin with parametric values in Table 4.1 [22–25].

Dealing with the above set of parametric values, we observe the system to be locally asymptotically stable at endemic equilibrium $E^*(35000, 4406, 81, 22)$ where $R_0 = 1.2698 > 1$ (cf. Figure 4.2(a)).

TABLE 4.1
A Set of Parameter Values

Parameter	Definition	Value
A	Immigration rate	400
β	Contact rate of aware susceptible and infected class	0.00002
β_1	Fraction part of β	0.2
λ	Dissemination rate of awareness by social media among susceptible	0.0002
λ_0	Transfer rate from aware to unaware susceptible class	0.02
γ	Limit of the effect through social media	0.001
α	Disease induced death rate from infective class	0.02
d	Natural death rate of all classes	0.01
μ_0	Depletion rate of awareness by social media d	0.06
k	Proportionality constant of awareness	0.8
m	Density level of social media focusing on the disease from outside areas	0.05
a	Positive constant due to saturated treatment rate	0.6
b	Positive constant due to saturated treatment rate	0.00005

4.5.1 System Behaviour Changes for A

The endemic equilibrium is seen as the immigration rate crosses the critical value $A = 316$. Taking $A = 300$, we observe that the system exhibits disease-free equilibrium, E_0, which satisfies our analytical finding (cf. Figure 4.2(b)). Thus, it signifies that as we reduce immigration rate, the infected population also decreases. Figure 4.2(c) illustrates the oscillatory behaviour of each class for a high value of A (viz. $A = 450$). Biologically, it signifies when immigration rate increases, and the disease is likely to outbreak. Now, for clear understanding of dynamic change, we plot a bifurcation diagram with respect to A (cf. Figure 4.2(d)). Here we see as the immigration rate increases after a certain point, the system outbreaks.

4.5.2 Dynamical Changes due to k and β

Taking $k = 2.8$, the system becomes unstable (cf. Figure 4.3(a)). It is observed that a high value of the contact rate of unaware susceptible to infective class ($\beta = 0.00004$) leads the system to oscillate (cf. Figure 4.3(b)). Further, we have displayed suitable bifurcation diagrams when k and β are treated as free parameters simultaneously (cf. Figure 4.3(c–d)). Biologically speaking, the bifurcation of k depicts that as the awareness by social media increases the infected decreases, but after a certain point (threshold value of k) the system outbreaks.

4.5.3 Impact of A on the Infected Population

Figure 4.4(a) represents the effect of A on the infected population. It is observed that the infected population decreases with a decrease of A. Here, a branch point (BP) is

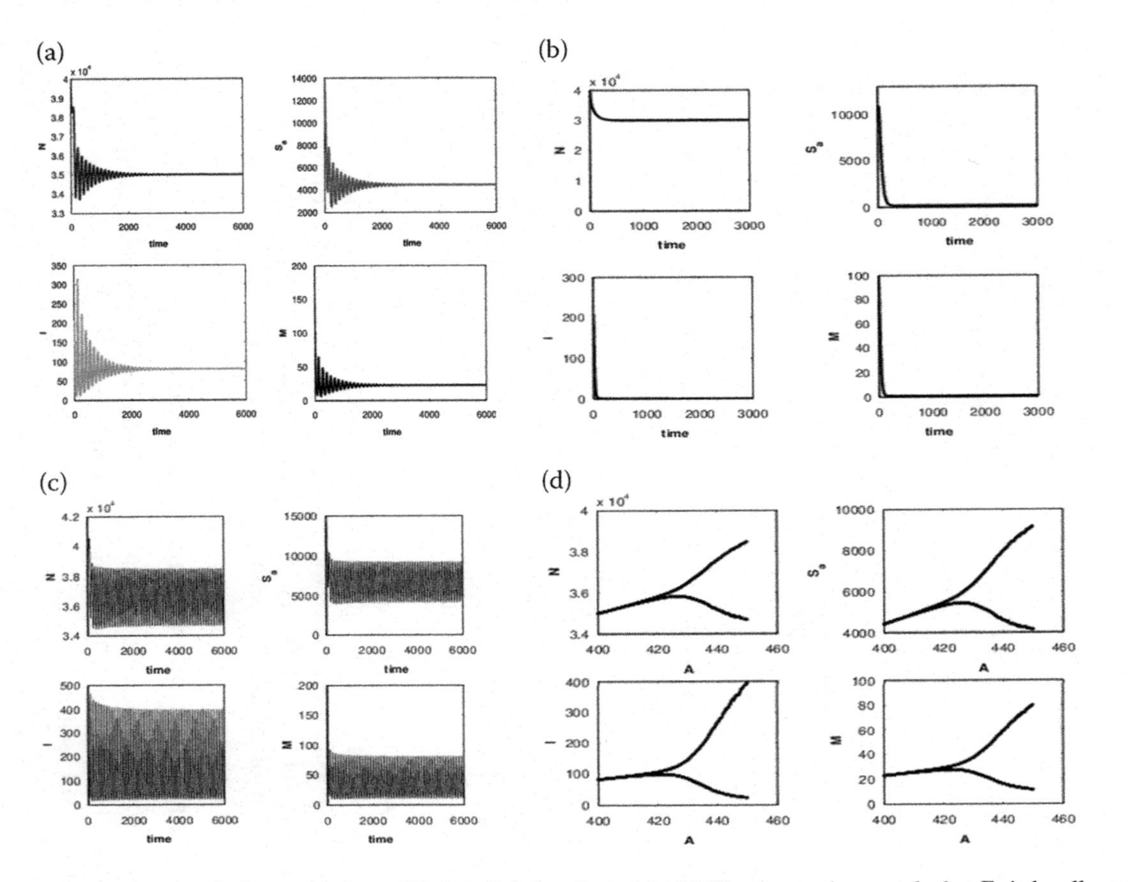

FIGURE 4.2 (a) The time series reveals that endemic equilibrium E^* is locally stable. (b) The time series reveals that E_0 is locally stable for $A = 300$. (c) Exhibit oscillatory behaviour of each population of system (1) for $A = 450$. (d) Bifurcation diagram for A.

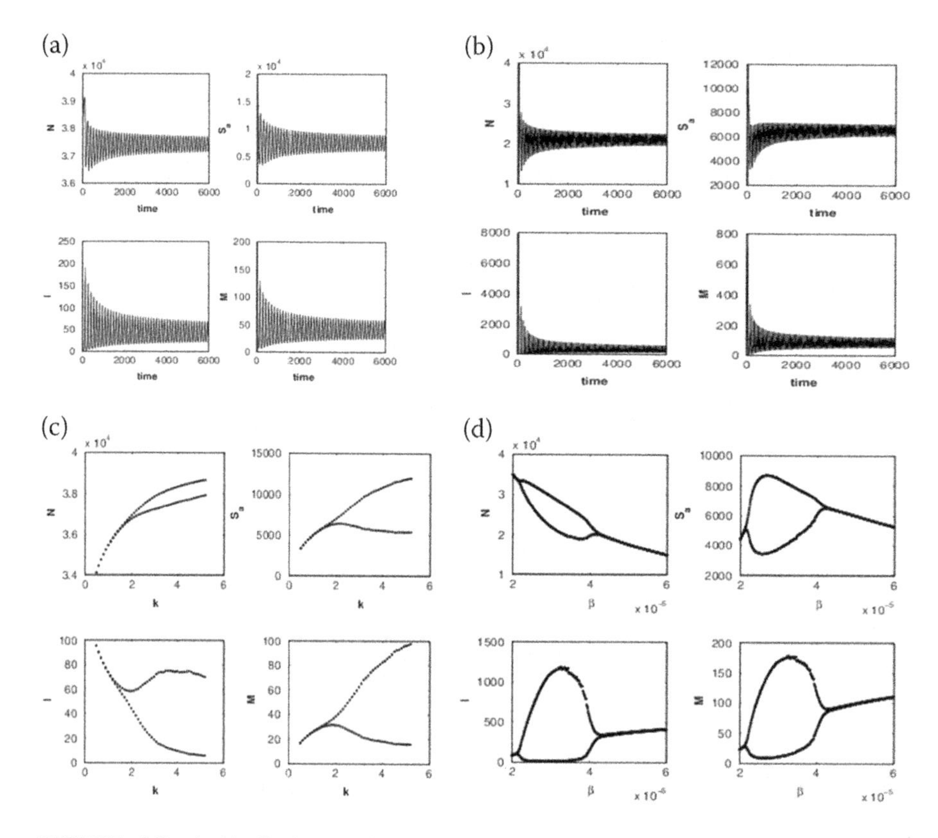

FIGURE 4.3 (a–b) Each population shows fluctuating behaviour for $k = 2.8$ and $\beta = 0.00004$, respectively. (c) Bifurcation diagram for k. (d) Bifurcation diagram for β.

situated at $A = 316$ with eigenvalues $-0.06, -0.03, -0.01, 0$ and the transcritical bifurcation occurs where the infected population goes to extinction. It is notified that the infected population increases with an increase of A. In this case, we have a Hopf bifurcation point H at $A_c = 433$ with first Lyapunov coefficient $-3.040463e^{-10}$. We draw a family of stable limit cycles bifurcating from H points.

4.5.4 Impact of k on the Infected Population

Figure 4.4(b) follows that the infected population decreases gradually as the value of k increases and after k crosses a certain value $k = k_c = 2.55$, the infected population will oscillate.

4.5.5 Effect of β

When we vary the parameter β as a free parameter, Figure 4.4(c) depicts the infected population exhibits oscillatory behaviour in between $0.000022 \leq \beta \leq 0.000040$. It clearly indicates that the system will be disease free for a low value of contact rate of unaware population with the infected population.

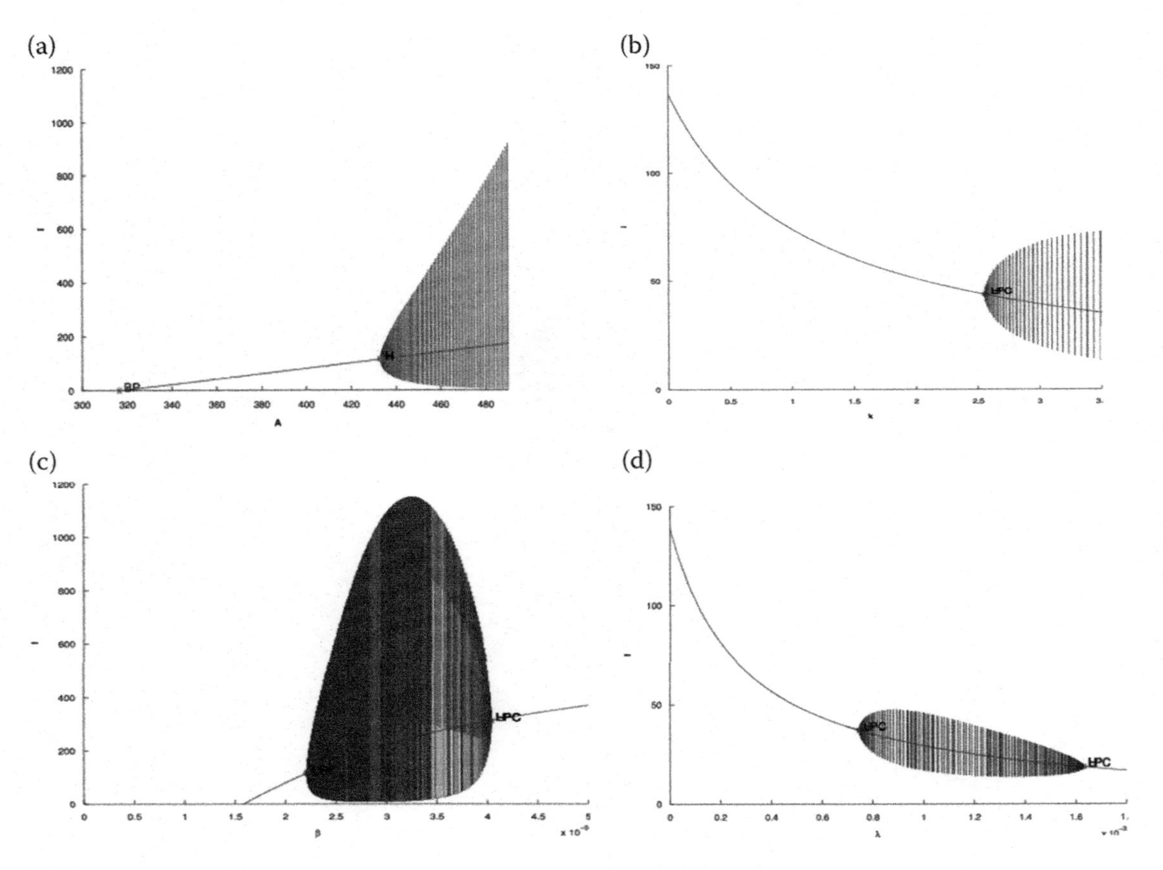

FIGURE 4.4 (a–d) The figures reveal different natures of infected class for A, k, β and λ, respectively.

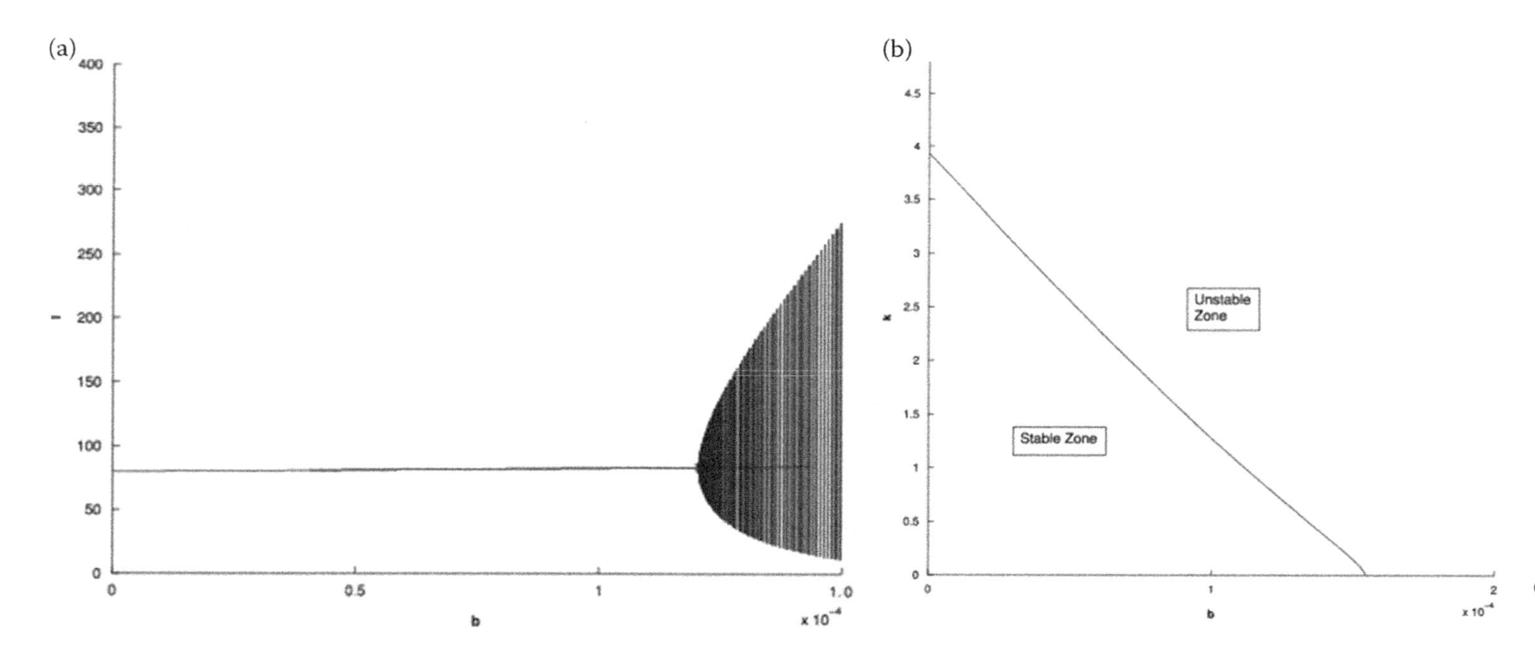

FIGURE 4.5 (a) Different characters of infected class for b. (b) Two parameters bifurcation diagram for $b - k$.

4.5.6 Effect of λ

Figure 4.4(d) follows that the infected population will oscillate in between $0.000747 \leq \lambda \leq 0.001630$. Therefore, dissemination rate of awareness among the susceptible population makes a big impact on the infected population.

4.5.7 Impact of Treatment (b) on the Infected Population

To study the impact of treatment on the infected population, we plot Figure 4.5(a). It follows that for high values of b, the infected population will oscillate i.e., disease can spread quickly due to low rate treatment.

4.5.8 Two-Parameter Bifurcation Diagram

Further, we study the combined effect of treatment and implementation of awareness by social media by plotting two parameters bifurcation diagram for $b - k$ (cf. Figure 4.5(b)). Finally, to find the combined effect of two parameters in proposed system bifurcation diagrams for $A - k$, $A - \beta$, $A - \lambda$ and $\beta - \lambda$ (cf. Figure 4.6(a–d)), respectively, are plotted. Biologically speaking, in the stable zone, the disease is under

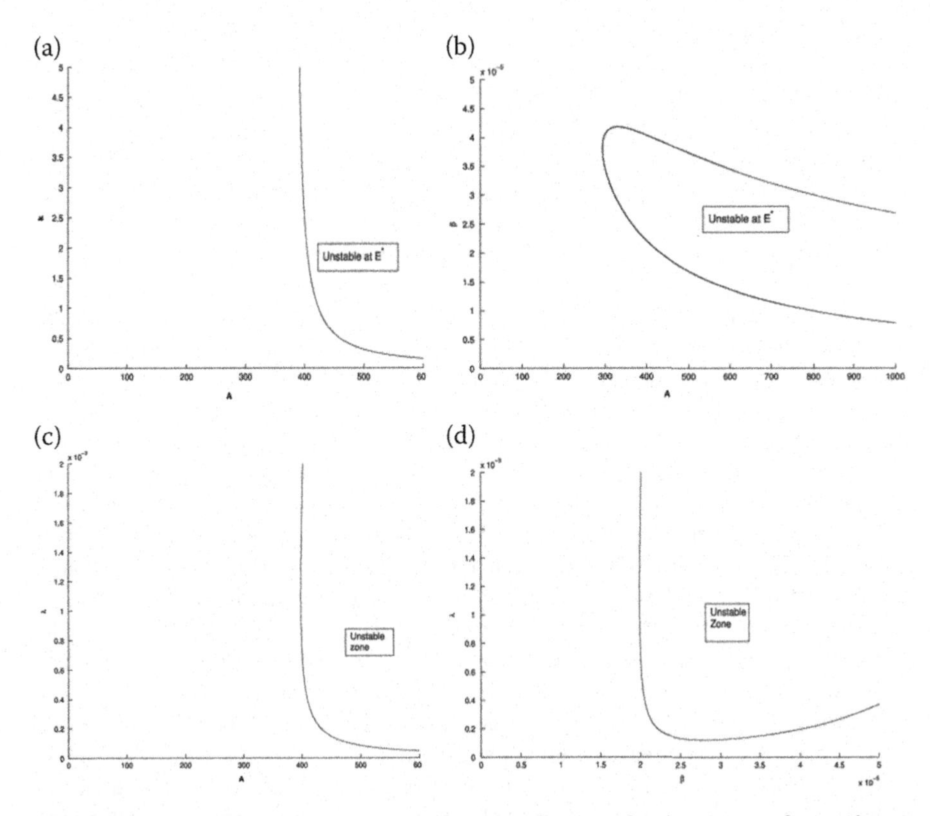

FIGURE 4.6 (a–d) The two parameter bifurcation diagrams for $A - k$, $A - \beta$, $A - \lambda$ and $\beta - \lambda$.

TABLE 4.2
Nature of Equilibrium Points

Parameters	Values	Eigenvalues	Equilibrium Points
A	433	$(-0.0890896,\ -0.0163409,\ \pm0.0541472i)$	Hopf (H)
	316	$(-0.06,\ -0.03,\ -0.01,\ 0)$	Branch Point (BP)
k	2.55	$(-0.0944078,\ -0.0126601,\ \pm.0499686i)$	Hopf (H)
β	0.000022	$(-0.0890093,\ -0.0167726,\ \pm0.0555492i)$	Hopf (H)
	0.000040	$(-.0996873,\ -.021768,\ \pm0.0951406i)$	Hopf (H)
λ	0.000747	$(-0.0954191,\ -0.0122348,\ \pm0.0498602i)$	Hopf (H)
	0.001630	$(-0.0981213,\ -0.0111113,\ \pm0.0496384i)$	Hopf (H)
b	0.000120	$(-0.0843235,\ -0.0162784,\ \pm0.046957i)$	Hopf (H)

control but in an unstable zone the disease may outbreak. Summarizing the observations, natures of equilibrium points are displayed in Table 4.2.

4.6 DISCUSSION

Social media is becoming the undisputed weapon in epidemics and pandemics for spreading awareness through health information. Keeping this aspect in mind, we have analyzed a five-compartment mathematical model. Then, we have evaluated two equilibria like E_0 and E^* under certain conditions. Analytic studies reveal that when $R_0 < 1$, the system exhibits E_0. The existence and stability of E^* will occur for $R_0 > 1$. They are related to each other by transcritical bifurcations when $R_0 = 1$. In particular, the disease-free equilibrium can be obtained from endemic equilibrium if the immigration rate fall below a critical threshold $R_0 < 316$. The biological significance of our study highlights various interesting facts. It shows that by increasing implementation of awareness by social media, the infected cases decline. But this social media is effective up to a certain extent, after crossing that threshold the system becomes unstable i.e, there may be disease outbreak. Immigration may be held responsible for such results. Monotonous information, political barriers, social and psychological barriers, prolonged time, etc. are some of the other reasons. Immigration also plays a big role in the disease outbreaks. When the immigration is low, the disease will be under control but a high rate of immigration may lead to an epidemic or pandemic. Further, we observe that the contact rate of unaware susceptible with infected class play a key tool for controlling the epidemic. We also find that when the treatment rate is high, then infected individuals decrease. Therefore, it clearly indicates that disease can be controlled and even eradicated when there is enough awareness by social media among the susceptible, enough treatment is available and immigration rate is low. Therefore, lacking at least one of these things may not be enough for disease control or eradication.

Recently, humanity is fighting against the global pandemic of Coronavirus at present, which is an emerging infectious disease. Our findings from the study correlate strongly with the COVID-19 scenario. Social media and the awareness it spreads had a big impact on our study. We are witnessing the same situation worldwide where social media has become an important tool for raising awareness, sharing health information, etc. in our fight against Coronavirus. Throughout the study, we have focused on applying our mathematical model in a real field scenario.

4.7 CONCLUSION

This paper formulates a model for studying the effect of awareness on emerging diseases. Awareness among the public and correct health information together forms the strong shield in our fight against these emerging diseases. Social media carries out this role of spreading awareness perfectly. This motivated us for this research and through our study we conclude that there is a decline in infected cases with increased awareness spread by social media. This proves the effectiveness of social media. The role of immigration is also vital. Its increase may lead to an epidemic or pandemic while its decrease keeps the system stable. Another major finding of our study focuses on reducing the infected cases with proper treatment. We are presently dealing with an emerging infectious disease i.e., COVID-19. This model may also be applied in the present COVID-19 scenario as its findings are highly relatable with the current situation.

REFERENCES

[1] Tang, L., Bie, B., Park, S. E., and Zhi, D. "Social media and outbreaks of emerging infectious diseases: A systematic review of literature." *American Journal of Infection Control*, 46, no. 9 (2018): 962–972. 10.1016/j.ajic.2018.02.010

[2] Freberg, K., Palenchar, M. J., and Veil, S. R. "Managing and sharing H1N1 crisis information using social media bookmarking services." *Public Relations Review*, 39, no. 3 (2013): 178–184. 10.1016/j.pubrev.2013.02.007

[3] Slovic, P. E. *The perception of risk.* Earthscan publications, (2000).

[4] Liu, Y., and Cui, J. A. "The impact of media coverage on the dynamics of infectious disease." *International Journal of Biomathematics*, 1, no. 01 (2008): 65–74. 10.1142/S1793524508000023

[5] Cui, J. A., Tao, X., and Zhu, H. "An SIS infection model incorporating media coverage." *The Rocky Mountain Journal of Mathematics*, 38, no. 5 (2008): 1323–1334. 10.1216/RMJ-2008-38-5-1

[6] Cui, J., Sun, Y., and Zhu, H. "The impact of media on the control of infectious diseases." *Journal of Dynamics and Differential Equations*, 20, no. 1 (2008): 31–53. 10.1007/s10884-007-9075-0

[7] Funk, S., Gilad, E., Watkins, C., and Jansen, V. A. "The spread of awareness and its impact on epidemic outbreaks." *Proceedings of the National Academy of Sciences*, 106, no. 16 (2009): 6872–6877. 10.1073/pnas.0810762106

[8] Misra, A. K., Sharma, A., and Shukla, J. B. "Modeling and analysis of effects of awareness programs by media on the spread of infectious diseases." *Mathematical and Computer Modelling*, 53, no. 5-6 (2011): 1221–1228. 10.1016/j.mcm.2010.12.005

[9] Misra, A. K., Sharma, A., and Singh, V. "Effect of awareness programs in controlling the prevalence of an epidemic with time delay." *Journal of Biological Systems*, 19, no. 02 (2011): 389–402. 10.1142/S0218339011004020

[10] Zakary, O., Rachik, M., and Elmouki, I. "On the impact of awareness programs in HIV/AIDS prevention: an SIR model with optimal control." *International Journal of Computer Applications in Technology*, 133, no. 9 (2016): 1–6. 10.5120/ijca2016908030

[11] Zakary, O., Larrache, A., Rachik, M., and Elmouki, I. "Effect of awareness programs and travel-blocking operations in the control of HIV/AIDS outbreaks: a

multi-domains SIR model." *Advances in Difference Equations*, 2016, no. 1 (2016): 1–17. 10.1186/s13662-016-0900-9

[12] Kumar, S., Bhusan, B., Singh, D., and kumar Choubey, D. (2020, July). "Classification of diabetes using deep learning." In *2020 International Conference on Communication and Signal Processing (ICCSP)* (pp. 0651–0655). IEEE. 10.1109/ICCSP48568.2020.9182293

[13] Khamparia, A., Singh, P. K., Rani, P., Samanta, D., Khanna, A., and Bhushan, B. (2020). "An internet of health things-driven deep learning framework for detection and classification of skin cancer using transfer learning." *Transactions on Emerging Telecommunications Technologies*, e3963. 10.1002/ett.3963

[14] Jindal, M., Gupta, J., and Bhushan, B. "Machine learning methods for IoT and their future applications." In *2019 International Conference on Computing, Communication, and Intelligent Systems (ICCCIS)* (pp. 430–434). IEEE. (2019), October. 10.1109/ICCCIS48478.2019.8974551

[15] Goyal, S., Sharma, N., Bhushan, B., Shankar, A., and Sagayam, M. "IoT enabled technology in secured healthcare: Applications, challenges and future directions." In *Cognitive Internet of Medical Things for Smart Healthcare* (pp. 25–48). Springer, Cham, (2021). 10.1007/978-3-030-55833-8_2

[16] Sharma, N., Kaushik, I., Bhushan, B., Gautam, S., and Khamparia, A. "Applicability of WSN and biometric models in the field of healthcare." In *Deep Learning Strategies for Security Enhancement in Wireless Sensor Networks* (pp. 304–329). IGI Global, Hershey, Pennsylvania, (2020). 10.4018/978-1-7998-5068-7.ch016

[17] Pattnayak, P., & Jena, O. P. "Innovation on machine learning in healthcare services—An introduction." *Machine Learning for Healthcare Applications*, 1. (2021). 10.1002/9781119792611.ch1

[18] Paramesha, K., Gururaj, H. L., & Jena, O. P. "Applications of machine learning in biomedical text processing and food industry." *Machine Learning for Healthcare Applications*, 151, (2021). 10.1002/9781119792611.ch10

[19] Panigrahi, N., Ayus, I., & Jena, O. P. "An expert system-based clinical decision support system for Hepatitis-B prediction & diagnosis." *Machine Learning for Healthcare Applications*, 57, (2021). 10.1002/9781119792611.ch4

[20] Ruan, S., and Wolkowicz, G. S. "Bifurcation analysis of a chemostat model with a distributed delay." *Journal of Mathematical Analysis and Applications*, 204, no. 3 (1996): 786–812. 10.1006/jmaa.1996.0468

[21] Pal, S., and Chatterjee, A. "Role of constant nutrient input and mortality rate of planktivorous fish in plankton community ecosystem with instantaneous nutrient recycling." *Canadian Applied Mathematics Quarterly*, 20, (2012): 179–207.

[22] Samanta, S., Rana, S., Sharma, A., Misra, A. K., and Chattopadhyay, J. "Effect of awareness programs by media on the epidemic outbreaks: A mathematical model." *Applied Mathematics and Computation*, 219, no. 12 (2013): 6965–6977. 10.1016/j.amc.2013.01.009

[23] Zuo, L., and Liu, M. "Effect of awareness programs on the epidemic outbreaks with time delay." In *Abstract and Applied Analysis* (Vol. 2014). Hindawi, (2014), January. 10.1155/2014/940841

[24] Zuo, L., Liu, M., and Wang, J. "The impact of awareness programs with recruitment and delay on the spread of an epidemic." *Mathematical Problems in Engineering*, 2015, (2015). 10.1155/2015/235935

[25] Purwati, U. D., & Amalia, N. "A mathematical model of social media popularity with standard incidence rate." In *IOP Conference Series: Materials Science and Engineering* (Vol. 546, No. 5, p. 052086). IOP Publishing, Malang, Indonesia, (2019), June. 10.1088/1757-899X/546/5/052086

5 Prediction of Diabetes Mellitus Using Machine Learning

Salliah Shafi Bhat and Gufran Ahmad Ansari
B.S. Abdur Rahman Crescent Institute of Science and Technology, Vandalur, Tamil Nadu, India

CONTENTS

5.1 INTRODUCTION

Disease is a complex condition associated with increasing blood glucose levels [1]. One of the causes of death among people around the world is a disorder that leads to severe heart attacks and affects blood vessels, eyes, kidneys, and nerves [2]. Diabetes mellitus is one of the most serious diseases under both developed as well as developing countries. Data on medical records consists of the number of examinations required for the diagnosis of a serious disease. The treatment is based on the doctor's knowledge and experience. A less experienced doctor or physician can incorrectly diagnose a problem. From machine learning, stakeholders benefit

DOI: 10.1201/9781003189053-5

tremendously in the area of healthcare. In the world of healthcare, there is a large number data and records available and the knowledge has no disciplinary importance to transform into awareness and facts, which can help to limit prices, raise earnings and sustain high-quality treatment for patients.

The primary objective of this work is the detection of diabetes using the classification of a hybrid approach consisting of Bayesian and multilayer classifications, support vector machine and classifies the information as hypoglycemic and non-diabetic. Generally, most diabetes is classified into two types i.e. type 1 and type 2 diabetes, and these are all the hypertension types [3]. High blood pressure is studied as a key significant health problem in which it is difficult to regulate the measurement of the sugar content. High blood pressure is not only caused by different variables such as age, gender, genetic factor and glucose, but also a sugar accumulation among all variables is the key explanation considered. The only alternative remaining is preventative medicine, which is much more complicated [4]. In both classification and forecasting algorithms, authors used machine learning, which has distinct abilities [5].

A small amount of work has been done to improve the performance and overall results. Precision for all diseases provides the optimum utility in a given data set and other techniques for other disorders approach. The rest among others are illnesses. Classification and analysis of diabetes mellitus (DM), overcoming the problem of single or entity classifiers, one of the most important decision-making methods is grouping, as shown in Figure 5.1.

Type 1 Diabetes: Type 1 diabetes is also referred to as diabetes mellitus, or glucose. Diabetes is a disease in which there is little insulin generated by the pancreas. Insulin is a hormone that is required to allow sugar (glucose) to reach energy-producing organisms. Diabetes mellitus develops a direct effect of the insulin factor not being produced by the pancreas. It can control normal glucose in normoglycemic disorder. Hypertension is a glucose resistance in prediabetes. In hyperglycemia, diabetes requires only demands glucose for function and gets survival needs of insulin.

Type 2 Diabetes: Type 2 diabetes is a pre-diabetic disorder of diabetes in which we can control the diabetes; it is insulin deficiency. In type 2 diabetes, it is caused by obesity, overweight, not physically active or a sedentary lifestyle, etc. It can cause hypertension or high blood pressure.

5.2 MACHINE LEARNING

The research field that deals with the way in which a machine adapts to changes is called machine learning. The term "artificial intelligence" is similar to the word machine learning for many researchers since the probability of studying is the main feature of an object is known as intelligent in the best possible way. A designed electronic system that would adjust and learn from their experiences is the purpose of machine learning. Mitchel provides a more comprehensive and systematic description of machine learning with regard of the certain classes of the tasks T and performance measures P, a programming language is set to learn from the knowledge [6]. We have to find the potential to find an answer with the emergence

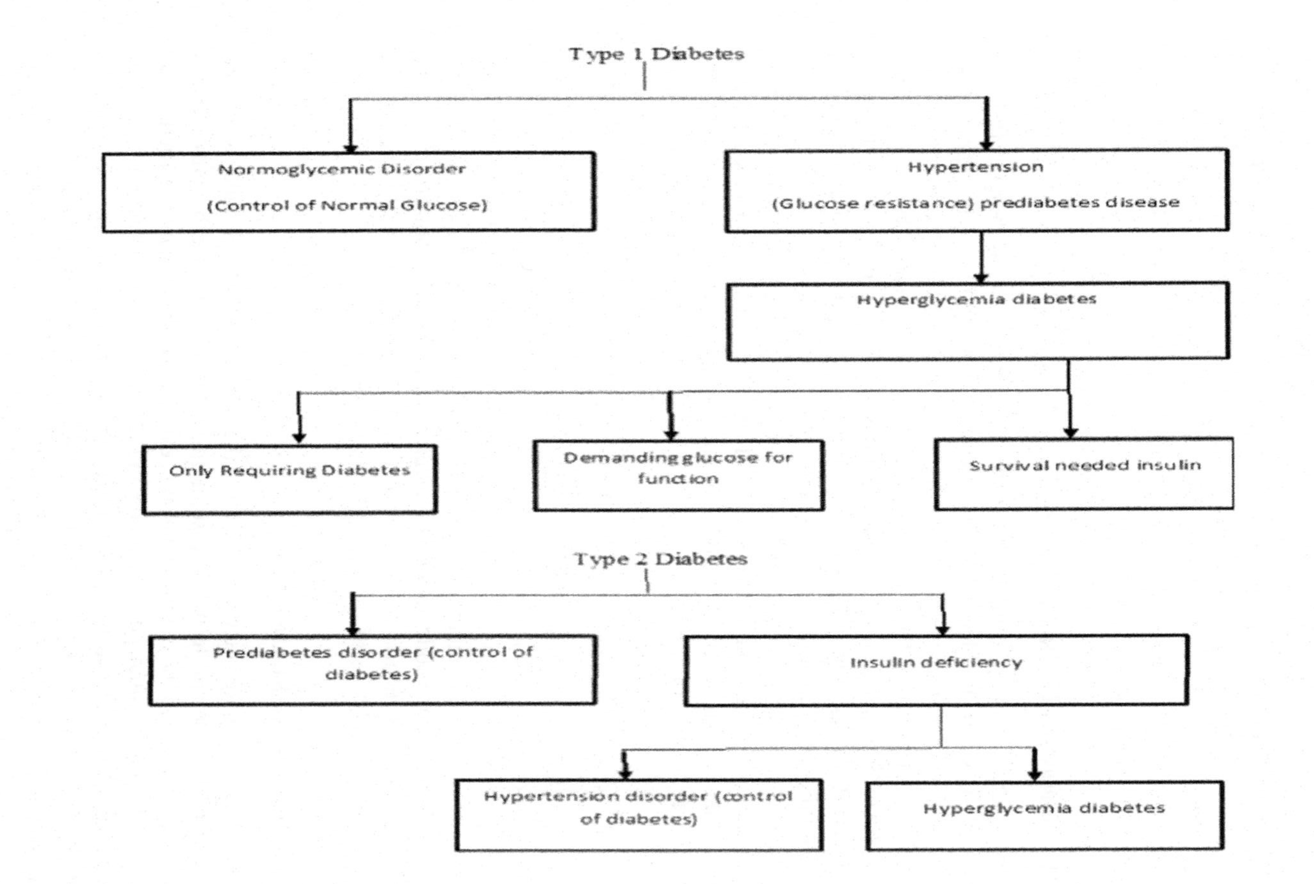

FIGURE 5.1 Phases in type 1 diabetes and type 2 diabetes.

of machine learning methods. Authors have to build a model using a data collection that can be determined whether or not the patient has diabetes mellitus. In addition, early disease prediction leads to the treatment of patients until it becomes crucial. Machine learning is capable of removing the secret insights from a vast volume of information linked to diabetes mellitus research and it has an important role more than ever before. The goal of this study is used to build a method that can estimate the level of diabetes mellitus risk to patients with greater precision. This is a study focus on designing a structure on several classifications, namely SVM, KNN, NB, DT and model of integrated algorithm.

5.2.1 Supervised Learning

In supervised learning, the model must learn a function called the goal function empirically in supervised learning, which is an example of the model representing data. In order to estimate the value, a parameter is called a dependent value or an independent variable. The optimal solution is used to predict the vector from a set of possibilities called independent variables or input variables or attributes of the feature. Provided a training range, the learning system takes into the account alternate functions called observations and this is defined by H in order to identify the best goal feature. There are two types of instructional functions in machine learning, i.e. classification and regression. In the classification method, our aim is to simulate separate classes. Some of the most popular methods are KNN, decision tree and SVM.

5.2.2 Unsupervised Learning

In unsupervised learning, the machine seeks to determine the secret structure of data or relation amongst the variations in unlabeled data. Learning data in any case consists of instances without any associated name mining, emerged much later than machine learning and is more influenced by the database in the research field. The process of organizing a collection of products in such a way that objects in the same group are called a structure are more related in one way or another to than that of those in the other classes of the database observation or grouping.

5.2.3 Reinforcement Learning

Reinforcement learning is the term given to the group of strategies under which the system aims to train and to increase some instances of collective benefits through direct interaction with the environment. It is essential to know that the structure has no basic idea of the atmosphere, attitude and the only way is to find out i.e. error, loss, disappointment. Reinforcement is applied to the system due to its environment, regardless of its equality for several real-life challenges and methods. In this chapter, authors focus on the following commitments given underneath:

- The classifications have been done using the support vector machine, Naïve-Bayes, decision tree and model of integrated algorithm.

- Proposed an integrated framework and workflow for prediction of diabetes mellitus using machine learning.
- The classification of precision is compared to find the best ensemble model to achieve the high precision, which is effective in computing.

The remaining part of this chapter is structured as follows. Section 5.2 is literature review. Section 5.3 is related to the workflow for prediction of diabetes mellitus using machine learning. Section 5.4 is discussing the proposed framework model. Section 5.5 is followed by methods of classification and evolution. Section 5.6 is about the symptoms of type 1 and type 2 diabetes. Section 5.7 uses results and discussion. Section 5.8 discusses the conclusion and future work.

5.3 LITERATURE REVIEW

Proper diet plan, exercise and sound sleep are the main ingredients of a healthy life. Most people are now more succeptible to infections due to heavy work demands and dietary behavior. People will no longer do any heavy exercises as a result of technological changes and as an effect, they are becoming obese and disease-prone [7]. By using distinct algorithms, different algorithms were explained. Parameters such as sugar levels, cholesterol, body size, glucose, hypertension, average body weight, feature of pedigree and gender. Not all of the factors are inclusive [8]. Not all parameters are included; only small sample data used. ANN, EM, and GMM on diabetes, logistic regression and SVM were added to the ANN (artificial neural network) data set were better supplied for precision and efficiency relative to other algorithms [9]. Techniques such as data mining were used to forecast the insulin-dependent disorders using data sets from the real world by gathering by transmitting interviewer results. Software for descriptive statistics and WEKA data interpretation and estimation were used, respectively [10]. A different algorithm for machine learning has been used in insulin disease prediction with better precision provided by the RF algorithm techniques of extraction [11]. Cross validation with tenfold different algorithms have been used as an assessment tool and regression logistics, Naïve-Bayes and SVM. Out of that, higher accuracy and precision were provided by numerous SVM algorithm quality relative to other approaches [12]. KNN, Naïve-Bayes, random forest, decision tree, and logistics regression have been used for the purpose of glucose prediction. At an early stage, hyperglycemia was based on filtering [13]. KNN and DISKR were used and storage was carried out and size has been limited. An example of a lower factor was abolished. Anomaly elimination improves all output correctness and precision [14]. K-nearest neighbor (KNN) accuracy value of 73 percent precision was introduced and given [15]. Different studies have been conducted in diabetic disease. Specific prediction algorithms are used for statistical models. Improved and successful output was not provided by the collective method and addresses the constraint of different solution and classification algorithms to help deal with consistency by combining them into the one. The typical overview or main observation of recent findings are described as follows in Table 5.1.

TABLE 5.1
Overview Findings of Methods for Prediction of Diseases

Ref.	Methodology	Findings
[12]	Naïve-Bayes, decision tree, random forest	Focused on the precision and improved results of the replacement, phasing of requirements may be expanded.
[16]	Naïve-Bayes, SVM, logistic regression	SVM provided a high precision of 82% from the three algorithms
[17]	ID3, Naïve-Bayes, random forest	Methods of classification algorithm best compared to other. In comparisons ID3 less precision than other was provided.
[13]	KNN, DISKR	A feature with a lower element should be removed. Accuracy is possible to improve the rise by eliminating outliers, spatial complexity reduced.
[8]	ANN, SVM, linear regression	Lower quality of used data set. The implementation comparisons were performed. Neural Network provides greater precision from such techniques compared to all classifiers.
[18]	Fuzzy rule	Using the ambiguous law and advice wrong care was minimized a framework for surgeon has been developed.
[19]	KNN, Simple CART, Zero R, NB	Different data bases that contain glucose, Frame work are implemented not cover the risk of implemented NB showed high precision by offering 76.02%.
[20]	Decision tree, J48	The strong quality supplier technique is designed as J48 range of features has increased function in the prediction.
[21]	J48, bagging SVM, decision tree	Improved precision was seen in J48 than in other approaches.
[22]	Genetic algorithm SVM, KNN	Embedded classification application aggregation and software classification is given better result.
[23]	SVM, KNN, J48, decision tree	By having 71.83% accuracy than J48 provides sufficient precision preprocessing. Some clusters and random Forest on the opposite given in efficient precision after immediate post.
[24]	CART, ID3	Two insulin databases were covered by the given algorithm
[25]	J48, KNN, logistic regression	Using this process 76.21% precision was determined.
[26]	KNN, CART, SVM	60% and 78% precision calculated in software test 1 and software test 2
[27]	J48, CART, SVM, KNN	With the average accuracy J48, CART, SVM, KNN were added and seen 62.15%, 52.39%, 64.05%
[28]	Naïve-Bayes, network, CART	73.1% precision calculated by the loop of the Ad boost.
[29]	Decision tree,SVM	79.168% Precision was seen.
[30]	SVM, KNN, Naïve-Bayes	71% precision calculated.
[31]	KNN, Naïve-Bayes, SVM	Specific purposes was seen for C3.5 than for others with an average gain of 79.251%
[32]	CART, logistic regression	75% precision was given.
[33]	Decision tree, SVM, NB, decisions tamp	The precision of 81.73% was calculated by decision stump.

(*Continued*)

TABLE 5.1 (Continued)
Overview Findings of Methods for Prediction of Diseases

Ref.	Methodology	Findings
[34]	ANN, decision tree, boosting, Naïve-Bayes, CART	Using the random forest 84.518% precision was calculated. The precision calculated by the HMV algorithm is reported as greater precision.
[35]	KNN, LR, SVM, RF, NB	78% were analyzed based on multiple diseases including diabetes. The precision calculated by the HMV algorithm is reported as greater precision
[36]	SVM	This methodology produced better results with an accuracy value of 79%.
[37]	Random rorest and decision tree	The quality of the random forest was superior to that of the decision tree.
[38]	NB, logistic regression and anthropometry	Dieting blood glucose prediction is the aim of this study. Anthropometry measured 75.1% efficiency and precision.
[39]	fuzzy rule, GA, and KNN	The rule has been generated.
[40]	Expert system and fuzzy rule	These are built with a concentrate on the expert method and for the purpose of care.
[41]	SVM	Using SVM 80% precision is considered higher.
[42]	KNN, C4.5	C4.5 had a greater precision of 90.43%, while KNN had a greater precision of 90.43%, 76.96% precision.

The information gathered would assist in treating diseases, and a personal analysis of an improved lifestyle is performed with a lot of toxic and remote control [43]. The comparison is used for the prediction of diabetes mellitus using a machine learning approach like Naïve-Bayes, support vector machine, and decision tree [44,45].

5.4 WORKFLOW

This work flow starts a process for diabetes mellitus for the diabetic patient. The recommended system used the knowledge based on the diabetes mellitus approach where the patients are recommending the profile and knowledge base of weight, height, obesity and we can predict the steps are as follows and are outlined in Figure 5.2.

In Figure 5.2, the author first starts the process of diabetes mellitus for the patients in which the author takes the input of patients by using the different machine learning algorithms and makes different optimizations of the diabetes mellitus on the process of weight, height and obesity. After that, the author is going to predict and update the parameters and then the author can do the tenfold cross validation. If an error occurs, then the author has to stop the training of the networks' hidden layer, momentum factors, etc. But if it working, then we have to obtain a parameter and the network is ready for the prediction of diabetes mellitus. Then, we stop and we will get the output.

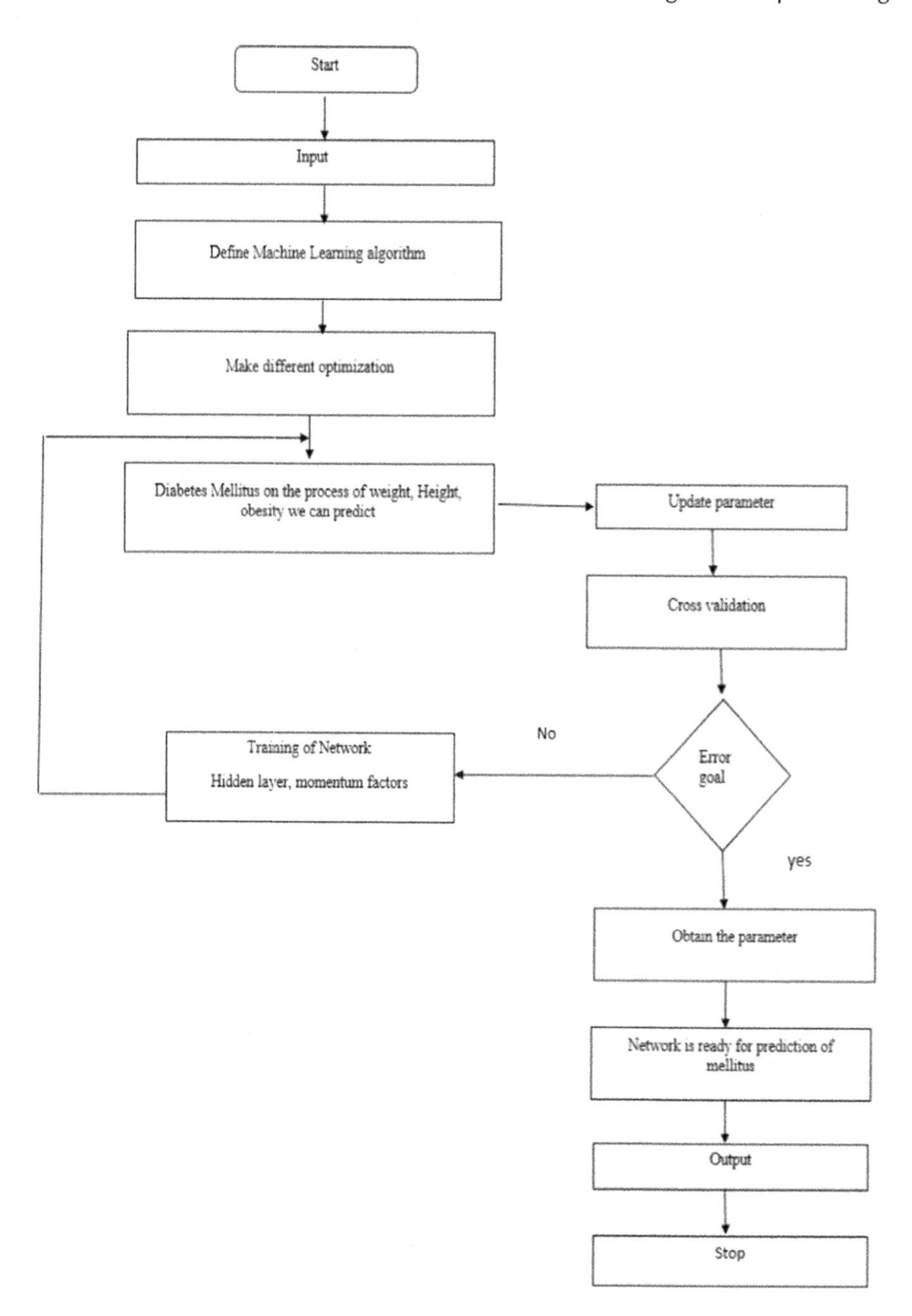

FIGURE 5.2 Work flow of diabetes mellitus.

5.5 PROPOSED FRAMEWORK MODEL

In Figure 5.3, the proposed framework model comprises of the data set in which the authors have done the collection of data that corresponds to one or more database. The author pre-processed the data in which they take the missing values and remove duplicate data. After that, the author uses the training data set in which author takes diabetic and non-diabetic data sets. Subsequent, the author applies the machine learning algorithm in which a different algorithm is used, such as SVM, Naïve-Bayes and decision tree.

In the machine learning algorithm, SVM is a supervised algorithm that can be used for classification. It is sometimes used to solve classification problem and the goal of SVM is to classify data points in a multidimensional space using an acceptable decision boundary. Naïve-Bayes classification is a Bayes' theorem based deterministic machine learning algorithm explained in terms of probability. Decision tree is based on a choice concept. It is tree shaped and offers a variety of services like high precision and consistency. After that, we do the testing set and apply the cross validation for SVM prediction, Naïve-Bayes prediction and decision tree prediction. Also, the authors compared the individual prediction and the meta classifier and finally do predictions and find the result.

5.6 METHODS OF CLASSIFICATION AND EVALUATIONS

On the basis of the scope of research, the authors set out to employ four of the most recognized algorithms for estimating such as Naïve-Bayes, support vector machine (SVM), decision tree and model of integrated ensemble machine learning algorithms will create the model for our data set based on the problem [46]. In this chapter, four algorithms were picked for the data set that is given:

- Support vector machine
- Naïve-Bayes
- Decision tree
- Model of integrated ensemble

5.6.1 Support Vector Machine

A SVM algorithm is a classification algorithm. Based on the segregation process, it works. It is a supervised learning algorithm. One of the most popular vector machines, it helps algorithms and is a commonly used technique of machine learning.

Step 1. Define the proper support vectors first.
Step 2. The second phase of the first step is to optimize the gap between the sample point's neighbors.
Step 3. Add a function to a feature ($Z = x^3 + y^3$). It reveals that the problem is solved by a support vector machine.
Step 4. To define the class, add the support vector machine classifier and the class is binary (0, 1).

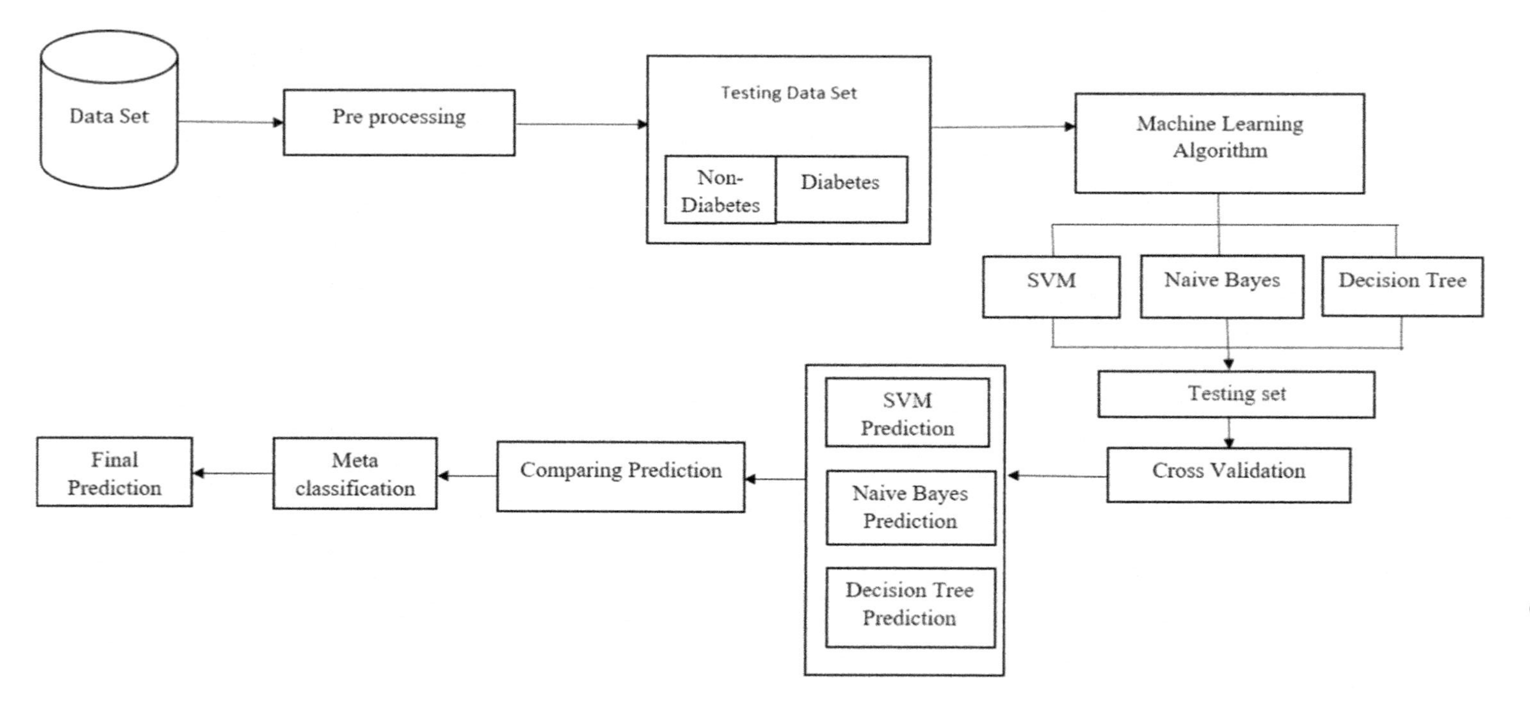

FIGURE 5.3 Proposed framework model.

5.6.2 Naïve-Bayes

The Naïve-Bayes algorithm uses the Bayes' law to define the data set. The classification is performed using all the features on the basis of the possibility observed from the training results. It is a supervised algorithm for learning. This technique's time complexity is short and computes using the likelihood formula, dependent on chance. Using it maximizes the possibility cost function = PR (class | characteristic).

Step 1. Change the data in a frequency table.
Step 2. Identify probability.
Step 3. The Naïve-Bayes equation in the third stage. Here, the planning is finished. It implies PR (class | feature).

5.6.3 Decision Tree (DT)

It is one of the most common classifications for machine learning algorithms that imputes meaning.

5.7 SYMPTOMS OF TYPE 1 DIABETES AND TYPE 2 DIABETES

High blood pressure is characterized by the following symptoms as well anxiety, mood swings and weight loss or weight gain and can also be encountered by individuals with type 1 or type 2 diabetes. There could also be restlessness and pins and needles in one's arms or legs in people with type 2 diabetes. According to the Diabetes Association, great glycogen practice and experience helps in preventing loss of sensation in someone effected with type 1 diabetes. For several years, many patients with type 2 diabetes will not have side effects and their diagnoses will often develop gradually over time. Some people with type 2 diabetes have no symptoms at all and do not find out till complications arise that they will have the condition. To detect hypertension, bloodwork and X-rays are used to search for diabetes. The most widely used measures for assessing whether the patient has the disease or not are oral glucose tolerance test (OGTT), A1C Test and fasting plasma glucose (FPG) test. The risk of developing type 2 diabetes can't be cured but they can be regulated and treated with special foods, exercise and insulin injections. Hypertension, leg mutilations, retinopathy, cataracts, an elevated risk of liver disease, heart attack and stroke are only a few of the disease's complications [47].

5.7.1 The Risk Factors for Type 1 and Type 2 Diabetes

Family history: People who have type 1 diabetes with a family member have a greater chance of having it themself.

Age: Diabetes can appear at any time, but among teenagers, it is most common.

Geography: The occurrence of prediabetes grows the farther away from earth we live.

Genetics: The existence of such genes indicates a higher risk of type 1 diabetes while the risk factors in type 2 diabetes are insulin resistance or highly raised levels in the blood sugar carry excess weight or overweight, a great deal of stomach fat, insufficiently active and over 45 years of age are active representatives of a family with type 2 diabetes [48].

5.8 RESULTS AND DISCUSSION

In this experiment, we have used Java code libraries that are available in WEKA tool. In this experiment, the authors used methods of classification and evaluation models using machine learning techniques. The analysis of models is done in different steps using machine learning algorithms such as SVM, NB, decision tree and model of integrated ensembles. Partitions of data play an important role in accuracy, as shown in Figure 5.4.

Figure 5.4 shows the overall data set performance precision of a model in which authors take different tasks such as support vector machines consist of 87.6% precision, Naïve-Bayes consists of 87.52%, decision tree consists of 82.70% and ad boost consists of 84.66%. Our proposed model contains precision of 91.26%. Analysis and results showed that our proposed model contains the better result when compared with the other algorithms. The experiment also shows that the proposed model has an accuracy of 91.26% compared to other algorithms.

5.9 CONCLUSION AND FUTURE WORK

There are different techniques available for data processing and its implementation. By applying machine learning, a data set has been tested and evaluated. In the separate sets of medical records, the technique was used in the diabetic data set.

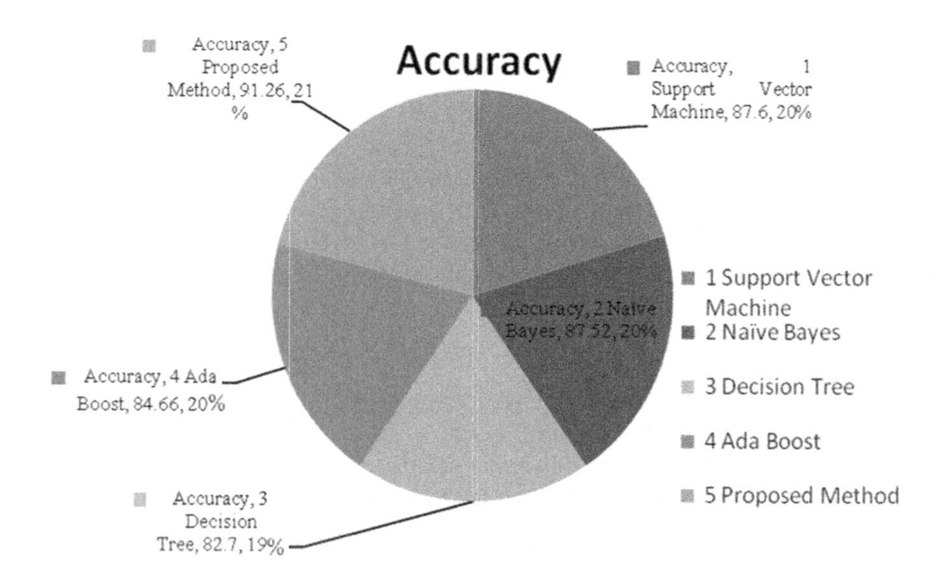

FIGURE 5.4 Overall data set performance of precision of model.

By using machine learning, we found that different data set methods have different abilities. We record the glucose data collection collected from UCI data set. The reference of suggested algorithm and the analysis method is performed. The validation done on the data set is tenfold cross validation for the performance of machine learning classification. In this study, we compared the algorithm and found the better result. The correctly classified instance and high precision with the precision value is 91.26% and the decision tree provides less precision of 82.70% accuracy and uses the aggregate process. It is used to have a better output of estimation or precision than a single one of our data set. We use the set of diabetes techniques in another method that can be generated in limited numbers of survey data and we can also implement the same model for a huge number of data with feature exapansions. For the estimation, multiple data sets may be used. It is also possible in the feature we have planned to do the classification for other algorithms with the missing data. This method can also help people to investigate a precise and efficient method that will provide patient assistance for better disease decision making.

REFERENCES

[1] Wu, Han, Yang Shangri, Huang Zhangqin, He Jian, and Wang Xiaoyi "Type 2 diabetes mellitus prediction model based on data mining," *Informatics in Medicine Unlocked* 10 (2018): 100–107.

[2] Kumar Dewangan, Amit, and Agrawal Pragati "Classification of diabetes mellitus using machine learning technique," *International Journal of Engineering and Applied Sciences* 2, no. 5 (2015): 257905.

[3] Mellitus, Diabetes "Diagnosis and classification of diabetes mellitus", *Diabetes Care* 28, no. S37 (2005): S5–S10.

[4] Vijayan, V. Veena, and Anjali C. "Prediction and diagnosis of diabetes mellitus a machine learning approach," In *IEEE Recent Advances in Intelligent Computational Systems (RAICS)*, IEEE, (2015): 122–127.

[5] Bashir, Saba, Qamar Usman, Khan Farhan Hassan, and Yuns Javed M. "An efficient rule-based classification of Diabetes using ID3,C4. 5& CART ensembles," In *2014 12th International Conference on Frontiers of Information Technology*, IEEE, (2014): 226–231.

[6] https://en.wikipedia.org/wiki/Tom_M._Mitchell. (12-3.2021).

[7] Sharma Nikhil, Kaushik Ila, Bhusan Bharat, Gautama Siddharth and Khamparia Aditya "Applicability of WSN and biometric models in the field of healthcare", (2020): 1–6.

[8] Komi, Messan, Li Jun, Zhai Yongxin, and Zhang Xingu. "Application of data mining methods in diabetes prediction," in *2017 2nd international conference on image, vision and computing (ICIVC)*, IEEE, (2017): 1006–1010.

[9] Meng, Xue-Hui, Huang Yi-Xiang, Rao Dong-Ping, Zhang Qiu, and Liu Qing. "Comparison of three data mining models for predicting diabetes or prediabetes by risk factors," *The Kaohsiung Journal of Medical Sciences* 29, no. 2 (2013): 93–99.

[10] Xu, Weifang, Zhang Jianxin, Zhang Qiang, and Wei Xiaopeng. "Risk prediction of type II diabetes based on random forest model," In *2017 Third International Conference on Advances in Electrical, Electronics, Information, Communication and Bio-Informatics (AEEICB)*, IEEE, (2017): 382–386.

[11] Kavakiotis, Ioannis, Tsave Olga, Salifoglou Athanasios, Calaveras Nicos, Vlahos's Ioannis, and Chouvarda Ioanna. "Machine learning and data mining methods in diabetes research," *Computational and Structural Biotechnology Journal* 15 (2017): 104–116.

[12] Zheng, Tao, Xie Wei, Xu Liling, He Xiaoying, Zhang Ya, You Mingrong, Yang Gong, and Chen You. "A machine learning-based framework to identify type 2 diabetes through electronic health records," *International Journal of Medical Informatics* 97 (2017): 120–127.

[13] Song, Yunsheng, Liang Jiye, Lu Jing, and Zhao Xing Wang. "An efficient instance selection algorithm for k nearest neighbor regression," *Neurocomputing* 251 (2017): 26–34.

[14] Rani, A. Swarupa, and Jyothi S. "Performance analysis of classification algorithms under different datasets," In *2016 3rd International Conference on Computing for Sustainable Global Development (INDIACom)*, IEEE, (2016): 1584–1589.

[15] Meza-Palacios, Ramiro, Aguilar-Lasserre Alberto A., Ureña-Bogarín Enrique L., Vázquez-Rodríguez Carlos F., Posada-Gómez Rubén, and Trujillo-Mata Armín. "Development of a fuzzy expert system for the nephropathy control assessment in patients with type 2 diabetes mellitus," *Expert Systems with Applications* 72 (2017): 335–343.

[16] Kavakiotis, Iohannis, Tsave Olga, Salifoglou Athanasios, Maglaveras Nicos, Vlahavas Ioannis, and Chouvarda Ioanna. "Machine learning and data mining methods in diabetes research," *Computational and Structural Biotechnology Journal* 15 (2017): 104–116.

[17] Xu, Weifang, Zhang Jinxing, Zhang Qiang, and Wei Xiaopeng. "Risk prediction of type II diabetes based on random forest model." In *2017 Third International Conference on Advances in Electrical, Electronics, Information, Communication and Bio-Informatics (AEEICB)*, IEEE, (2017): 382–386.

[18] Meza-Palacios, Ramiro, Aguilar-Lasserre Alberto A., Ureña-Bogarín Enrique L., Vázquez-Rodríguez Carlos F., Posada-Gómez Rubén, and Trujillo-Mata Armín. "Development of a fuzzy expert system for the nephropathy control assessment in patients with type 2 diabetes mellitus," *Expert Systems with Applications* 72 (2017): 335–343.

[19] Rani, A. Swarupa, and Jyothi S. "Performance analysis of classification algorithms under different datasets", in *2016 3rd International Conference on Computing for Sustainable Global Development (INDIACom)*, IEEE, (2016): 1584–1589

[20] Pradeep, K. R., and Naveen N. C. "Predictive analysis of diabetes using J48 algorithm of classification techniques," In *2016 2nd International Conference on Contemporary Computing and Informatics (IC3I)*, IEEE, (2016): 347–352.

[21] Perveen, Sajida, Shahbaz Muhammad, Guergachi Aziz, and Keshavjee Karim. "Performance analysis of data mining classification techniques to predict diabetes," *Procedia Computer Science* 82 (2016): 115–121.

[22] Santhanam, T. and Padmavathi M. S. "Application of K-means and genetic algorithms for dimension reduction by integrating SVM for diabetes diagnosis," *Procedia Computer Science* 47 (2015): 76–83.

[23] Bashir, Saba, Qamar Usman, Khan Farhan Hassan, and Younus Jived M. "An efficient rule-based classification of Diabetes using ID3, C4. 5& CART ensembles," In *2014 12th International Conference on Frontiers of Information Technology*, IEEE, (2014): 226–231.

[24] Meng, Xue-Hui, Huang Yi-Xiang, Rao Dong-Ping, Zhang Qiu, and Liu Qing. "Comparison of three data mining models for predicting diabetes or prediabetes by risk factors", *The Kaohsiung Journal of Medical Sciences* 29, no. 2 (2013): 93–99.

[25] Saxena, Krati, Khan Zubair, and Singh Shefali. "Diagnosis of diabetes mellitus using k nearest neighbor algorithm," *International Journal of Computer Science Trends and Technology (IJCST)* 2, no. 4 (2014): 36–43.
[26] Saravananathan, K. and Velmurugan T. "Analyzing diabetic data using classification algorithms in data mining," *Indian Journal of Science and Technology* 9, no. 43 (2016): 1–6.
[27] Guo, Yang, Bai Guohua, and Hu Yan. "Using bayes network for prediction of type-2 diabetes," In *2012 International Conference for Internet Technology and Secured Transactions*, IEEE, (2012): 471–472.
[28] Al Jarullah, Asma A. "Decision tree discovery for the diagnosis of type II diabetes", In *2011 International conference on innovations in information technology*, IEEE, (2011): 303–307.
[29] Negi, Anjli, and Jaiswal Varun. "A first attempt to develop a diabetes prediction method based on different global datasets." In *2016 Fourth International Conference on Parallel, Distributed and Grid Computing (PDGC)*, IEEE, (2016): 237–241
[30] Kaur, Prableen, and Sharma Manik. "Analysis of data mining and soft computing techniques in prospecting diabetes disorder in human beings: a review," *International Journal of Pharmaceutical Sciences and Research* 9 (2018): 2700–2719.
[31] Anand, Ayush, and Shakti Divya. "Prediction of diabetes based on personal lifestyle indicators," In *2015 1st International Conference on Next Generation Computing Technologies (NGCT)*, IEEE, (2015): 673–676.
[32] Vijay An, V. Veena, and Anjali C. "Prediction and diagnosis of diabetes mellitus—A machine learning approach," In *2015 IEEE Recent Advances in Intelligent Computational Systems (RAICS)*, IEEE, (2015): 122–127.
[33] Nai-Arun, Nongyao, and Moungmai Rungruttikarn. "Comparison of classifiers for the risk of diabetes prediction," *Procedia Computer Science* 69 (2015): 132–142. classifiers for disease prediction. *Journal of Computational Science* 13 (2016): 10–25.
[34] Bashir, Saba, Qamar Usman, Khan Farhan Hassan, and Waseem Lubna "HMV: a medical decision support framework using multi-layer classifiers for disease prediction," *Journal of Computational Science* 13 (2016): 10–25.
[35] Kamari, V. Anuja, and Chitra R. "Classification of diabetes disease using support vector machine," *International Journal of Engineering Research and Applications* 3, no. 2 (2013): 1797–1801.
[36] Prajwala, T. R. "A comparative study on decision tree and random forest using R tool," *International Journal of Advanced Research in Computer and Communication Engineering* 4, no. 1 (2015): 196–199.
[37] Lee, Bum Ju, Ku Boncho, Nam Jiho, Pham Duong Duc, and Kim Jong Yeol. "Prediction of fasting plasma glucose status using anthropometric measures for diagnosing type 2 diabetes," *IEEE Journal of Biomedical and Health Informatics* 18, no. 2 (2013): 555–561.
[38] Pavate, Aruna, and Ansari Nazneen. "Risk prediction of disease complications in type 2 diabetes patients using soft computing techniques," In *2015 Fifth International Conference on Advances in Computing and Communications (ICACC)*, IEEE, (2015): 371–375.
[39] Mekruksavanich, Sakorn. "Medical expert system based ontology for diabetes disease diagnosis." In *2016 7th IEEE International Conference on Software Engineering and Service Science (ICSESS)*, IEEE, (2016): 383–389.
[40] Kang, Seokho, Kang Pilsung, Ko Taehoon, Cho Sungzoon, Rhee Su-In, and Yu Kyung-Sang. "An efficient and effective ensemble of support vector machines for anti-diabetic drug failure prediction," *Expert Systems with Applications* 42, no. 9 (2015): 4265–4273.

[41] Kandhasamy, J. Pradeep, and Balamurali S. "Performance analysis of classifier models to predict diabetes mellitus," *Procedia Computer Science* 47 (2015): 45–51.
[42] Patel, Bankat M, Joshi Ramesh Chandra, and Toshniwaln Durga "Hybrid prediction model for type-2 diabetic patients", *Expert Systems with Applications* 37, no. 12 (2010): 8102–8108.
[43] Jindal Mansi, Gupta Jatin and Bhushan Bharat. "Machine learning methods for IoT and their future applications" *International Conference on Computing, Communication and Intelligent Systems (ICCCIS)*, IEEE, Greater Noida, India, (2019).
[44] Kumar Santosh, Bhusan Bharat, Singh Debabrata and Choubey Dilip Kumar, "Classification of diabetes using deep learning" International Conference on Communication and Signal Processing, IEEE, Kerala, India, (2020).
[45] Pattnayak, Parthasarathi, and Jena Om Prakash "Innovation on machine learning in healthcare services—An introduction", *Machine Learning for Healthcare Applications* 1 (2021): 1–14. https://doi.org/10.1002/9781119792611.ch1
[46] Paramecia, K., Guru Raj H. L., and Jena Om Prakash, "Applications of machine learning in biomedical text processing and food industry" *Machine Learning for Healthcare Applications* 1 (2021): 151–167. https://doi.org/10.1002/9781119792611.ch10
[47] Sivakani, R., and Ansari Gufran Ahmad. "Imputation using machine learning techniques." In *2020 4th International Conference on Computer, Communication and Signal Processing (ICCCSP)*, IEEE, (2020): 1–6.
[48] Panigrahi, Niranjan, Ayus Ishan and Jena Om Prakash "An expert system-based clinical decision support system for Hepatitis-B prediction & diagnosis", *Machine Learning for Healthcare Applications* 1 (2021): 57–75. https://doi.org/10.1002/9781119792611.ch4

6 Spectrogram Image Textural Descriptors for Lung Sound Classification

Bhakti Kaushal and Mukesh D. Patil
Department of Electronics and Telecommunication Engineering, Ramrao Adik Institute of Technology, Nerul, Navi Mumbai, India

Smitha Raveendran and Gajanan K. Birajdar
Department of Electronics Engineering, Ramrao Adik Institute of Technology, Nerul, Navi Mumbai, India

CONTENTS

DOI: 10.1201/9781003189053-6

6.1 INTRODUCTION

The diseases of the respiratory system are a tremendous burden on public health, and they are the third major cause of death in the world [1]. Chronic respiratory diseases (CRD) are the diseases of the lungs, their other structures, and airways. The most common CRDs are chronic obstructive pulmonary disease (COPD) and asthma [2]. As part of the global burden of diseases (GBD) 2016, it is reported that the CRDs in India have increased from 4.5% in 1990 to 6.4% in 2016 [3]. Out of the global deaths and disability-adjusted life years (DALYs), 32% took place in India due to CRDs in 2016 [3]. The 75.6% and 20% of the CRD DALYs in India occurred due to COPD and asthma in 2016 [3]. This percentage is increasing every day, and the major causes include smoking tobacco, air pollution, occupational dust, chemicals, etc.

Due to the above reasons, it is a burden and significant problem for the public health systems. As CRDs are not completely curable, routine examination of patients helps in timely detection. A proper treatment plan is then determined for the patient, which can help control the symptoms and increase the quality of life.

Let us understand some diseases of the respiratory system:

- **Upper respiratory tract infections (URTI):** It is also known as the common cold. These infections are contagious and commonly caused by viruses. They occur in the upper air passages, which include the larynx, pharynx, nasal passages, and cavity. The symptoms of URTI include sore throat, cough, sneezing, nasal congestion, mild fever, runny nose, excess mucus, etc. [4].
- **Lower respiratory tract infections (LRTI):** These infections occur in the airways below the voice box as well as in the alveolar sacs and the trachea. The acute infections that affect the airways lead to acute bronchitis, influenza, and bronchiolitis, affecting the alveolar sacs leading to pneumonia. These infections are most commonly caused by bacteria or viruses, and they are contagious in nature. The symptoms are similar to that of the common cold that includes cough, fever, headache, chest pain, difficulty in breathing, etc. [5].
- **Pneumonia:** It occurs when the alveoli are filled with pus or fluid due to infections. A person suffering from it has difficulty breathing, as enough oxygen doesn't reach the bloodstream. Individuals over the age of 65 and younger than the age of 2 are at higher risk as their immune systems are weak. They are most commonly caused by bacteria, fungi, or viruses [6].
- **COPD:** It occurs when the walls of alveoli are destroyed and are merged in one big air sac, which causes less oxygen absorption such that it doesn't reach the bloodstream. The springiness of the lungs is lost such that the air is trapped inside it, and it gets difficult to breathe out for an individual

suffering from it. The most common causes are tobacco smoking and breathing secondhand smoke. Long-time exposure to air pollution, dust, or some chemicals can also cause COPD [6].

- **Asthma:** It occurs when the air-carrying tubes to the lungs come in contact with a trigger and get narrow, inflamed, and clogged up with mucus such that it gets difficult for the air to move freely, causing breathlessness to an individual suffering from it. The symptoms vary from person to person, but the most common include shortness of breath, coughing, wheezing, tightness in the chest, etc. [6].
- **Bronchiolitis:** It occurs when the bronchioles (small breathing tubes) are infected and filled with mucus such that the air cannot move in and out of it. It usually happens in infants or children younger than two years of age and rarely affects adults. The most common cause is a viral infection, and they are contagious in nature. The first symptoms are similar to a cold and later include fast breathing and labored breathing, wheezing, dehydration, vomiting, constant coughing, difficulty in swallowing and drinking [6].
- **Bronchiectasis:** It affects the bronchi (the tube carrying air in and out of the lungs) as they become thick and damaged. It causes severe breathing problems and is a long-term disease that gets worse with time. The major causes are inflammation in bronchial walls and infections. Also, gastroesophageal reflux disease (GERD), which may cause acid reflux into the lungs, can damage them. The most common symptoms are coughing up blood or phlegm, fatigue, chest pain, wheezing, and frequent respiratory infections [6].
- **Cystic fibrosis (CF):** It is a genetic disorder. The individuals suffering from CF have thick mucus, which clogs up the tubes and ducts, making it difficult to breathe. The thick mucus can catch germs, which can lead to viral or bacterial infections. As the name suggests, it can severely damage the lungs with cysts and fibrosis. The symptoms are greasy stools, trouble breathing, frequent lung infections, salty skin, and difficulty in gaining weight [6].

Various respiratory conditions are assessed through lung auscultation and spirometry [1]. Spirometry is one of the simple and useful lung function measurement techniques. It helps in measuring the time taken and the volume of the air inhaled and exhaled by an individual. One major limitation of this technique is the cooperation provided by an individual, and there is a chance of high potential error if the effort put by the individual is substandard. Also, due to its high cost and the challenges faced by clinicians to guide patients, not many clinical settings can use it [1]. Lung auscultation is another method to assess respiratory sounds, measured with the help of a stethoscope. It is placed on the patient's anterior and posterior chest by a trained expert clinician so that they can listen and understand the sounds, which can help in correct detection between normal and abnormal sounds. The main limitation of the conventional auscultation method is that it does not continuously monitor the respiratory sounds. It requires an expert clinician to understand the findings, which can vary individually [1]. These limitations can be overcome by an automated diagnostic system for respiratory sounds [7]. Hence, we have used the International Conference on Biomedical and Health Informatics (ICBHI) 2017 challenge data set [1] and built an algorithm in this work such that digital auscultation can also be used at primary care centers and homes.

Lung diseases are fatal and lead to death in the case of delay in diagnosis and treatment. Conventional methods are dependent on factors like skilled and well-trained health providers and also on the cooperation of the patients. Automated diagnostic systems with good accuracy rates can help overcome such healthcare challenges to a great extent [8–10]. Hence, we have proposed the algorithm for lung sound detection, which will be able to detect the abnormality in the lungs in reduced time and with better precision.

The algorithm used in this work incorporates spectrogram time-frequency images, textural descriptors for feature extraction, dimensionality reduction technique as feature selection, and decision tree as classifiers for lung sound classification. The ICBHI 2017 challenge data set used in this work comprises lung sound recordings. These audio recordings are then converted into three different spectrograms: conventional spectrogram, constant-Q transform (CQT) spectrogram, and Mel-Scale spectrogram. Further, local binary pattern (LBP), completed local binary pattern (CLBP), and local phase quantization (LPQ) features are extracted from these spectrogram time-frequency images. The feature vector dimensionality is then reduced using neighbourhood component analysis. Finally, the reduced features are fed to a decision tree classifier for lung sound classification.

Feature extraction is an essential step for classification. The common features for audio classification include temporal, harmonic, perceptual, and spectral features; MFCCs (Mel-frequency cepstral coefficients); and energy descriptors as they provide acoustic motivation. But lately, it has been observed that these audio signals exhibit fascinating patterns in the visual domain when they are represented in their time-frequency spectrograms [11,12]. Some particular patterns are observed frequently in these spectrograms of normal and abnormal audio signals [12]. On this basis, it gets easier to distinguish between normal and abnormal (pneumonia) lung sounds. Hence, in this work, we have utilized the audio recordings of respiratory sounds from the ICBHI challenge data set and converted them into the spectrogram time-frequency images so that they can be easily classified into lung sounds of normal and pneumonia samples.

The following are the main contributions of this chapter:

- The classification of respiratory sounds into normal and abnormal lung sounds using the ICBHI 2017 challenge data set with better accuracy.
- This method employs three types of spectrograms, i.e., conventional spectrogram, constant-Q transform (CQT) spectrogram, and Mel-Scale spectrogram, as time-frequency images which are generated by converting the lung sounds from the data set. The LBP, CLBP, and LPQ as textural descriptors, neighbourhood component analysis (NCA) as a feature selection technique, and decision tree as the classifier.

The experimental results are assessed by the performance evaluation parameters, i.e., accuracy, precision, sensitivity, specificity, and F1 score, which shows that the proposed method performs comparatively better than the existing methods.

This chapter is organized in the following manner: The literature is reviewed in Section 6.2. The proposed algorithm is discussed in Section 6.3. The pre-processing techniques are described in Section 6.4. Feature extraction, feature selection, and classification are explained in Section 6.5. The experimental results are analyzed in Section 6.6, and finally, the conclusion of the chapter is drawn in Section 6.7.

6.2 LITERATURE SURVEY

Many techniques are present in the literature for the binary and multi-class classification of lung sounds into normal and abnormal. Some common methods used are spectral features, MFCC, wavelet transform for feature extraction and support vector machine (SVM), k-nearest neighbor (KNN), and artificial neural networks (ANN) for classification.

Islam et al. [13] suggested a method to discriminate normal and asthmatic patients based on lung sounds of a total of 60 subjects; out of this, 30 are asthmatic and 30 are normal. They have developed feature extraction and classification technique based on spectral sub-band, ANN, and SVM classifiers. The performance is evaluated using classification accuracy and achieved 89.2(±3.87)% with ANN and 93.3(±3.10)% with SVM. Nabi et al. [14] recommended a detection method for asthmatic patients based on the following: the spectral integrated (SI) features, univariate and multivariate statistical analysis and ensemble, KNN, and SVM classifiers. It is a multi-class prediction method with three mild, moderate, and severe classes based on the severity level of the patient's condition. The best positive predictive values (PPV) proposed from this work for the mild, moderate, and severe samples were 95% (ENS), 88% (ENS), and 90% (SVM), respectively. Binary classification, as well as detection of wheezes present in the lung sounds, was proposed by Pramono et al. [15] using averaged PSD, wavelet transform, MFCC, LPC coefficients, percentile frequency ratio, entropy-based, power ratio, ASE flux, tonality index, mean crossing irregularity, and other time and spectral features. It employed a linear classifier for a single feature and logistic regression (LR) for multiple features. They worked on discriminating between 202 normal and 223 wheezing respiratory sounds out of 425 lung sound recordings. The F1 score of 82.67% was obtained from the third MFCC coefficient in their proposed work.

For the detection of COPD in subjects based on lung sounds, Haider et al. [16] proposed a combination of relevant lung sound parameters, i.e., linear predictive coefficient and median frequency and spirometry parameters, i.e., forced expiratory volume in 1 s (FEV1) and forced vital capacity (FVC) for binary classification of normal and COPD using SVM and logistic regression (LR). The data of a total of 55 subjects were recorded, out of which 25 were healthy and 30 had COPD. The total lung sound and spirometry features were 39 and 3, respectively. The accuracy of 100% was achieved. Ulukaya et al. [17] proposed a time-scale resolution method that employs rational dilation wavelet transform (RADWT) for discriminating wheeze types. They used peak energy ratio (PER) to select the features, and support vector machine (SVM), k-nearest neighbor (k-NN), and extreme learning machine (ELM) classifiers for the classification of different wheeze types. The SVM earned the highest accuracy of 82.9% with leave-one-subject-out (LOSO) and 86% with leave-one-out (LOO) cross-validation techniques.

The wheeze sound classification of healthy or asthmatic patients using time-frequency features was proposed by Nabi et al. [18]. The mean and quartile frequencies, as well as average power, were used as features, and the behavior of these features was analyzed by univariate statistical analysis. The data were grouped into nine data sets taken from 55 asthmatic patients based on three severity levels, i.e., mild, moderate, and severe. The results show that the tracheal wheeze sounds predict the severity levels more specifically. Naqvi and Choudhry [19] employed a technique for diagnosing COPD and pneumonia using ICBHI 2017 challenge lung sound database. The de-noising and segmenting of the pulmonic signal was done using empirical mode decomposition (EMD) and discrete wavelet transform (DWT). The time domain, cepstral, and spectral features were fused together, and the back-elimination method was utilized for feature selection. The selected features were fed to the quadratic discriminate classifier, and an accuracy of 99.70% was achieved. The telemedicine framework to classify normal and six different types of respiratory sounds such as squawk, roughness, stridor, coarse crackling, polyphonic wheeze, and monophonic wheeze was suggested by Jaber et al. [20]. The R.A.L.E. (Respiration Acoustics Laboratory Environment) Lung Sounds database was utilized, and the features were obtained using wavelet transform and MFCC.

The classification approaches were trained using bagging and boosting algorithms. The features were fed to the improved random forest classifier and two ensemble learning techniques, i.e., Gradient Boosting and AdaBoost. The classification accuracy of 99.04% is achieved from this proposed work. Meng et al. [21] proposed an approach that uses 705 lung sound recordings acquired from 130 patients to detect normal, crackles, and rhonchus respiratory sounds by dividing them into five groups. A 15-dimensional feature vector was obtained by employing relative wavelet energy, wavelet entropy, and Gaussian kernel functions with seven, one, and seven dimensions, respectively. The classifiers, namely SVM, KNN, and ANN, are used in their proposed method. The classification accuracy of 85.43% was provided by ANN, which was the highest amongst the three classifiers [22,23]. Messner et al. [24] used a multi-channel approach to classify lung sound recordings into healthy and pathological (person with IPF, i.e., idiopathic pulmonary fibrosis). They developed a 16-channel recording device to record lung sounds, and spectrogram features were extracted from it. They used different architectures of deep neural network for classification and have accomplished a 92% F-score using a convolutional recurrent neural network for this proposed work.

Jayalakshmy and Gnanou [25] proposed a method that is based on Alexnet CNN, which is pre-trained to predict the lung sounds of four classes, namely, normal, wheezes, low-pitched wheezes, and crackles. They used intrinsic mode functions (IMFs) of empirical mode decomposition (EMD) to convert lung sounds into Bump and Morse scalograms. The accuracy of 83.78% is achieved by the proposed method. To distinguish and classify between healthy and five-different respiratory diseases, García-Ordás et al. [26] proposed the Variational Convolutional

Autoencoder with a convolutional neural network (CNN) architecture. There are 920 lung sounds present in the data set, out of which 35 are healthy, 810 are chronic, and 75 are non-chronic. Two types of multi-class classifications were performed, and it was observed that the F1 score of three- and six-label classification achieved 99.3% and 99%, respectively. Acharya and Basu [27] suggested a method that is built using Mel spectrograms to extract features and hybrid CNN-RNN to train and classify breathing sound abnormality (wheeze, crackle) to detect respiratory diseases. They used the ICBHI'17 data set. The memory required was reduced using local log quantization. In this method, 66.31% F1 score was achieved initially, and after re-training the model, 71.81% F1 score was achieved with LOO validation.

To detect pulmonary diseases and classify them, Demir et al. [28] employed a method using spectrogram images, short-time Fourier transform (STFT), and two deep learning-based approaches. In the first method, CNN was utilized for feature extraction and SVM for classification. The accuracy of 65.5% was obtained using the first approach. In the second method, CNN was used again, but it was fine-tuned with the help of spectrogram images and provided an accuracy of 63.09%. Demir et al. [29] used a pre-trained CNN for deep feature extraction and classification of lung sound signals. The performance was increased by connecting a max-pooling layer in parallel with an average-pooling layer. The deep features were utilized and given as the input to the linear discriminant analysis (LDA) classifier, which makes use of the random subspace ensembles (RSE) method. The accuracy produced from this proposed work is 71.15% [30,31]. For the detection of pulmonary diseases, Shuvo et al. [32] suggested a CNN model on the basis of hybrid scalogram features and continuous wavelet transform (CWT). The accuracy of 99.20% and 99.05% was achieved for three-class and six-class classification, respectively, from this proposed work. Fraiwan et al. [13] suggested a method for multi-class lung sound classification of various diseases. A total of 1,176 and 308 recordings from the ICBHI challenge data set and clinically acquired recordings of the lung sound were used, respectively. The features were obtained using logarithmic energy entropy, Shannon entropy, and spectrogram-based spectral entropy. The best overall accuracy of 98.27% was provided by boosted decision trees, and an accuracy of 98.20% was obtained using SVM. Table 6.1 briefs about the existing methods present in the literature for lung sound classification.

6.3 PROPOSED APPROACH FOR LUNG SOUND CLASSIFICATION USING TIME-FREQUENCY TEXTURAL FEATURES

This book chapter presents a lung sound classification approach developed using time-frequency representations and textural descriptors. The abnormalities present in abnormal (pneumonia) sound samples are represented using spectrogram visualization and extracted using different textural features. The detailed lung sound classification architecture is shown in Figure 6.1.

Firstly, the input lung sound samples (healthy and pathological) are converted into spectrogram time-frequency representations. In this work, three types of spectrogram visualization are used: (a) conventional spectrogram, (b) Mel scale

TABLE 6.1
The Comparison between the Feature Extraction, Feature Reduction, and Classification Techniques of Existing Methods with Their Accuracy as well as F1 Score Present in the Literature

Author	Feature Extraction Method	Feature Reduction Method	Classification	Accuracy/F1 Score
Islam et al. [13]	spectral sub-band based features	–	ANN and SVM	89.2(±3.87)% and 93.3(±3.10)%
Nabi et al. [14]	spectral integrated (SI) features	–	ENS, KNN and SVM	95% (PPV), 88% (PPV) and 90% (PPV)
Pramono et al. [15]	averaged PSD, wavelet transform, MFCC, LPC coefficients, percentile frequency ratio, entropy-based, power ratio, ASE flux, tonality index, mean crossing irregularity and other time and spectral features	–	logistic regression	82.67% (F1-score)
Haider et al. [16]	lung sound and spirometry features	–	SVM and LR	100% and 100%
Ulukaya et al. [17]	Rational Dilation Wavelet Transform (RADWT)	peak energy ratio (PER)	SVM with LOSO and SVM with LOO	82.9% and 86%
Naqvi and Choudhry [19]	time domain, cepstral, and spectral features	back-elimination method	quadratic discriminate classifier	99.70%
Jaber et al. [20]	wavelet transform and MFCC	symmetrical uncertainty and correlation-based feature selection (CFS)	improved random forest	99.04%
Meng et al. [21]	relative wavelet energy, wavelet entropy and Gaussian kernel functions	–	ANN	85.43%

(Continued)

Messner et al. [24]	spectrogram features	–	convolutional recurrent neural network	92% (F1-score)
Jayalakshmy and Gnanou [25]	Bump and Morse scalograms from IMFs of EMD	–	Alexnet CNN	83.78%
García-Ordás et al. [26]	Variational Convolutional Autoencoder	–	3-label and 6-label CNN	(F1-score) 99.3% and 99%
Acharya and Basu [27]	Mel spectrograms	–	hybrid CNN-RNN	71.81% (F1-score)
Demir et al. [28]	spectrogram images, STFT, CNN	–	SVM	65.5% And 63.09%
Demir et al. [29]	CNN	–	LDA (RSE)	71.15%
Shuvo et al. [32]	hybrid scalogram features and continuous wavelet transform (CWT)	–	CNN	99.20% (three-class) and 99.05% (six-class)
Fraiwan et al. [13]	logarithmic energy entropy, Shannon entropy, and spectrogram-based spectral entropy	–	boosted decision trees and SVM	98.27% and 98.20%

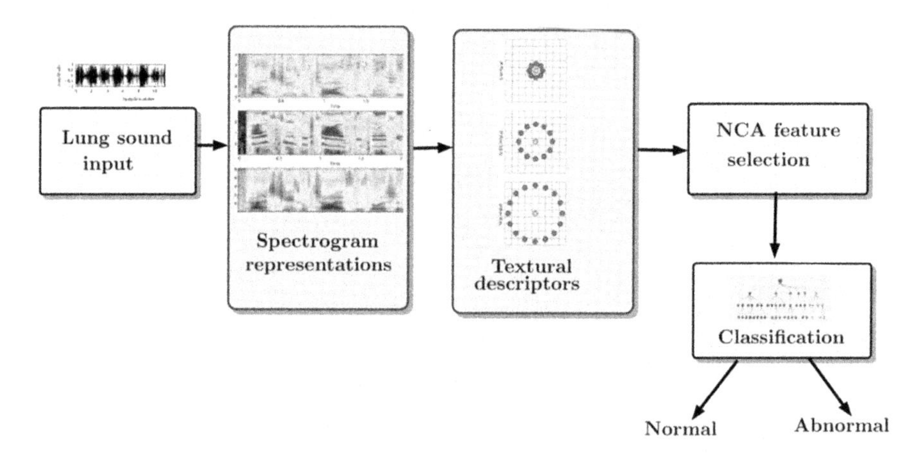

FIGURE 6.1 The proposed method for lung sound classification.

spectrogram, and (c) IIR-CQT. The three different spectrograms are exploited to produce discriminable variations in the normal and abnormal (pneumonia) sound signals. The textural variability present in these spectrogram images is effectively extracted using texture features. This study uses three different textural descriptors: (1) local binary pattern (LBP), (2) completed local binary pattern (CLBP), and (3) local phase quantization (LPQ).

These features are predominantly utilized for a variety of time-frequency textural feature applications in the literature. The distinct patterns present in the spectrogram because of the abnormal (pneumonia) lung sound are effectively captured using these textural features. The dimensionality of the combined feature vector is large and may affect the complexity of the proposed algorithm in terms of training and testing times of the classification algorithm.

To minimize the feature vector dimensionality and to eliminate the less contributing features, the proposed algorithm employs the neighbourhood component analysis (NCA) technique. The NCA is a filter feature selection approach useful to identify and determine prominent features during the classification stage. Finally, the subsets of features are fed to a classification method to label the input sample as healthy or pathological. A decision tree algorithm is used for the classification task.

The proposed algorithm for the lung sound classification method is presented in Algorithm 6.1. It is evaluated using the ICBHI 2017 Scientific Challenge Database, which is available publicly. Different valuation parameters such as precision, specificity, sensitivity, F1 score, and accuracy are computed using the database to prove the improved performance.

6.4 PRE-PROCESSING TECHNIQUES

Time-frequency representations of lung sound signals bear a resemblance to texture images. By treating the representations as texture images, an array of features can be extracted, thereby helping to build a robust classification system. The time-frequency representations of audio signals such as lung sounds contain remarkable

ALGORITHM 6.1 THE PROPOSED ALGORITHM FOR THE LUNG SOUND CLASSIFICATION METHOD

THE ALGORITHM OF THE PROPOSED LUNG SOUND CLASSIFICATION

Input data –
N = total audio recordings in the data set
M = total number of segments
P = number of selected NCAs
Output –
accuracy, precision, specificity, sensitivity and F1 score

```
for i ← 1 to N perform
   a. len ← total length of audio file
   b. seg1, seg2,... ← divide the signal into '7' seconds segments

   for j ← 1 to M perform
   c. Spect, mel, cqt ← compute the conventional, log-Mel and IIR-CQT
      spectrograms for all the segments

   for k ← 1 to 3 perform
   d. LBP, CLBP, LPQ ← extract the three types of texture features
   e. NCA[1:P] ← compute NCA
   f. Save the feature data set

   end for
  end for
 end for

   g. [Train, test] ← divide the feature data set into training and testing
   h. ctree ← provide the decision tree classifier with NCA feature and
      labelled data set for training
   i. confusion matrix ← predict the test set to get the confusion matrix
   j. Accuracy, precision, specificity, sensitivity and F1 score ← calculate
      the parameters from confusion matrix for performance assessment.
```

patterns in the visual domain. The distinctive patterns obtained from the time-frequency representations are found to exhibit important features of the audio signals as they contain whole information of the audio signal.

6.4.1 Conventional Spectrogram

The first step consists of converting the lung sound signals to a graphical representation such as a spectrogram. The features extracted from the spectrogram image provide important information required for the classification of sound. The amount of energy content present at a given frequency and time instant is decided by the intensity level at each point of the spectrogram image [33]. The information related to the audio signal is present in the spectral and temporal directions of the spectrogram image. To generate a spectrogram image, the input audio signal $x(n)$ is segmented into frames of fixed window length N. Discrete Fourier transform is applied to each segment [34] of length $0 < N - 1$, as shown in equation (6.1):

$$X_K = \sum_{n=0}^{N-1} x(n)\omega(n)e^{\frac{-2\pi ikn}{N}}, \quad K = 0, \ldots\ldots\ldots, N - 1 \tag{6.1}$$

X_K represents the *kth* harmonic frequency corresponding to $f(k)$. For a given frame, $f(k)$ is represented as shown in equation (6.2):

$$f(k) = KF_s/N \tag{6.2}$$

and F_s is the sampling frequency for the given hamming window. Log-spectrogram is used in the spectrogram image, as the perception of audio signals by humans is logarithmic. X_K is used to determine the log values and is given by equation (6.3) as

$$S_{log}(k) = log|X(k)| \tag{6.3}$$

Normalization of the log values in the range [0, 1] helps to generate the spectrogram image. The information about the fundamental frequency, the bandwidth of frequency, and pitch period can be extracted from the spectrogram.

6.4.2 Log-Mel Spectrogram

Features from the time and frequency domain that determine the power of a signal are obtained from a Mel-spectrogram image. The strength of the signal at various frequencies can be obtained with the help of this time-frequency representation. Fast Fourier transform is utilized in order to generate a Mel-scale spectrogram [35]. The transform is applied to a pre-processed input sound signal with time-domain samples $x_i(n)$ and an analysis window $h_\omega(n)$ of length N samples. If $X_i(p)$ represents the samples in the frequency domain, then it is expressed as shown by the equation (6.4):

$$X_i(p) = \sum_{n=1}^{N} x_i(n)h_\omega(n)e^{\frac{-j2\pi np}{N}} \tag{6.4}$$

Mel filter bank is used to convert the amplitude of the spectrum obtained from FFT to Mel-scale. Mel frequency is given by equation (6.5):

$$mel(frequency) = 1125 \times \ln\left(1 + \frac{frequency}{700}\right) \tag{6.5}$$

A logarithmic conversion of the energy obtained from the filter bank will facilitate the generation of the log-Mel spectrogram [36].

6.4.3 Constant-Q Transform (CQT)

The transformation from the time-domain to the time-frequency domain can be achieved with the help of the constant-Q transform. The geometrically spaced frequency bins generated in the spectra of CQT make it a complex and time-consuming task to compute the features. Due to computational efficiency, short-time Fourier transform (STFT) is employed for evaluating the CQT [37].

The IIR-CQT spectrogram is widely used in the audio signal analysis as it provides good spectral and temporal resolution at lower and higher frequency values, respectively. Multi-resolution FFT is employed for the computation of IIR-CQT. The spectrum is estimated by filtering the FFT of the sound signal in a recursive manner. IIR-CQT can be derived with the help of equation (6.6):

$$X_{CQT}(k) = \frac{1}{N_k} \sum_{m=0}^{N_k-1} x(n)\omega(n, k)e^{\frac{-j2\pi Q_n}{N_k}} \tag{6.6}$$

where n and k represent the time and frequency index, $\omega(n)$ is the analysis window of size N_k with the quality factor of Q.

Initially, an IIR filter bank is designed by maintaining the Q value constant. The location of poles in the filter bank is adjusted to retain the non-uniform width of the time window. At lower frequency values, a broad window length is used, while for higher frequency values, a narrow window is utilized. In the subsequent step, an efficient linear time-variant IIR (LTV-IIR) filter bank is designed, which involves the selection of poles of the filter bank corresponding to the frequency bin [36]. The recursive equation in order to approximate an LTV IIR filter bank is expressed by equation (6.7):

$$Y(m) = X(m) + X(m+) + P(m)Y(m-1) \tag{6.7}$$

X(m) denotes the DFT of the sound segment, the pole at m-th frequency bin is denoted as *P(m)*, and *Y(m)* is the IIR-CQT spectrum of the audio signal.

6.5 FEATURE EXTRACTION, FEATURE SELECTION, AND CLASSIFICATION

Features are extracted from the time-frequency representations with the help of local binary pattern, completed local binary pattern, and local phase quantization texture descriptors.

6.5.1 Local Binary Pattern (LBP)

The LBP texture descriptor, due to its illumination invariant property and computational efficiency, plays a promising role in texture analysis. The local binary pattern (LBP) is used for feature extraction from the spectrogram images. This method basically works on the differences between the central pixel and its neighbouring pixels. It encodes the information present in the textured images. The images are scanned by sampling the gray level pixels at a central position CP00 and n points that are spaced at equidistant points across a circle of radius r. In the conventional approach, the pixels are designated a binary number by using a threshold between the center pixel and its neighbouring pixels. The feature vector that is obtained finally matches the occurrence of all binary patterns that occur in the image [38,39].

6.5.2 Completed Local Binary Pattern (CLBP)

The completed local binary pattern is a general version of the local binary pattern. CLBP has proven to be very useful as a texture descriptor. It comprises three main components: CLBP_S, CLBP_M, and CLBP_C, respectively. CLBP_S represents the positive or negative sign of the resulting vector, CLBP_M is the difference in magnitude of the central pixel and the local neighboring pixel. CLBP_C denotes the difference between the average value of the central pixel and the local pixel in the neighbourhood. It computes the threshold value using the average gray level of the textured input. The feature vector for the entire image is created by solving the equations used for generating CLBP_S, CLMP_M, and CLBP_C [40].

6.5.3 Local Phase Quantization (LPQ)

The LPQ texture descriptor uses the local phase information extracted from a short-term Fourier transform (STFT) which is computed on a rectangular *N-by-N* neighbourhood. LPQ technique depends upon the blur invariance property and a point spread function (PSF). The local phase details evaluated over a rectangular neighbourhood *k* of size N- by-N at each pixel point *p* of the image *f(p)* is expressed by equation (6.8):

$$F(y, p) = \sum_{l \in K} f(p - k) e^{-j2\pi u^T l} \tag{6.8}$$

In LPQ representation, all the coefficients are quantized and mapped to the integer values using the process of binary coding. The generated binary codes are accumulated in a histogram, which is then used as a feature vector [41].

In order to minimise the feature vector dimensionality, a non-parametric method of feature selection, neighbourhood component analysis is used in order to maximise the prediction accuracy of the proposed algorithm.

6.5.4 Neighbourhood Component Analysis (NCA)

In the feature selection method using neighbourhood component analysis, the finest features are selected by maximising the objective function. NCA is used for the measurement of Mahalanobis distance that is used in the classification algorithm using KNN. Neighbourhood component analysis (NCA) is actually a non-parametric method that is used for feature selection and fulfills the objective of maximising the accuracy of prediction in classification and regression algorithms. NCA linearly transforms the data set used for training to a space that maximises the average leave-one-out classification accuracy [42]. If Z is the feature vector that has to be learned, the probability that Nj being selected as a reference point for Ni, from the available samples is defined mathematically by equation (6.9):

$$P_{ij} = \begin{cases} \dfrac{-\exp(-\|ZN_i - ZN_j\|^2, \quad j \neq i}{\Sigma_k \|ZN_i - ZN_k\|^2} \\ 0, \quad j = i \end{cases} \tag{6.9}$$

The probability of accurately classifying N_i as a true class is given by equation (6.10):

$$P_i = \frac{1}{F} \sum_{j=1, j \neq i}^{F} P_{ij} T_{ij} \tag{6.10}$$

where T_{ij} returns the value one when $T_i = T_j$, for other values else its value is considered zero [43].

This equation characterises the average leave-one-out accuracy in classification that is evaluated under the training data set. As we have to achieve good classification accuracy, the transformation matrix Z has to be solved such that the equation is maximised. A regularisation parameter lambda is used in the objective function in order to prevent over-fitting of the model. The objective function is given by equation (6.11) as

$$D = \sum_{l=1}^{n} P_i - \lambda \sum_{m=1}^{r} Z_m^2 \tag{6.11}$$

This is also known as RNCA or regularised NCA. A conjugate gradient approach is used to maximise the objective function D. If D is a diagonal matrix, then the diagonal values give the weight of each of the features. Based on the outcome of the weights, the finest subset of features is selected [43].

During the process of feature selection, prominent features are identified and determined. The subsets of features are fed to a classification method in order to label the input sample as healthy or pathological. A decision tree algorithm is employed for the task of classification.

6.5.5 Decision Tree

The decision tree prediction model is one of the intelligent learning models used in the domain of machine learning. These models are used for the purpose of classification tasks. The decision tree model incorporates a tree structure with various node points like roots, branches, and leaf nodes. The training data is used to construct a well-defined tree structure where the root nodes characterise a feature, and the leaf node represents the class labels. A well-constructed model leads to the high performance of the decision tree models. These models can efficiently predict the labels of new unknown samples. They are easier to interpret and low in terms of usage of memory. They offer good prediction speeds. The depth of the decision trees can be controlled with the aid of splits setting. Coarse tree, medium tree, and fine tree classifier types are supported by decision tree models. Few leaves make a coarser distinction between the classes, and an increase in the number of leaves leads to finer distinctions between the classes [44,45].

6.6 EXPERIMENTAL RESULTS AND DISCUSSION

The experiments are performed on a computer with 2.30 GHz Pentium(R), a 2 GB size RAM, a processor with dual-core configuration, and with a 64-bit Windows 7 operating system using 'MATLABR2014a'. The performance of the proposed algorithm is assessed using the below metrics, and they are defined using eq. 6.12 to 6.16:

$$\text{Accuracy} = \frac{\text{TN} + \text{TP}}{\text{TP} + \text{TN} + \text{FP} + \text{FN}} \cdots \tag{6.12}$$

$$\text{Sensitivity}(\text{S}) = \frac{\text{TP}}{\text{FN} + \text{TP}} \cdots \tag{6.13}$$

$$\text{Specificity} = \frac{\text{TN}}{\text{FP} + \text{TN}} \cdots \tag{6.14}$$

$$\text{Precision}(\text{P}) = \frac{\text{TP}}{\text{TP} + \text{FP}} \cdots \tag{6.15}$$

$$\text{F1 score} = 2 * \frac{\text{P} * \text{S}}{\text{P} + \text{S}} \cdots \tag{6.16}$$

where

True Negative (TN) = correctly predicted pneumonia recordings
True Positive (TP) = correctly predicted normal recordings
False Positive (FP) = incorrectly predicted normal recordings
False Negative (FN) = incorrectly predicted pneumonia recordings

6.6.1 DATABASE

The audio recordings for this experiment are procured from the ICBHI 2017 challenge respiratory sound database [1], an open-access database. It has lung sound recordings of a total of '126' individuals, out of which '26' are healthy, and '100' are patients suffering from various respiratory diseases. The lung sounds were taken from various chest locations, i.e., lateral right, trachea, lateral left, posterior left, anterior left, posterior right, and anterior right. The two types of acquisition modes used were sequential/single-channel and simultaneous/multichannel. They used four types of recording equipment, namely AKG C417L Microphone, 3M Litmmann 3200 Electronic Stethoscope, 3M Littmann Classic II SE Stethoscope, and WelchAllyn Meditron Master Elite Electronic Stethoscope [1].

We used two data sets in our proposed method; the first data set, 'Db1', contains audio recordings of lung sounds, and these were further converted into spectrograms to get the second data set, 'Db2'. The 'Db1' data set has a total of '72' lung sound recordings; out of that, '35' are 'normal' recordings, and '37' are of 'pneumonia' recordings as given in Table 6.2. The average length of these recordings is 19–20 seconds. They are divided into two segments of 7 seconds each to get a total of '144' segments; out of that, '70' are 'normal' recordings, and '74' are of 'pneumonia' recordings as given in Table 6.2. Figure 6.2 shows the plot of normal and pneumonia lung sound samples and their 7-second segments.

The obtained segments of audio recordings were further converted into three types of time-frequency representations, i.e., conventional spectrogram, log-Mel spectrogram, and IIR-CQT spectrogram, which stand close to the texture images to obtain a data set 'Db2', as shown in Table 6.2. Figure 6.3 shows the samples of all three types of spectrograms of normal and pneumonia. It contains a total of '144' spectrograms of each type, as shown in Table 6.2.

6.6.2 Pre-processing

The audio recordings of the lung sounds of Db1 are further divided into 7-second segments, and they are converted into three types of spectrograms to generate two segments each from one.wav file. The first spectrogram used in this experiment is the conventional spectrogram, which uses short-time Fourier transform (STFT) and divides the signal '*x*' into exact eight segments with 50% overlap and a sampling frequency of '*fs*'. If it cannot divide the signal into exact eight segments, it gets truncated. All the segments are windowed with the Hamming window. The total frequency points used are equal to the length of FFT, i.e., 'nfft', and it is either the

TABLE 6.2
The Number of Normal Samples, Pneumonia-Related Samples and Total Audio Recordings, as well as Spectrograms Used in db1 and db2

Data Sets	Normal Samples	Pneumonia Samples	Total Samples
Db1_audio (Audio/Lung Sound recordings)	35	37	72
Db1_seg (Audio/7-second segments)	70	74	144
Db2_conv (Conventional spectrogram)	70	74	144
Db2_mel (log-Mel spectrogram)	70	74	144
Db2_cqt (IIR-CQT spectrogram)	70	74	144

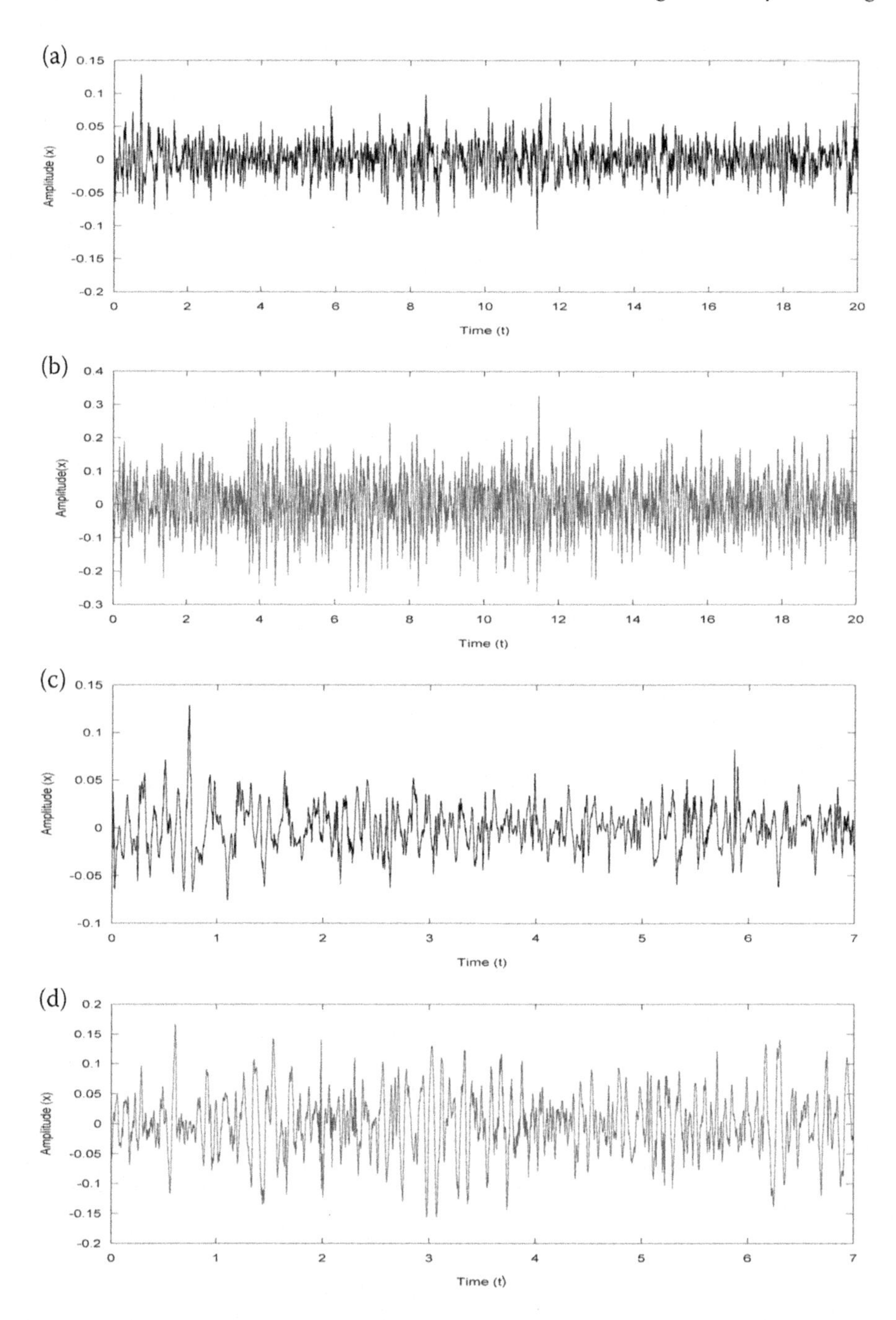

FIGURE 6.2 (a) Normal lung sound sample. (b) Pneumonia sample of lung sound. (c) Seven-second segment of normal sample. (d) Seven-second segment of pneumonia sample.

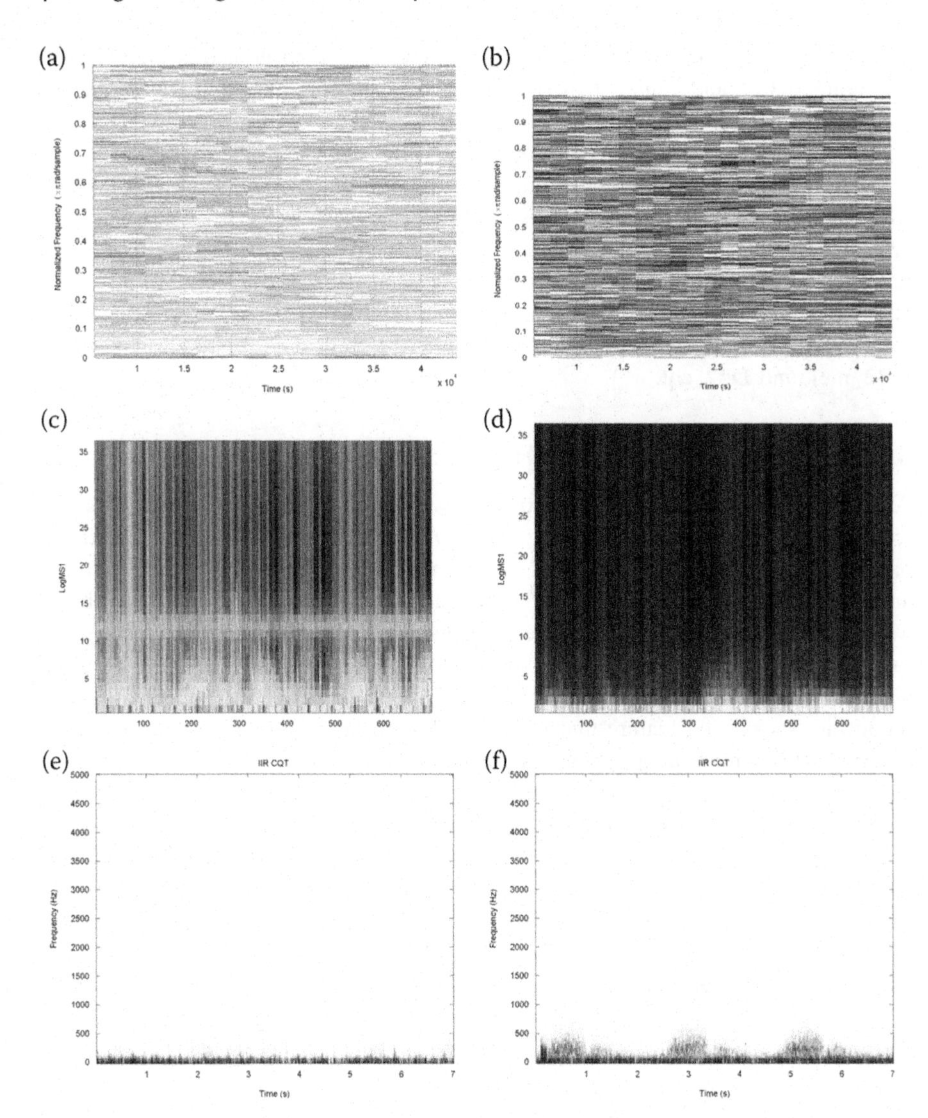

FIGURE 6.3 (a) Normal sample of conventional spectrogram. (b) Pneumonia sample of conventional spectrogram. (c) Normal sample of log-Mel spectrogram. (d) Pneumonia sample of log-Mel spectrogram. (e) Normal sample of IIR-CQT spectrogram. (f) Pneumonia sample of IIR-CQT spectrogram.

maximum of 256 or the next power of 2 greater than the length of each segment of signal 'x'. The difference between normal and pneumonia samples of conventional spectrograms is as shown in Figure 6.3(a) and Figure 6.3(b).

The second type is logarithmically scaled Mel-spectrograms or simply log-Mel spectrograms, which are spectral-temporal representations of audio signals. The Hamming window is used as a windowing function for each segment. The window length used is 25 ms, and the window shift is taken as 10 ms. The frequency range is from 64Hz to fs/2 (or maximum 12 KHz). The visual difference is clearly seen in Figure 6.3(c) and Figure 6.3(d) between a normal and pneumonia sample of log-Melspectrograms.

The third type is IIR-CQT spectrogram, i.e., IIR (LTV) Q spectrogram or multi-resolution constant quality spectrogram, which are calculated by varying an IIR filter of the DFT. The length of the window is denoted by 'nfft' and is taken as *'1024'* samples. The hop size of *'64'* samples and a quality factor of *'13'* are provided to compute these spectrograms. The visual difference between a normal and pneumonia sample of IIR-CQT is shown in Figure 6.3(e) and Figure 6.3(f). The three types of spectrograms are stored in three different data sets, i.e., Db2_conv, DB2_mel, and Db2_cqt.

6.6.3 Feature Extraction and Feature Selection

After generating the different spectrograms and storing them in a data set, the textural features are extracted using three types of feature extraction techniques, namely LBP, CLBP, and LPQ for all three types of spectrograms. The LBP features are extracted using uniform mapping with a radius of '1' and '8' neighbors to obtain a total of '59' features. The CLBP features were also computed by considering the radius of '1' and '8' neighbors with uniform mapping. A total of '256' LPQ features were extracted by considering a window size of '5'. The features of all the techniques are stored in a feature matrix. The different parameters and values used for feature extraction are as given in Table 6.3.

The classifier takes an immense amount of time for predicting the output if the size of the feature matrix is large. It is necessary to feed the classifier with a selected number of features to reduce the computation time to provide better efficiency and accuracy while predicting the outputs. So, the dimensionality reduction is performed using NCA, which is based on neighbourhood components (NC). The normalisation with zero mean is required before implementing NCA to reduce the feature matrix dimensionality. The number of features or components is reduced to

TABLE 6.3
The Parameters of Three Feature Extraction Techniques, Its Values and the Total Number of Features Extracted

Feature Extraction Technique	Total No. of Features	Parameter	Value
LBP	59	Radius	1
		Neighbours	8
		mapping	uniform
CLBP	59	Radius	1
		Neighbours	8
		mapping	uniform
LPQ	256	Window size	5

'10' and '20' to obtain a feature matrix with the selected number of NCs, and they are a result of trial and error.

6.6.4 Classification Using Decision Tree and Performance Evaluation

As the experiment is implemented using a supervised learning approach, the reduced feature matrix along with the labeled data is provided as input to the decision tree classifier. In the proposed algorithm, the features are divided into training samples and test samples by a percentage of 70% ($0.7 \times M$) and 30% ($0.3 \times M$), respectively, where M is the total number of spectrograms in the data set Db2, that is, Mdb2 = 144. The classification decision tree uses 'gdi' (or Gini's diversity index) split criteria, one of the best optimisation criteria. The binary splits lead to child nodes with a minimum leaf size of '1'. The stopping rule uses a minimum parent size of '10' and a maximum number of splits of '10' nodes to stop the splitting. For classification, the splitting is also stopped when the node is pure such that it consists of the samples of only one labeled class. Table 6.4 explains all the setup parameters used to grow the decision trees.

The data set with test samples is used to assess the performance of the trained decision tree classifier. The various plots of accuracy versus the three types of spectrograms, i.e., conventional, log-Mel, and IIR-CQT, versus the three feature extraction techniques, i.e., LBP, CLBP, and LPQ, are shown in Figure 6.4. Figure 6.4(a) shows the accuracy percentage computed without using the NCA feature reduction technique. The accuracy of 100% is achieved using the conventional spectrogram with LBP and LPQ and the log-Mel with LBP. After implementing the feature reduction technique, NCA with '10' number of NCs, the log-Mel with LPQ provided an accuracy of 100%, as shown in Figure 6.4(b). Also, it is observed that the accuracy increased slightly for IIR-CQT with all the feature extraction techniques. Figure 6.4(c) shows the implementation using NCA with '20' number of NCs. The accuracy for conventional and log-Mel spectrograms with LBP and LPQ again achieved the maximum of 100%. It is also observed that the accuracy is slightly increased for IIR-CQT with different feature extraction techniques when the number of features for NCA is increased from '10' to '20'.

TABLE 6.4
The Parameter Setup for Decision Tree Classifier

Parameters	Value
Optimization criterion or split criterion	gdi (or Gini's diversity index)
Minimum leaf size	1
Minimum parent size	10
Maximum number of splits	10
Prune	on
Merge leaves	on

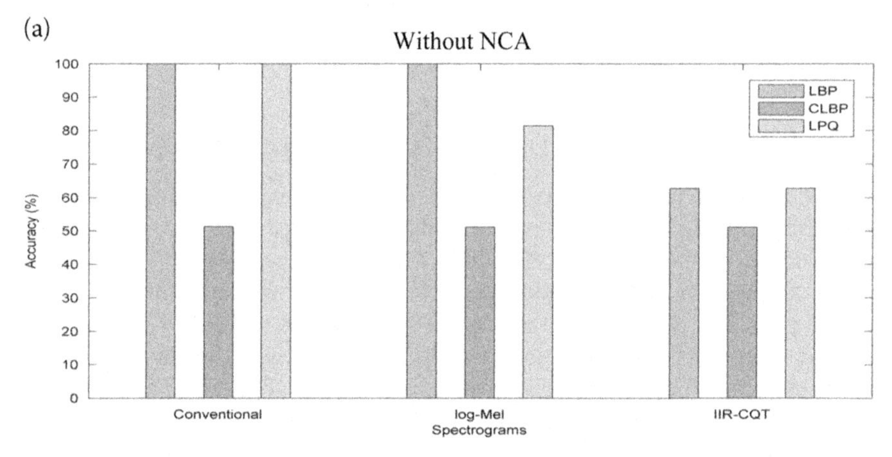

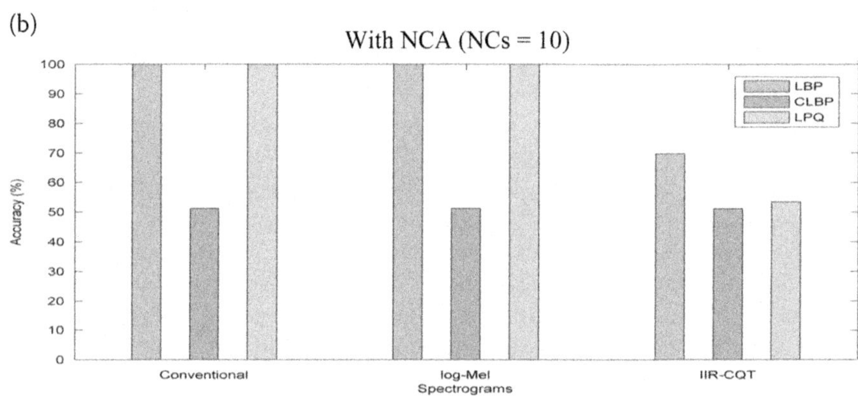

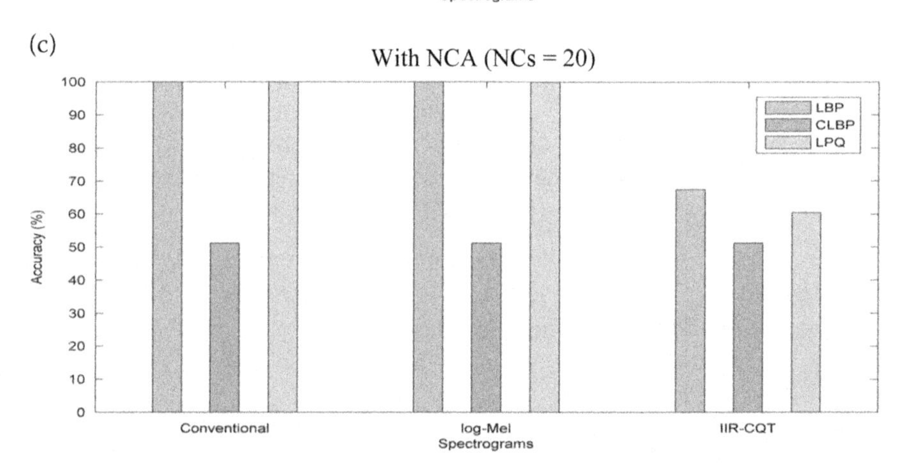

FIGURE 6.4 Plot of accuracy versus three types of spectrograms versus feature extraction techniques.

TABLE 6.5
Comparison between Various Performance Evaluation Parameters and Proposed Methods without Using NCA

Technique	Accuracy	Sensitivity	Specificity	Precision	F1 Score
Spect + LBP	100	1	1	1	1
Spect + CLBP	51.16	1	0.51	1	1
Spect + LPQ	100	1	1	1	1
Mel + LBP	100	1	1	1	1
Mel + CLBP	51.16	1	0.51	1	1
Mel + LPQ	81.4	1	0.73	0.62	0.77
CQT + LBP	62.79	0.73	0.59	0.38	0.50
CQT + CLBP	51.16	1	0.51	1	1
CQT + LPQ	62.79	0.65	0.62	0.52	0.58

TABLE 6.6
Comparison between Various Performance Evaluation Parameters and Proposed Methods When NCA Is Used with NCs = 10

Technique	Accuracy	Sensitivity	Specificity	Precision	F1 Score
Spect + LBP	100	1	1	1	1
Spect + CLBP	51.16	1	0.51	1	1
Spect + LPQ	100	1	1	1	1
Mel + LBP	100	1	1	1	1
Mel + CLBP	51.16	1	0.51	1	1
Mel + LPQ	100	1	1	1	1
CQT + LBP	69.77	0.67	0.74	0.76	0.71
CQT + CLBP	51.16	1	0.51	1	1
CQT + LPQ	53.49	0.54	0.53	0.33	0.41

Table 6.5 shows the comparison between all the techniques implemented in this work based on the performance evaluation parameters, i.e., accuracy, sensitivity, specificity, precision, and F1 score, without using NCA. It is observed that log-Mel with LBP and conventional spectrogram with LBP and LPQ performs better by achieving an F1 score of 1 when NCA is not used. Table 6.6 shows the comparison between different methods and their performance evaluation parameters when NCA is used with '10' NCs. It is seen that the accuracy for log-Mel with LBP and conventional spectrogram with LBP and LPQ remains unchanged. The accuracy, specificity, and F1 score for log-Mel with LPQ are

TABLE 6.7
Comparison between Various Performance Evaluation Parameters and Proposed Methods When NCA Is Used with NCs = 20]

Technique	Accuracy	Sensitivity	Specificity	Precision	F1 Score
Spect + LBP	100	1	1	1	1
Spect + CLBP	51.16	1	0.51	1	1
Spect + LPQ	100	1	1	1	1
Mel + LBP	100	1	1	1	1
Mel + CLBP	51.16	1	0.51	1	1
Mel + LPQ	100	1	1	1	1
CQT + LBP	67.44	0.64	0.72	0.76	0.70
CQT + CLBP	51.16	1	0.51	1	1
CQT + LPQ	60.47	0.59	0.62	0.62	0.60

increased from 81.4% to 100%, 0.73 to 1, and 0.77 to 1, respectively. It is also observed that the performance of IIR-CQT with LBP is slightly increased. Table 6.7 shows the comparison between different methods and their performance evaluation parameters when NCA is used with '20' NCs. The results remain unchanged for log-Mel and conventional spectrograms with LBP and LPQ. It can be observed that IIR-CQT with LPQ performs better in this case. Table 6.8 shows the comparison of some existing methods with our proposed method.

6.7 CONCLUSION

In this book chapter, a lung sound detection method is proposed on the basis of time-frequency representations using three different types of spectrograms, i.e., conventional, log-Mel, and IIR-CQT spectrograms, and three textural-based feature extraction techniques, namely, LBP, CLBP, and LPQ. We have extended the approach of one-dimensional audio lung sound signals to two-dimensional time-frequency representations. The features are reduced using NCA, and a decision tree classifier is employed to classify lung sound signals.

The parameters, i.e., sensitivity, accuracy, precision, specificity, F1 score, are used to evaluate the performance of the proposed method. The audio recordings of the lung sounds are acquired from the ICBHI 2017 challenge respiratory sound database, an open-access database. The results of three types of spectrograms are compared with the feature extraction and selection techniques. It is observed that the log-Mel and conventional spectrogram with LBP and LPQ are better in terms of IIR-CQT. The results show improvement when NCA is used as a feature reduction technique.

TABLE 6.8
Comparison of the Proposed Method with Other Existing Methods

Author	Dataset	Feature Extraction/ Reduction Method	Classification Method	Accuracy
Naqvi and Choudhry [19]	ICBHI 2017 challenge	Time domain, cepstral, and spectral features and back-elimination method	quadratic discriminate classifier	99.70%
Demir et al. [28]	ICBHI 2017 challenge	Spectrogram images, STFT, CNN	SVM	65.5% and 63.09%
Shuvo et al. [32]	ICBHI 2017 challenge	Hybrid scalogram features and continuous wavelet transform (CWT)	CNN	99.20% (three-class) and 99.05% (six-class)
Fraiwan et al. [13]	ICBHI 2017 challenge	Logarithmic energy entropy, Shannon entropy, and spectrogram-based spectral entropy	boosted decision trees and SVM	98.27% and 98.20%
Proposed Method	ICBHI 2017 challenge	**Spect + LPQ Spect + LBP Mel + LBP Without NCA**	Decision tree	100%
Proposed Method	ICBHI 2017 challenge	**Spect + LBP Spect + LPQ Mel + LBP Mel + LPQ with NCA**	Decision tree	100%

REFERENCES

[1] Rocha, Bruno M., Filos Dimitris, Mendes Luís, Serbes Gorkem, Ulukaya Sezer, Kahya Yasemin P., Jakovljevic Nikša et al. "An open access database for the evaluation of respiratory sound classification algorithms." *Physiological Measurement* 40, no. 3 (2019): 035001.
[2] https://www.who.int/health-topics/chronic-respiratory-diseases#tab=tab_1
[3] Salvi, Sundeep, Anil Kumar G., Dhaliwal R. S., Paulson Katherine, Agrawal Anurag, Koul Parvaiz A., Mahesh P. A. et al. "The burden of chronic respiratory diseases and their heterogeneity across the states of India: the Global Burden of Disease Study 1990–2016." *The Lancet Global Health* 6, no. 12 (2018): e1363–e1374.
[4] https://www.medicalnewstoday.com/articles/323886#summary
[5] https://www.templehealth.org/services/conditions/lower-respiratory-tract-infections
[6] https://www.webmd.com/lung/understanding-pneumonia-basics
[7] Hassanien, Aboul Ella, Khamparia Aditya, Gupta Deepak, Shankar K., and Slowik Adam. "Cognitive internet of medical things for smart healthcare.", Springer Publisher, ISBN 978-3-030-55832-1. https://doi.org/10.1007/978-3-030-55833-8

[8] Pattnayak, Parthasarathi, and Jena Om Prakash. "Innovation on machine learning in healthcare services—An introduction." *Machine Learning for Healthcare Applications*, 1 (2021): 1–14. https://doi.org/10.1002/9781119792611.ch1

[9] Paramesha, K., Gururaj H. L., and Jena Om Prakash. "Applications of machine learning in biomedical text processing and food industry." *Machine Learning for Healthcare Applications* (2021): 151.

[10] Panigrahi, Niranjan, Ayus Ishan, and Jena Om Prakash. "An expert system-based clinical decision support system for Hepatitis-B prediction & diagnosis." *Machine Learning for Healthcare Applications* 1 (2021): 57–75. https://doi.org/10.1002/9781119792611.ch4

[11] Birajdar, Gajanan K., and Mukesh D. Patil. "Speech/music classification using visual and spectral chromagram features." *Journal of Ambient Intelligence and Humanized Computing* 11, no. 1 (2020): 329–347.

[12] Yu, Guoshen, and Slotine Jean-Jacques. "Audio classification from time-frequency texture." In 2009 IEEE International Conference on Acoustics, Speech and Signal Processing, pp. 1677–1680. IEEE, 2009.

[13] Fraiwan, Luay, Hassanin Omnia, Fraiwan Mohammad, Khassawneh Basheer, Ibnian Ali M., and Alkhodari Mohanad. "Automatic identification of respiratory diseases from stethoscopic lung sound signals using ensemble classifiers." *Biocybernetics and Biomedical Engineering* 41, no. 1 (2021): 1–14.

[14] Nabi, Fizza Ghulam, Sundaraj Kenneth, Lam Chee Kiang, and Palaniappan Rajkumar. "Characterization and classification of asthmatic wheeze sounds according to severity level using spectral integrated features." *Computers in Biology and Medicine* 104 (2019): 52–61.

[15] Pramono, Renard Xaviero Adhi, Imtiaz Syed Anas, and Rodriguez-Villegas Esther. "Evaluation of features for classification of wheezes and normal respiratory sounds." *PloS One* 14, no. 3 (2019): e0213659.

[16] Haider, Nishi Shahnaj, Singh Bikesh Kumar, Periyasamy R., and Behera Ajoy K. "Respiratory sound based classification of chronic obstructive pulmonary disease: A risk stratification approach in machine learning paradigm." *Journal of Medical Systems* 43, no. 8 (2019): 1–13.

[17] Ulukaya, Sezer, Serbes Gorkem, and Kahya Yasemin P. "Wheeze type classification using non-dyadic wavelet transform based optimal energy ratio technique." *Computers in Biology and Medicine* 104 (2019): 175–182.

[18] Nabi, Fizza Ghulam, Sundaraj Kenneth, Lam Chee Kiang, and Palaniappan Rajkumar. "Analysis of wheeze sounds during tidal breathing according to severity levels in asthma patients." *Journal of Asthma* 57, no. 4 (2020): 353–365.

[19] Naqvi, Syed Zohaib Hassan, and Choudhry Mohammad Ahmad. "An Automated System for Classification of Chronic Obstructive Pulmonary Disease and Pneumonia Patients Using Lung Sound Analysis." *Sensors* 20, no. 22 (2020): 6512.

[20] Jaber, Mustafa Musa, Abd Sura Khalil, Mohamed Shakeel P., Burhanuddin M. A., Mohammed Mohammed Abdulameer, and Yussof Salman. "A telemedicine tool framework for lung sounds classification using ensemble classifier algorithms." *Measurement* 162 (2020): 107883.

[21] Meng, Fei, Yan Shi, Na Wang, Maolin Cai, and Zujing Luo. "Detection of respiratory sounds based on wavelet coefficients and machine learning." *IEEE Access* 8 (2020): 155710–155720.

[22] Sharma, Nikhil, Ila Kaushik, Bharat Bhushan, Siddharth Gautam, and Aditya Khamparia. "Applicability of WSN and biometric models in the field of healthcare," in *Deep Learning Strategies for Security Enhancement in Wireless Sensor Networks*, pp. 304–329. IGI Global, Hershey, Pennsylvania, 2020.

[23] Jindal, Mansi, Jatin Gupta, and Bharat Bhushan. "Machine learning methods for IoT and their future applications," in *2019 International Conference on Computing, Communication, and Intelligent Systems (ICCCIS)*, pp. 430–434. IEEE, Greater Noida, India, 2019.

[24] Messner, Elmar, Melanie Fediuk, Paul Swatek, Stefan Scheidl, Freyja-Maria Smolle-Jüttner, Horst Olschewski, and Franz Pernkopf. "Multi-channel lung sound classification with convolutional recurrent neural networks." *Computers in Biology and Medicine* 122 (2020): 103831.

[25] Jayalakshmy, S., and Gnanou Florence Sudha. "Scalogram based prediction model for respiratory disorders using optimized convolutional neural networks." *Artificial Intelligence in Medicine* 103 (2020): 101809.

[26] García-Ordás, María Teresa, José Alberto Benítez-Andrades, Isaías García-Rodríguez, Carmen Benavides, and Héctor Alaiz-Moretón. "Detecting respiratory pathologies using convolutional neural networks and variational autoencoders for unbalancing data." *Sensors* 20, no. 4 (2020): 1214.

[27] Acharya, Jyotibdha, and Arindam Basu. "Deep neural network for respiratory sound classification in wearable devices enabled by patient specific model tuning." *IEEE Transactions on Biomedical Circuits and Systems* 14, no. 3 (2020): 535–544.

[28] Demir, Fatih, Abdulkadir Sengur, and Varun Bajaj. "Convolutional neural networks based efficient approach for classification of lung diseases." *Health Information Science and Systems* 8, no. 1 (2020): 1–8.

[29] Demir, Fatih, Aras Masood Ismael, and Abdulkadir Sengur. "Classification of lung sounds with CNN model using parallel pooling structure." *IEEE Access* 8 (2020): 105376–105383.

[30] Khamparia, Aditya, Prakash Kumar Singh, Poonam Rani, Debabrata Samanta, Ashish Khanna, and Bharat Bhushan. "An internet of health things-driven deep learning framework for detection and classification of skin cancer using transfer learning." *Transactions on Emerging Telecommunications Technologies* (2020): e3963.

[31] Kumar, Santosh, Bharat Bhusan, Debabrata Singh, and Dilip kumar Choubey. "Classification of Diabetes using Deep Learning." In *2020 International Conference on Communication and Signal Processing (ICCSP)*, pp. 0651–0655. IEEE, Chennai, India, 2020.

[32] Shuvo, Samiul Based, Shams Nafisa Ali, Soham Irtiza Swapnil, Taufiq Hasan, and Mohammed Imamul Hassan Bhuiyan. "A lightweight cnn model for detecting respiratory diseases from lung auscultation sounds using emd-cwt-based hybrid scalogram." *IEEE Journal of Biomedical and Health Informatics* 25, no. 7 (2020): 2595-2603. 10.1109/JBHI.2020.3048006

[33] Ghosal, Arijit, Rudrasis Chakraborty, Bibhas Chandra Dhara, and Sanjoy Kumar Saha. "Song/instrumental classification using spectrogram based contextual features." In Proceedings of the CUBE International Information Technology Conference, pp. 21–25. 2012.

[34] Sharan, Roneel V., and Tom J. Moir. "Audio surveillance under noisy conditions using time-frequency image feature." In 2014 19th International Conference on Digital Signal Processing, pp. 130–135. IEEE, 2014.

[35] Oo, Mie Mie, and Lwin Lwin Oo. "Fusion of Log-Mel Spectrogram and GLCM feature in acoustic scene classification." In International Conference on Software Engineering Research, Management and Applications, pp. 175–187. Springer, Cham, 2019.

[36] Hao, Man, Wei-Hua Cao, Zhen-Tao Liu, Min Wu, and Peng Xiao. "Visual-audio emotion recognition based on multi-task and ensemble learning with multiple features." *Neurocomputing* 391 (2020): 42–51.

[37] Birajdar, Gajanan K., and Mukesh D. Patil. "Speech and music classification using spectrogram based statistical descriptors and extreme learning machine." *Multimedia Tools and Applications* 78, no. 11 (2019): 15141–15168.

[38] Felipe, Gustavo Z., Rafael L. Aguiar, Yandre MG. Costa, Carlos N. Silla, Sheryl Brahnam, Loris Nanni, and Shannon McMurtrey. "Identification of infants' cry motivation using spectrograms." In 2019 International Conference on Systems, Signals and Image Processing (IWSSIP), pp. 181–186. IEEE, 2019.

[39] Sharma, Garima, Deepak Prasad, Karthikeyan Umapathy, and Sridhar Krishnan. "Screening and analysis of specific language impairment in young children by analyzing the textures of speech signal." In 2020 42nd Annual International Conference of the IEEE Engineering in Medicine & Biology Society (EMBC), pp. 964–967. IEEE, 2020.

[40] Chowdhury, Amit A., Vaibhav S. Borkar, and Gajanan K. Birajdar. "Indian language identification using time-frequency image textural descriptors and GWO-based feature selection." *Journal of Experimental & Theoretical Artificial Intelligence* 32, no. 1 (2020): 111–132.

[41] Ojansivu, Ville, and Janne Heikkilä. "Blur insensitive texture classification using local phase quantization." In International Conference on Image and Signal Processing, pp. 236–243. Springer, Berlin, Heidelberg, 2008.

[42] Malan, N. S., and S. Sharma. "Motor imagery EEG spectral-spatial feature optimization using dual-tree complex wavelet and neighbourhood component analysis." *IRBM* (2021), ISSN 1959-0318. https://doi.org/10.1016/j.irbm.2021.01.0 02

[43] Malan, Nitesh Singh, and Shiru Sharma. "Feature selection using regularized neighbourhood component analysis to enhance the classification performance of motor imagery signals." *Computers in Biology and Medicine* 107 (2019): 118–126.

[44] Chambres, Gaëtan, Pierre Hanna, and Myriam Desainte-Catherine. "Automatic detection of patient with respiratory diseases using lung sound analysis." In 2018 International Conference on Content-Based Multimedia Indexing (CBMI), pp. 1–6. IEEE, 2018.

[45] Chekhovych, M. G., A. S. Poreva, V. I. Timofeyev, and P. Henaff. "Using of the machine learning methods to identify bronchopulmonary system diseases with the use of lung sounds." *Вісник Національного технічного університету України Київський політехнічний інститут. Серія: Радіотехніка. Радіоапаратобудування* 73 (2018): 55–62.

7 Medical Image Analysis Using Machine Learning Techniques

A Systematic Review

Mustafa A. Al-Asadi and Sakir Tasdemir
Department of Computer Engineering, Selçuk University, Konya, Turkey

CONTENTS

DOI: 10.1201/9781003189053-7

7.1 INTRODUCTION

Machine learning (ML) is a relatively recent area of study that refers to learning computers from past experiences (past information) to improve future implementation [1]. For example, if you have a model that consists of parameters, optimizing the model's parameters based on training data or experience is called learning or training. The learned model can then predict the outcome from new data that has not been used during the learning process [2]. Machine learning applications range from household to healthcare, local applications to enterprise applications, as well as military, agricultural and all walks of life [3]. There are multiple and endless machine learning applications in healthcare. Therefore, machine learning helps simplify the administrative work in hospitals. In addition, machine learning plays a very dominant role in clinical decision support and influences physician and hospital decisions [4]. Medical imaging is one of the essential tools for diagnosing and treating patients used in modern medicine. However, due to the large amount and complexity of data, it is challenging to interpret objects such as human body structure and pathology in medical images. Therefore, machine learning plays an essential role in medical image analysis like image registration, image segmentation, image search, and image-based surgery, which have been widely used to improve computer-aided detection and diagnosis (CAD) that collects computer-aided detection (CADe) and computer-aided diagnosis (CADx) that also has been rapidly developed as a reliable tool for assisting and assisting doctors by automatically reading and interpreting medical images [5]. As a result, machine learning can be used in managing and sharing health information and improving the administrative process. Thus, facilitating access to clinical data and updating workflow regularly [4]. In this chapter, we highlight the role of machine learning algorithms in raising competence in medical imaging. In particular, we address the major studies on the application of machine learning methods to biomedical image segmentation, image registration, computer-assisted diagnostic systems (CADx, CADe). As well, we review traditional machine learning algorithms like artificial neural networks that are applied in content-based image retrieval, K-nearest neighbours, a genetic algorithm, and ant colony optimization. We discuss the successes and challenges of each machine learning model and offer some experimental approaches to address these challenges.

This chapter is organized as follows: Section 7.2 presents the methodology of work. Section 7.3 reviews the history and principles of various medical images. Section 7.4 explains how machine learning is applied in medical imaging via an artificial neural network used in content-based image retrieval, a combination of k-nearest neighbours, genetic algorithm, and ant community optimization. As well, the section presents some improvements for previous models. Finally, discussion and conclusions are made in Section 7.5.

7.2 METHODOLOGY

As a first step, the history, principle, and applications of different medical images were researched. The research was conducted using Google Scholar's database

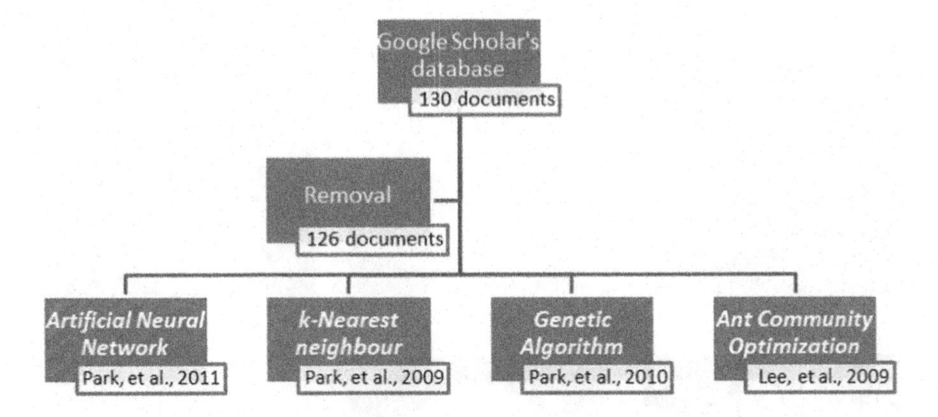

FIGURE 7.1 Flow chart of the selection process of articles.

during December 2020. The following keywords have used for the search: "history of medical images". Subjects returned in searches also refer to the applications and principles of medical images.

As a second step, Google Scholar's database was used for the same previous period (December 2020), to highlight the role of machine learning algorithms in raising competence in medical imaging. The following keywords were used for the search: "machine learning for medical image analysis". The initial search resulted in 130 documents (articles and books). Then, filters were applied concerning the knowledge area of the articles, which limited the following areas: machine learning application methods to biomedical image segmentation, image registration, computer-assisted diagnostic systems (CADx, CADe), artificial neural networks in content-based image retrieval, K-nearest neighbours, a genetic algorithm, and ant colony optimization. The remainder documents had their titles and abstracts evaluated. Finally, we ended up with four papers after excluding non-target studies. Figure 7.1 shows the flow chart of the selection process.

7.3 HISTORY AND CHARACTERISTICS OF MEDICAL IMAGES

Medical images (Figure 7.2) differ in their uses and the process of their historical development. Therefore, some images' acquisition methods are different from other images because of each image's characteristics and can be useful for specific medical subjects. These medical images include plain radiography, computed tomography (CT), ultrasound imaging, magnetic resonance imaging (MRI), and positron emission tomography (PET) (Table 7.1). X-ray refers to the form of electromagnetic waves in a region of shorter wavelength than ultraviolet light. The X-ray was first unexpectedly discovered in 1895 by a German physicist, Wilhelm Conrad Röntgen, who experimented with current flow through a tube. He named X-ray, which means a new type of radiation that is not known. It is also called the Röntgen line and his name [6]. Flatbed radiography using X-rays in medical imaging is the most basic and most widely used medical image acquisition method, even though it is the oldest. Using this method, images are recorded on the

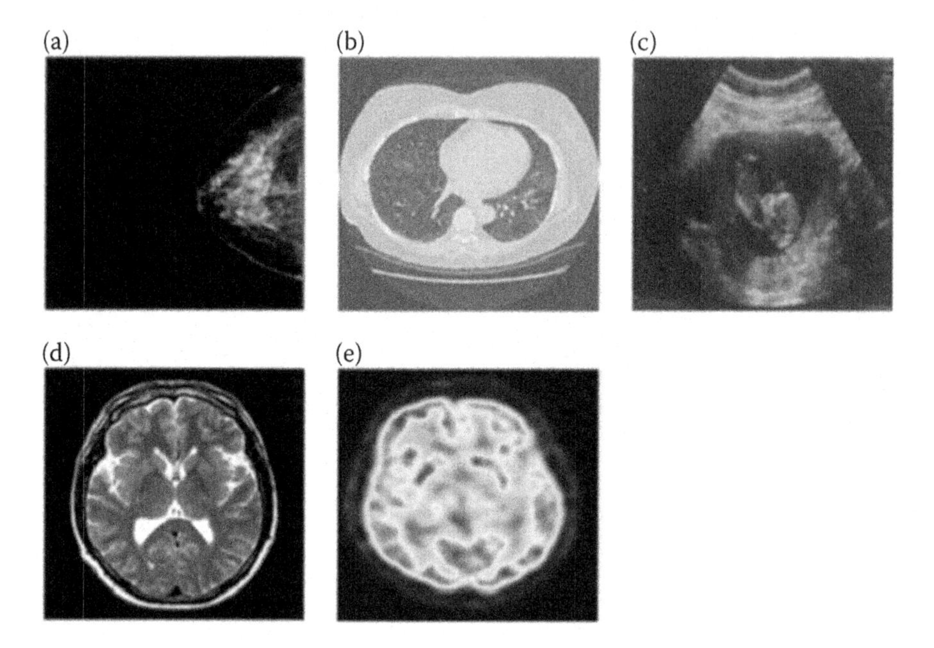

FIGURE 7.2 Various medical images: (a) mammography, (b) computed tomography, (c) ultrasound, (d) magnetic resonance imaging, and (e) positron emission tomography.

recording plate by exposing a recording plate to the back of the area of interest and exposing a small amount of ionizing radiation to the body area of interest to acquire images of the body. Chest radiography (CXR) is a typical application of flat plate radiography used to photograph bones of the heart, lung, bronchial, blood vessels, and vertebrae. Another application of plate radiography is mammography. Breast cancer is a common disease in middle-aged women aged 40 or older [7]. In general, the World Health Organization notes that the incidence of cancer has increased over the past decades. Therefore, detection and classification of cancer at an early stage of development enables patients to be diagnosed and treated properly. Also, earlier diagnosis and treatment can significantly reduce mortality [8]. Mammography has been the most cost-effective way to diagnose early breast cancer, including breast mass and micro-calcification cluster [9]. The information obtained from the transmitted energy by emitting light to an object is called a projection. Tomography refers to a technique of imaging an object's monolayer using a projection obtained from various directions [10]. Radon solved the problem of reconstructing a function in the projection in 1917, and the current CT diagnostic technique was developed by Godfrey Hounsfield. In 1972, Godfrey Hounsfield invented the first commercially viable CT scanner [11]. When the patient lies on a table of tomography equipment to take a CT image, he slides into the round bar attached to the table. It transmits X-rays at various angles to the human body in the tube and measures the number of X-rays that are reduced while passing through the human body in the form of electrical signals. Analyze the measured signals using a computer and reconstruct the inner surface of the human body. General x-ray images are displayed on a

TABLE 7.1
Characteristics and Application Fields of Medical Images

	Discoverer	Discover Year	Characteristic	Applications
X-ray	roentgen	1895	• The shape of electromagnetic waves in a region of shorter wavelength than ultraviolet. • Because it is represented on a two-dimensional projection plate.	• Shooting bones of chest X-ray, heart, lung, bronchus, blood vessels and spine, mammography
CT	Guard Free	1972	• Measure the number of X-rays in the form of electrical signals. • Show the shape of the selected section.	• Diagnosis of tumours, cancer, internal organs such as liver or kidney
Ultrasound image	Spallanzani	1794	• Higher than the audible frequency • Convert ultrasound back into the image	• Muscles, tendons, and various internal organs, their size, structure, and pathological damage are displayed in real-time as cross-sectional images
MRI	Damadian	1969	• The human body is put in the vital magnetic field area, and the high frequency is generated. Then the distribution of the waveform is classified. • Benefits and high resolution without using X-rays	• Early diagnosis of cancer disease, determination of therapeutic effect, and discovery of recurrence
PET	Gordon et al.	The 1950s	• Detection of extinction radiation generated by the interaction between the positron and the substance after injecting radiopharmaceuticals emitting the positron into the blood vessels in vitro • Morphological changes and biochemical changes of lesions can be confirmed more accurately in 3-D images	• Diagnosis of brain diseases such as Alzheimer's disease, Parkinson's disease, epilepsy, and some cardiovascular diseases in addition to cancer and brain tumours

two-dimensional projection plate, so there is a limitation in representation. CT, on the other hand, shows all the features of the selected section. It is possible to accurately diagnose various facts that are difficult to find out with conventional X-ray images. Because of this, CT is being used to acquire various medical images [12].

Ultrasound has a higher frequency than the audible frequency. Lord Rayleigh first published the mathematical expression of sound waves that underpin the practical study of acoustics' future. Then, in 1794, Spallanzani published the theory that bats can move in dark places through the reflections of sounds that humans cannot hear. By 1930, ultrasound began to be used in England and Germany for therapeutic purposes [13]. The process of acquiring an ultrasound image first places a producer probe at the patient's site to be imaged. Apply a gel to the probe and the diagnostic area to obtain a clearer image. The computer converts the returned ultrasound into an image. Ultrasonography using this method is useful for real-time diagnosis and detection of fetal development or wound or cancer of the body's internal organs. Also, ultrasound imaging in early breast cancer detection is more useful than mammography to detect small masses in dense breast, which is frequently seen in young women [14].

The initial name of the MRI was NMRI (nuclear magnetic resonance imaging). Still, it became commercially available as a medical diagnostic device and became an MRI except for the "N" because of nuclear's negative meaning. The basic principle of MRI was discovered by Bloch and Purcell in 1946 and was proposed in 1969 by Damadian for medical purposes, particularly for the detection of cancer [15]. Unlike MRI, which obtains images from externally excised or ultrasonic waves, the human body is placed in a strong magnetic field area to generate high-frequency waves. Then the distribution of the waveforms is classified and imaged. Unlike other X-ray-based images, it is used for various medical image acquisition and diagnosis because of the advantage of not using X-ray and high resolution.

The use of radiation in medicine is now widespread and routine. Recently, the techniques of diagnostic radiology, nuclear medicine and radiotherapy have developed and are considered essential tools in all branches and specialties of medicine [16]. Nuclear medical imaging uses electromagnetic signals emitted from inside the body and is known as the only way to image the body's inside without sending signals from outside. PET using radioactive isotopes developed in the nuclear medicine field injected radiopharmaceuticals that emit positron into several essential metabolites and then detected annihilation radiation generated by the interaction between the positron and the material in vitro is one of the imaging methods to diagnose diseases. Most diseases are characterized by functional changes and biochemical changes before anatomic changes occur. Positron emission tomography (PET) is a health technology that belongs to a medical specialty called nuclear medicine and is widely used for the diagnosis, prediction and control of tumours. PET is useful for the early diagnosis of various diseases. PET is commonly used in clinical practice, especially in early diagnosis of cancer, determination of the therapeutic effect and recurrence discovery [17]. Gordon Brownell et al. in the 1950s, had an enormous impact on PET technology development by introducing extinction radiation in medical imaging. A significant factor in applying PET imaging to a broader area is developing radiopharmaceuticals, first used by humans in 1976. PET/CT or PET/MRI, which combines PET technology with CT and MRI, can more accurately confirm morphological and biochemical changes in lesions in 3D space [18].

7.4 MACHINE LEARNING APPLICATION IN MEDICAL IMAGING

7.4.1 Artificial Neural Network

Interstitial lung diseases (ILD) is a group of about 120 different diseases associated with the lungs. ILD gradually diminishes the size of the lungs and shows an important mortality rate. Early ILD therapy is an essential step in preventing disease progression. Park et al. developed a system that initially detects ILD in CT images and helps the patient perform the appropriate treatment [19]. This system's essential role is to automatically split the lungs and then examine every lung's pixel to see if it is associated with the ILD. However, since inspecting all the lungs requires extensive computation, it is necessary to cover a specific size grid on a divided lung image to inspect the pixels where each texture is encountered, and if there is an ILD, growing. When examining a pixel, a predetermined region of interest (ROI) is extracted from a pixel and removed from the ROI with a minimum of 22 texture features and four histograms of grey level first-order statistics it is determined whether the pixel is an ILD-related pixel by an artificial neural network. The volume of the last detected ILD pixel and the divided lung volume are calculated, and their rate is used as the ILD detection score. If the detection score is greater than the specified threshold, it is determined that there is ILD in the CT image. Otherwise, it is judged as normal.

An artificial neural network is a learning method approaching an optimal global function by learning using a pair of input and result data [20]. The back-propagation algorithm is most often used for the training of neural networks. The training process calculates the output according to the input pattern and then calculates the error between the desired output and the output according to the input. To reduce the error, the weights of the output layer and the hidden layer are updated in the opposite direction to the neural network's processing direction [21]. The weight update phase to reduce error is called the weights update phase. This process is repeated until the error rate is reduced to the lowest value [22].

The modified rules of updating the weights are expressed as:

$$w_{ij}^{neu} = w_{ij}^{alt} + \Delta w_{ij} \tag{7.1}$$

$$\Delta w_{ij} = a. \ (t_j - o_j). \ x_i \tag{7.2}$$

Δw_{ij} = the change of the weight $\boldsymbol{ij}$ between the $\boldsymbol{i}$ (input) and $\boldsymbol{j}$ (output).

t_j = the desired output.

o_j = the real output.

x_i = neurons' input.

Artificial neural networks are widely used as a machine learning tool for CAD systems in various medical images because of their ability to optimize the relationship between input features and required output classes using some noise training data.

7.4.1.1 Analysis of Previous Methods

The neural network structure used in Park et al. [19] was composed of three layers: the input layer, hidden layer, and output layer. The input layer consisted of 12 neurons representing 11 excellent features and one bias among the 26 features extracted from the ROI, and the silver layer was determined by ten neurons experimentally [19]. Generally, the neural network output layer consists of one neuron to solve the two-class problems. However, another training procedure is required to select the cut-off value to judge the two classifications.

7.4.1.2 Proposed Solutions

To solve this problem, we used two neurons and left decision value to the training of data and neural networks. The learning and bias values used in the learning process were chosen as 0.05 and 0.95 by experience, and the sigmoid function was used as the activation function for each neuron. In the training process, the neurons' weight values are repeatedly learned by the back-propagation algorithm until there is no change in the total squared error or until the maximum specified number of iterations is reached. The training with limited data was overtraining, which affected the neural network's generalization, so the maximum number of training was limited to 500. For the evaluation of the proposed system, 19 CT images were selected by radiologists as light ILD symptoms. This study aimed to detect early ILD patients, and CT images with severe ILD symptoms were excluded from the study. Next, we selected randomly selected 19 CT images from the CT images database for lung cancer that did not affect ILD. Therefore, the database used in the experiment consisted of 38 CT images. The database was used for training and testing, in which CT images of normal and ILD patients were divided in half.

7.4.1.3 Results

Experimental results in the case of a slice thickness of 2.5 mm in the CT images, the segmented closed area consisted of 4,317,211 pixels. However, after applying the region growing method, the system visited only 280,292 pixels, reducing the number of pixels to be examined by about 93.5%, and the processing time was improved by about 15.6 times. After applying the neural network trained system to all test CT images, the AUC (area under ROC curve) was around 0.880 ± 0.060. As a result, the system showed a sensitivity of 80.0% and a specificity of 85.5%. In the normal CT image, the ILD detection score was constant in the narrow range from 0.91 to 4.60, while the detection system varied from 1.07 to 15.40 for the CT image, including the ILD. Therefore, it is shown that the proposed system can distinguish CT images, including normal and ILD, effectively. Figure 7.3 shows the interstitial lung disease detection system using the proposed model.

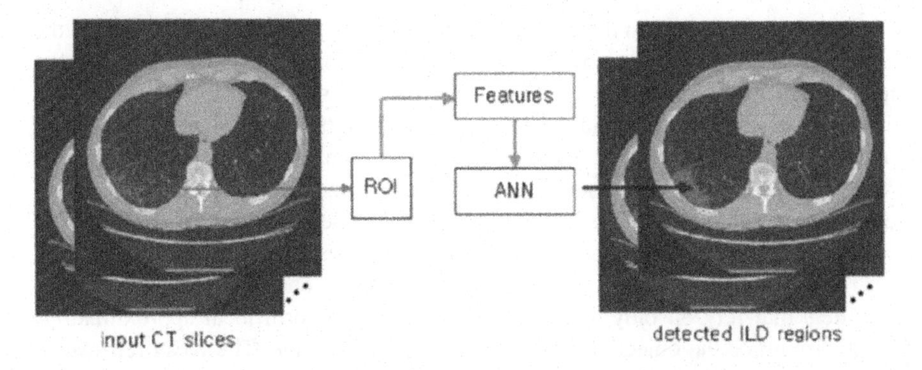

FIGURE 7.3 Interstitial lung disease detection system using neural network.

7.4.2 K-Nearest Neighbour Algorithm

The K-nearest neighbor (KNN) algorithm is one of the simplest and most popular algorithms in machine learning, used to solve classification and regression problems [23]. In the KNN algorithm, the entry consists of examples of k-training in the feature space. The KNN algorithm is considered the simplest algorithms of machine learning. K-nearest neighbours measure the distance de (qi, pj) among query points qi and a set of training pj to classify a new object mapped according to the majority of the KNN class of Y traits of the training samples (Equation 7.3):

Query point qi = q1, q2, q3 …. qn.

Training sample pj = pl, p2, p3 … pn.

$$d(p,q) = d(q,p) = \sqrt{(q_1 - p_1)^2 + (q_1 - p_1)^2 + \ldots + (q_1 - p_1)^2} \quad (7.3)$$

7.4.2.1 Analysis of Previous Methods

Park et al. [5] developed a system to classify whether a mammogram's partial image contains a breast mass, depending on the content-based search results. Specifically, the K-nearest neighbourhood algorithm (KNN) is applied as a tool for searching for similar images [5].

7.4.2.2 Proposed Solutions

For the same previous purpose, we extracted 3,000 ROIs (region of interest) from the mammograms using the previously developed CADe [24] and stored them in the reference database. In the region of interest extracted, 1,500 contained the actual breast mass, true-positive, and the remaining 1,500 have normal tissue as false-positive removed by the useful tool. Fourteen features are extracted from the extracted regions of interest, including morphological features and pixel brightness-based features. In detail, three mass-based features are used because the entire breast area's features can define the breast mass. For example, the average pixel brightness, the average fluctuation, and the standard deviation of the pixel brightness in the entire divided chest area. Eleven regional features are then calculated from the extracted mass and mass background. For example, the complicity of the region, the average of the radial length from the centre of mass to the border, the standard deviation of the radial distance, the skew of the radial distance, the circularity of the border, standard deviations of brightness, standard deviations of the gradient of border pixels, standard deviations of pixel background brightness, average variation of pixel background brightness, and centre of mass. Fourteen features representing each breast mass are stored in the reference database and the extracted breast mass ROI and used in the search phase. Also, one fractal feature was removed to show the visual similarity. The KNN is one of the local data-based classifiers that rely on only a few training samples to form local approximations that approximate the objective function—given a test image. The KNN retrieves k reference images that are most similar to the test image in the reference database. The distance between the test image and the reference image is calculated as the Euclidean distance between them. After applying the content-based retrieval system using KNN, we judge that the retrieved reference mass images are clinically identical to each other if they are of the same class (mass or mass) as the mass image. Since the search system using KNN is a machine learning technique for solving based on local instances, no pre-training process is required.

7.4.2.3 Results

The performance of the system was evaluated using a leave-one-case-out evaluation method. For example, 3,000 ROI images are used once as query images, and the remaining 2,999 images are considered reference images. When one ROI is selected as a test image (query image) in the iterative execution for system performance evaluation, it searches k similar images in the remaining reference databases. Depending on the system's retrieval score for mass and non-mass ROI, the ROC (receiver operating characteristic curve), including the AUC and the 95% confidence interval is calculated. Here, AUC was used as a measure to evaluate the performance of the system. As a result, the search system using all 15 features and KNN with 26 neighbours (k = 26) showed AUC = 0.866 at a 95% confidence interval.

7.4.3 Genetic Algorithm

Pulmonary embolism (PE), also called deep vein thrombi, occurs when a blood clot from a vein in the deep legs of a body falls from the vein wall. It passes through the right atrium, right ventricle, and it is caused by blocking the blood vessels of the lungs. Pulmonary embolism is a relatively easy-to-treat disease only when it is found at an appropriate time, but it is challenging to diagnose it because of the ambiguous and uncharacteristic early symptoms of respiratory distress, syncope, coughing, and haemoptysis. In the United States, computed tomography images are used to diagnose this. Physicians spend a lot of time adjusting the dark areas of the pulmonary artery, adjusting the intensity level, and selecting suspect areas [25]. Thus, the development and research of CAD systems that have helped radiologists assist in the interpretation of effective computed tomography images have attracted much attention over the past few years. Ultimately, the computer-aided detection system has been studied to be used as a stand-alone diagnostic tool. However, until now, the detection of pulmonary embolism from computed tomography has detected many positive errors, making it unable to perform the same role as a lane solver that supports radiation and physician interpretation.

7.4.3.1 Analysis of Previous Methods

Park et al. [26] proposed several approaches to eliminate false positives in a pulmonary embolism detection system. In the pre-processing process, the proposed system searches for pulmonary embolism candidates. It extracts 27 features (12 features based on contrast, 11 based on shape, and 4 based on candidate border) from the posterior feature. And KNN was applied at the stage of classifying the pulmonary embryo candidate area [26]. The reference database of the KNN is configured so that the affirmative error and the positive error are equal to each other in advance.

A genetic algorithm is a method for improvement and research by relying on biologically inspired factors such as mutation, crossover, and selection. This method can be classified as an evolutionary algorithm (EA) method [27]. In a genetic algorithm, a set of solutions (called individuals, creatures, or phenotypes) has been developed for the problem of optimization to arrive at better solutions. Each candidate solution contains a set of characteristics (chromosomes or genotype) that can be changed; traditionally, solutions are represented in binary from 0 and 1, but there are also other possible symbols. Evolution usually starts from a group of randomly formed individuals, an iterative process in which the population in each iteration is called a generation. In each generation, the fitness of each member of the population is assessed; usually, fitness is the objective function value in the improvement problem being solved. The fittest individuals are randomly selected from the current population, and each individual's genome is modified to form a new generation. Then the new generation of candidate solutions is used in the next iteration of the algorithm. Generally, the algorithm ends when the maximum number of generations is produced, or a fitness level satisfactory for the population has been reached [28].

7.4.3.2 Proposed Solutions

Regarding the study presented by Park et al. [26], genetic algorithms (GA) were applied to improve the classification ability by reducing false positives and increasing sensitivity and selecting an optimal feature that is an important feature of classification by KNN among the 27 features. GA also selects the number of images (k) most similar to the reference database's test image. Specifically, before applying GA for optimization, a binary coding method is used to generate the genetic algorithms chromosomes. Each selected feature corresponds to a chromosome of one gene. Therefore, for 27 features, the genetic algorithm has 27 genes. A value of 1 means that the feature is selected and a value of 0 do not participate in the best feature set. Also, for choosing an optimal outcome, we search from 5 to a maximum of 31 in this study. Therefore, an additional five genes are included in the chromosome for the selection of the optimal neighbours. For example, if $k = 7$, the optimal neighbours' five gene values would have 00111.

As a result, the chromosome has a total of 32 genes. To find the optimal gene, the system's performance with k corresponding to the combination of selected genes at each step of the GA is compared, and the characteristics and k of the system with high performance are preserved.

7.4.3.3 Results

In this experiment, 100 gene-chromosomes were evaluated to find the optimal gene combination. It can be said that the genetic algorithm defined 100 new gene combinations with cross-over and mutation operations. After applying the GA to find the optimal set of input features for the KNN classifier, the system has 15 features (six pixel brightness-based features, seven shape-based features, two border-based characteristics). To find the optimal neighbours of KNN, up to 31 nodes were searched, and finally, seven nodes were determined. Based on this, the system showed a performance of AUC = 0.918 ± 0.048 (p = 0.003).

7.4.4 Ant Community Optimization

In 1997, the ant system was first applied to the travelling salesman problem by Dorigo and Gambardella [29]. The following year, the same researchers modified the system to improve its performance and its application to other optimization problems [30]. The basic principle is that the ants, called agents, secrete pheromones in each path while they are moving toward their destination. The ants that pass by then use the heuristic search to select the next path using the pheromone information accumulated in the path (Figure 7.4). In other words, an algorithm suitable for probabilistic combinatorial optimization applied the habit of learning how real ants would be at home while feeding.

7.4.4.1 Analysis of Previous Methods

In Lee et al. [31], researchers applied an ant population optimization algorithm to the regionalization algorithm using brain MR images learning. The medical image segmentation method can search for similar pixels after pre-learning the pixels to be segmented in the image like the habit of remembering the way the ants are searching for food. Ants that find similar pixels accumulate pheromone in the pixel, affecting when the passing ants choose the next path. Then, at each iteration step, the image's position is changed according to the state transition rule to arrive at the final destination. Finally, the divided result is obtained through the analysis of the pheromone distribution.

7.4.4.2 Proposed Solutions

Ant colony optimization algorithm (ACO) was used to automatically and accurately separate white matter, and grey matter in a brain MRI for application to a computer-assisted diagnostic system for analysing brain volume change rate in the presence of brain disease. In MRI, the grey scale is directly related to the signal intensity. The high signal intensity structure appears bright, and the medium signal intensity and low signal intensity are grey and black. Thus, on T1-weighted images of brain MRI, brain tissue has moderate signal intensity. The cerebrospinal fluid appears black,

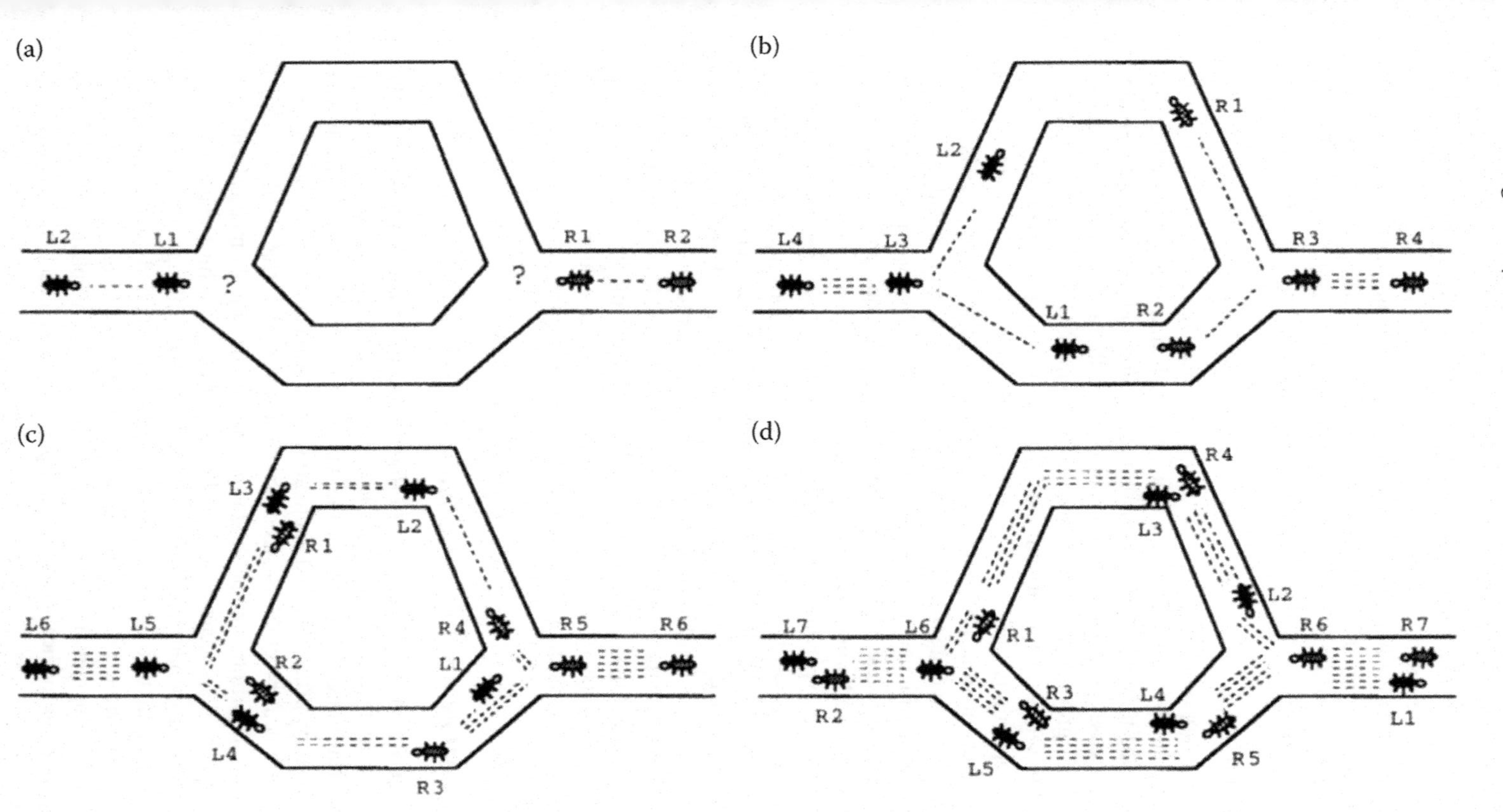

FIGURE 7.4 How ants can be the shorter path. (a) Ants reach the decision point. (b) Some ants select the lower path and some upper path. The option is random. (c) Because ants move at a roughly constant speed, the ants that determine the lower and shorter path reach the opposite resolution faster than those that choose the top and long path. (d) Pheromone accumulates at a higher rate on the shorter path. The number of intermittent lines approximates the number of pheromones deposited by ants.

and the brain parenchyma, such as fat, white matter and grey matter, appears relatively white. T2-weighted images are globally dark, but the cerebrospinal fluid distributed throughout the brain is relatively bright, and the brain parenchyma, such as white matter and grey matter, appears relatively dark. The database used for segmentation consisted of 20 MR images of 20 normal T1 and T2 images, 10 T1 and T2 images with brain disease, and 20 MR images.

7.4.4.3 Results

The results after applying the ant colony optimization algorithm are as follows. First, we set the number of iterations by focusing on obtaining the optimal threshold value. Suppose the number of repetitions is too low for both T1- and T2-weighted images. In that case, it is possible to confirm that the anatomical structures of white matter and grey matter are not correctly segmented. That white matter is more accurately segmented as the number of iterations increases. However, when the number of repetitions increases infinitely, the overtraining is performed, and the result is over-segmentation. Therefore, the maximum repetition frequency is limited to 200. In the AN algorithm system, each region of the anatomical structure's brightness to be partitioned was compared with the conventional various partitioning techniques by searching for the amount of pheromone and the number of repetitions accumulated when the ants moved.

As a comparative experiment, it was compared with Otsu, genetic algorithm, fuzzy method, etc. It was found that applying the ant colony optimization algorithm more accurately divides the structural part of white matter (see Figure 7.4 T1-weighted image and T2-weighted image). Also, Otsu and genetic algorithm results showed that the inside of the grey matter was hardly divided. In contrast, the result of using the fuzzy method showed that the inside of the grey matter was removed much (Figure 7.5). Therefore, in the result of the comparison experiment, the method using the ant colony optimization algorithm obtained more accurate division results than the basic methods and showed the performance of AUC = 0.9378.

7.5 DISCUSSION AND CONCLUSIONS

Medical images are an essential means of diagnosing a set of diseases and treating patients in modern medicine. Machine learning has played an essential role in automatic medical images analysis for the past decade. In this chapter, we briefly reviewed the history, principles, and applications of various medical images used as useful tools in clinical practice. Besides, we reviewed studies that used traditional machine learning algorithms in enabling efficiency in the field of medical imaging. As well, we discuss the successes and challenges of each machine learning model and offer some experimental approaches to address these challenges. We confirmed that machine learning techniques could be effectively applied to the automatic analysis of various medical images. Medical image analysis using machine learning can be a steady development because it can reduce the work of physicians who read and decode images in medical activities and play a role as a second reader to help detect lesions.

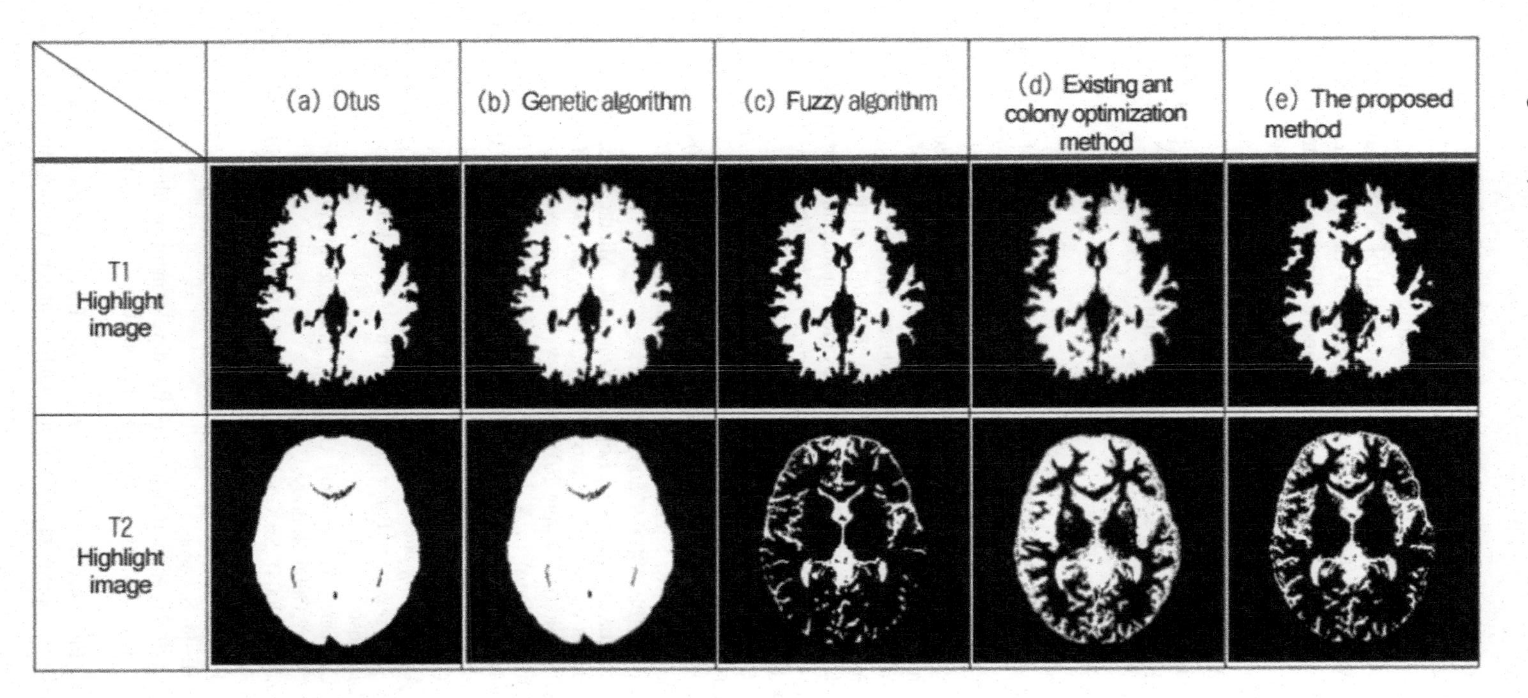

FIGURE 7.5 The proposed method and the division result of the existing method.

Google Scholar's database was used during December 2020. The following keyword has used for the search: "machine learning for medical image analysis". The initial search resulted in 130 documents (articles and books). Of these, only four articles were selected for analysis. The research of Park et al. [5,19,26] and Lee et al. [31] was identified as the main references of the area. It is important to note that none of the four works refers to more than two related papers. Also, no other articles with similar objectives were found, given the scientific foundations analyzed, which include "machine learning for medical image analysis". These facts demonstrate the relevance of this research to the environment analyzed, dealing with a significant problem recognized in one of the most popular applications in the medical field and standardizing its main references.

REFERENCES

[1] Rana, A. K., Salau, A., Gupta, S., & Arora, S. (2018). A survey of machine learning methods for IoT and their future applications. *Amity Journal of Computational Sciences*, *2*(2), 1–5.

[2] Alpaydin, E. (2014). Introduction to Machine Learning. Second Edition, MIT Press.

[3] Paramesha, K., Gururaj, H., & Jena, O. P. (2021). Applications of machine learning in biomedical text processing and food industry. *Machine Learning for Healthcare Applications*, 151–167. doi: 10.1002/9781119792611.ch10

[4] Pattnayak, P., & Jena, O. P. (2021). Innovation on machine learning in healthcare services—An introduction. *Machine Learning for Healthcare Applications*, 1–14. doi: 10.1002/9781119792611.ch1

[5] Park, S. C., Pu, J., & Zheng, B. (2009). Improving performance of computer-aided detection scheme by combining results from two machine learning classifiers. *Academic Radiology*, *16*(3), 266–274. doi: 10.1016/j.acra.2008.08.012

[6] Novelline, R. A., & Squire, L. F. (2005). *Squire's Fundamentals of Radiology*. La Editorial, UPR. ISBN 9780674057951.

[7] Kamińska, M., Ciszewski, T., Łopacka-Szatan, K., Miotła, P., & Starosławska, E. (2015). Breast cancer risk factors. *Przeglad menopauzalny = Menopause Review*, *14*(3), 196. doi: 10.5114/pm.2015.54346

[8] Panigrahi, N., Ayus, I., & Jena, O. P. (2021). An expert system-based clinical decision support system for Hepatitis-B prediction & diagnosis. *Machine Learning for Healthcare Applications*, 57–75. doi: 10.1002/9781119792611.ch4

[9] Park, S. C., Zheng, B., Wang, X.-H., & Gur, D. (2008). *Applying a 2D based CAD scheme for detecting micro-calcification clusters using digital breast tomosynthesis images: An assessment.* Paper presented at the Medical Imaging 2008: Computer-Aided Diagnosis.

[10] Kak, A. C., Slaney, M., & Wang, G. (2002). *Principles of Computerized Tomographic Imaging*. Wiley Online Library.

[11] Richmond, C. (2004). Sir Godfrey Hounsfield. *British Medical Journal Publishing Group*.

[12] Broder, J. S. (2011). *Diagnostic Imaging for the Emergency Physician E-Book*. Elsevier Health Sciences.

[13] Woo, J. (2002). A short history of the development of ultrasound in obstetrics and gynecology. *See* http://www. ob-ultrasound. net/history1. html (last checked 14 May 2011).

[14] Ikedo, Y., Fukuoka, D., Hara, T., Fujita, H., Takada, E., Endo, T., & Morita, T. (2007). Development of a fully automatic scheme for detection of masses in

whole breast ultrasound images. *Medical Physics*, *34*(11), 4378–4388. doi: 10.1118/1.2795825
[15] Filler, A. (2009). The history, development and impact of computed imaging in neurological diagnosis and neurosurgery: CT, MRI, and DTI. *Nature Precedings*, *7*(1), 1–85. doi: 10.1038/npre.2009.3267.2
[16] Donya, M., Radford, M., ElGuindy, A., Firmin, D., & Yacoub, M. H. (2015). Radiation in medicine: Origins, risks and aspirations. *Global Cardiology Science and Practice*, *2014*(4), 57. doi: 10.5339/gcsp.2014.57
[17] Verger, A., & Langen, K.-J. (2017). *PET Imaging in Glioblastoma: Use in Clinical Practice* (pp. 155–174). Exon Publications. doi: 10.15586/codon.glioblastoma.2017.ch9
[18] Guan, H., Kubota, T., Huang, X., Zhou, X. S., & Turk, M. (2006). Automatic hot spot detection and segmentation in whole body FDG-PET images. *2006 International Conference on Image Processing*, 85–88. 10.1109/ICIP.2006.312368
[19] Park, S. C., Tan, J., Wang, X., Lederman, D., Leader, J. K., Kim, S. H., & Zheng, B. (2011). Computer-aided detection of early interstitial lung diseases using low-dose CT images. *Physics in Medicine & Biology*, *56*(4), 1139. doi: 10.1088/0031-9155/56/4/016
[20] Bishop, C. M. (1994). Neural networks and their applications. *Review of Scientific Instruments*, *65*(6), 1803–1832. doi: 10.1063/1.1144830
[21] Lei, Y. (2017). Individual intelligent method-based fault diagnosis. *Intelligent Fault Diagnosis and Remaining Useful Life Prediction of Rotating Machinery* (pp. 67–174). Butterworth-Heinemann.
[22] Kumar, S., Bhusan, B., Singh, D., & Kumar Choubey, D. (2020). *Classification of Diabetes using Deep Learning*. Paper presented at the 2020 International Conference on Communication and Signal Processing (ICCSP).
[23] Kutyłowska, M. (2018). K-nearest neighbours method as a tool for failure rate prediction. *Periodica Polytechnica Civil Engineering*, *62*(2), 318–322. doi: 10.3311/PPci.10045
[24] Zheng, B., Chang, Y.-H., & Gur, D. (1995). Computerized detection of masses in digitized mammograms using single-image segmentation and a multilayer topographic feature analysis. *Academic Radiology*, *2*(11), 959–966. doi: 10.1016/S1076-6332(05)80696-8
[25] Budnik, I., & Brill, A. (2018). Immune factors in deep vein thrombosis initiation. *Trends in Immunology*, *39*(8), 610–623. doi: 10.1016/j.it.2018.04.010
[26] Park, S. C., Chapman, B. E., & Zheng, B. (2010). A multistage approach to improve performance of computer-aided detection of pulmonary embolisms depicted on CT images: Preliminary investigation. *IEEE Transactions on Biomedical Engineering*, *58*(6), 1519–1527. doi: 10.1109/TBME.2010.2063702
[27] Mitchell, M. (1998). *An Introduction to Genetic Algorithms*. MIT Press, Cambridge, MA, United States.
[28] Whitley, D. (1994). A genetic algorithm tutorial. *Statistics and Computing*, *4*(2), 65–85. doi: 10.1007/BF00175354
[29] Dorigo, M., & Gambardella, L. M. (1997). Ant colony system: a cooperative learning approach to the traveling salesman problem. *IEEE Transactions on Evolutionary Computation*, *1*(1), 53–66.
[30] Islam, T., Islam, M. E., & Ruhin, M. R. (2018). An analysis of foraging and echolocation behavior of swarm intelligence algorithms in optimization: ACO, BCO and BA. *International Journal of Intelligence Science*, *8*(01), 1. doi: 10.4236/ijis.2018.81001
[31] Lee, M.-E., Kim, S.-H., & Lim, J.-S. (2009). Region segmentation from MR brain image using an ant colony optimization algorithm. *The KIPS Transactions: Part B*, *16*(3), 195–202.

8 Impact of Ensemble-Based Models on Cancer Classification, Its Development, and Challenges

Barnali Sahu
Department of Computer Science and Engineering, Siksha 'O' Anusandhan University, Bhubaneswar, Odisha, India

Sitarashmi Sahu
Foundation for Technology and Business Incubation (FTBI), National Institute of Technology, Rourkela, Odisha, India

Om Prakash Jena
Department of Computer Science, Ravenshaw University, Cuttack, Odisha, India

CONTENTS

DOI: 10.1201/9781003189053-8

8.1 INTRODUCTION

The automated detection of diseases with a high accuracy rate is one of the most significant complications of health informatics. The word "cancer" refers to a group of diseases marked by irregular cell growth. Machine learning algorithms are widely used for the automatic detection of illnesses. Cancer is one of the most common diseases among humans and the leading cause of death worldwide. As a result, developing an efficient classifier for automatic cancer diagnosis is critical in order to improve the chances of early detection and more successful treatment. If the data label is skewed or the selected model is over-fitted with the corresponding data, the model will not show the proper output. Ensemble techniques are a form of machine learning technology that has emerged as a solution to these problems. It improves predictive accuracy by combining multiple learning algorithms. It's a promising area for improving base classifier efficiency.

These are supervised learning models that combine biomolecular and clinical data with computational functions. Every single model can be outperformed by committee approaches [1]. The concept also creates a predictive mechanism that combines two or more models and can improve bleak forecasts [2]. Accuracy and diversity are two important factors to consider when building a classifier ensemble. When creating an efficient ensemble, it is important to use as many different types of classifiers as possible. Ensembles normally produce better results when the models are more diverse [3]. It is a type of machine learning in which several models are trained to solve the same problem and then combined to improve performance. The basic concept is that by correctly combining weak models, more stable and/or robust models can be generated. When dealing with classification or regression in machine learning, the model we select is crucial. Several factors in the issue influence this decision, including the amount of data, the dimensionality of the space, and the distribution hypotheses. Low bias and low variance are the two most significant criteria for a model, and they often vary in opposite directions. We need enough degrees of freedom in our model to solve the underlying data uncertainty, but not too many to avoid high variance and increase accuracy. The definitions of bias and variation are well known to be mutually contradictory. In an ensemble learning system, weak learners (also known as base models) are models that can be combined to create more complex models. Most of the time, these simple models do not perform well on their own, either because they are biased or because there is too much variation for them to be accurate. By combining a large number of weak learners into a strong learner (or ensemble model) that performs better, ensemble methods seek to reduce the bias and/or variance of such weak learners. Stacking, sequential ensemble learning (boosting), and parallel ensemble learning (bagging) are the three types of ensemble learning. Other ensemble classifiers, such as Bayesian optimal classifier [4], Bayesian model average [5], Bayesian model combination [6], and bucket of models [7], rotation forest [8] has demonstrated superior performance when compared to state-of-the-art ensemble models.

In this paper, we propose a stack-based ensemble model for cancer microarray data classification that uses majority voting as the combination scheme. The model has used five state-of-the-art classifiers that are trained with a different subset of data. The models are trained with several relevant feature subsets selected by the MRMR feature selection technique. The proposed model results are compared with random forest, bagging, and boosting methods. Consistently, all of the classifiers are subjected to a tenfold cross-validation procedure, and it has been demonstrated that the proposed ensemble model outperforms stand-alone classifiers and state-of-the-art ensemble models.

The following is a breakdown of the chapter's structure. Section 8.2 discusses the different types of ensemble models and how they are used in cancer classification, Section 8.3 describes the proposed stacking model for cancer microarray data classification, Section 8.4 discusses the findings and discussion, and Section 8.5 concludes with some final thoughts.

8.2 TYPES OF ENSEMBLES AND THEIR APPLICATION ON CANCER CLASSIFICATION

Stacking, sequential ensemble learning (boosting), and parallel ensemble learning (bagging) are the three types of ensemble learning. Stacking is a form of ensemble learning in which various classifications or regression models are combined using a meta-classifier or a meta-regressor. After the base level models have been trained on a complete training set, the outputs of the base level model-like features are used to train the meta-model. The primary goal of stacking is to boost the committee's forecasts. Sequential ensemble, such as adaptive boosting, produces base learners in sequential order (AdaBoost). The dependency between base learners is promoted by the sequential generation of base learners. The model's efficiency is then enhanced by giving previously misrepresented learners higher weights. In parallel ensemble techniques, such as random forest, the base learners are created in a parallel format. The parallel generation of base learners is used in parallel methods to promote base learner independence. The independence of base learners decreases the error caused by the application of averages substantially. Bagging stands for 'bootstrap aggregation,' and it's a method for lowering the level of uncertainty in a prediction model. Bagging is a parallel strategy that caters to various, distinct learners while allowing them to be trained at the same time. Boosting is a sequential ensemble approach that changes the weight of observations based on the previous classification iteratively. If an observation is incorrectly classified, it increases the weight of that observation. In layman's words, boosting refers to algorithms that turn a weak learner into a stronger one. It reduces bias error and creates robust predictive models. To minimize bias, sequential ensemble models (boosting) are used, and parallel ensemble (bagging) learning is used to reduce variance.

A large amount of data related to cancer has been developed as a result of recent advances in high-throughput technologies (HTTs). The most recent predictive machines, according to the previous study, integrate a wide range of data types and databases, with genetic, medical, histological, image, socioeconomic, epidemiologic, and proteomic data [9]. Bagging and boosting are two of the most important advances in the area of ensemble learning [2,10,11]. Ensemble learning is a well-established principle [2,10,11], which were created in the 1990s, when the most commonly used ensemble methods were bagging and boosting [12]. When researching bagging methods in 1996, Breiman found that this technique would yield better precision when the basic base classifiers were inaccurate. The breast cancer data set was bagged using nearest neighbor classifiers in the same year [13,14]. The use of several ensemble approaches to analyze biomolecular, biological, and biomedical data is becoming more common. Sajid et al. [15] compares the output of six common EL methods, including bagging, Ada Boost, dagging, decorate, multi-boost, and random subspace, using 14 base learners, including Bayes Net, FURIA, K-nearest neighbors (KNN), C4.5, RIPPER, Kernel logistic regression (KLR), K-star, logistic regression (LR), multilayer perceptron (MLP), Naïve-Bayes (NB), random forest, simple cart (SC), support vector machine (SVM), and LMT for automatic detection of cancer. The experiential results show that EL can increase base learners' predictive output in the medical domain. Sheau-Ling Hsieh et al. [16] list the breast cancer medical diagnostic results. For feature selection, information gain has been reformed. For classifications, neural fuzzy (NF), K-nearest neighbor (KNN), and quadratic classifier (QC) models, as well as related ensemble models, have been established. Furthermore, a mixed ensemble model involving these three organizations was developed for additional validations. Ensemble learning outperforms individual learning, according to the findings of the experiments. Furthermore, of all models, the integrated ensemble model has the maximum precision for breast cancer.

For lung abnormality classification from chest X-rays, Liveris et al. [17] proposed a new ensemble learning model with a semi-supervised learning algorithm. The proposed algorithm makes use of a new weighted voting scheme that gives each ensemble component learner a vector of weights based on its precision on individual class. The proposed ensemble model was thoroughly tested on three well-known real-life standards: the Guangzhou Women and Children's Medical Center's Pneumonia Chest X-rays data set, Shenzhen Hospital's Tuberculosis data set, and the CT medical images of cancer data set. The proposed ensemble technique outperformed simple voting strategies and other conventional semi-supervised approaches in the numerical experiments presented. To minimise cancer patient heterogeneity within each subtype, Yi-Cheng Gao et al. [18] used a clustering algorithm to separate patients into various subtypes. Some members of the network have the ability to impact cancer patient prognosis, and all societies dealing with prognosis have the ability to fully expose cancer patient prognosis. They used an ensemble classifier built on the gene co-expression network of the particular subtype to predict the prognosis of cancer patients of individual subtypes. Three subtypes of ovarian cancer were discovered using gene expression data from patients in The Cancer Genome Atlas (TCGA). Patients in different subtypes have different mortality risks, according to a survival study. For each subtype, three ensemble classifiers were developed. The proposed method outperformed control and literature approaches in leave-one-out and independent validation studies. Table 8.1 shows the use of state-of-the-art ensemble models for cancer data classification.

Deep learning approaches for cancer classification, such as skin cancer, diabetes, and several IoT/ML base models for smart healthcare have recently evolved and are producing better results [29–35].

TABLE 8.1
Stacking, Sequential Ensemble Models, Parallel Ensemble Models Used for Cancer Data Classification

Method	Paper	Classifiers Used	Validation Technique Used	Dataset Used	Findings
Stacking	[19]	Deep neural network, gradient boosted model, distributed random forest, a generalized linear model	5-fold	Breast Cancer	For both sets of breast cancer results, using the GBM as a meta-learner resulted in higher accuracy, and using the GLM as a meta-learner resulted in a low root-mean-squared error.
	[20]	The base classifiers are Naïve-Bayes (NB), C4.5 decision tree (DT), and SVM, while SVM is used as a meta-classifier.	10-fold	Breast Cancer	The overall best performance was achieved by a stack ensemble model that used the NB and SVM as base classifiers and the DT as a meta-classifier.
	[21]	Random forest (RF), random tree (RT), sequential minimal optimization (SMO), and logistic regression (LR)	–	miRNA	In the second stage of the proposed model, the output improves due to the stack-based ensemble process.
	[22]	Decision tree, Naïve-Bayes, and neural network	10-fold cross-validation	Breast cancer data	combining all three algorithms using the stacking approach is the best approach for predicting breast cancer.
	[23]	Six deep learning models are used as level-0 learner models or sub-models in SGE, and logistic regression is used as a level-one learner or meta-learner model.	–	Histopathological breast cancer images	In terms of accuracy, precision, recall, and F1 calculation, the results show that the proposed methodology performed exponentially well in image classification.
Sequential Ensemble	[24]	XGBoost	5-fold	Multi-omics data	The results of this study also revealed that DNA methylation outperforms other molecular data (mRNA expression and miRNA expression) in terms of accuracy and stability for discriminating between early-stage and late-stage groups.

(*Continued*)

TABLE 8.1 (Continued)
Stacking, Sequential Ensemble Models, Parallel Ensemble Models Used for Cancer Data Classification

Method	Paper	Classifiers Used	Validation Technique Used	Dataset Used	Findings
	[25]	The RBF neural network and the ensemble boosting learning classifier are combined in the hybrid module.	10-fold	Diagnostic breast cancer (WDBC), breast cancer original (WBC), breast cancer, prognostic (BCP), and breast cancer diagnosis data sets from Wisconsin (BCD)	The general diagnosis accuracy for the WBC, BCD, BCP, and WBCD UCI data sets was 97.4 percent, 98.4 percent, 97.7 percent, and 97.0 percent, respectively, based on 10-fold cross-validation using the RBFNN process.
	[26]	Gradient boosting machine	–	Breast image data	The application section demonstrated that the GBM algorithm outperformed the other ones. The GBM algorithm had higher precision, accuracy, and sensitivity than the other algorithms.
Parallel Ensemble	[27]	Bagging, boosting, and random forest	10-fold	Breast cancer, lung cancer, lymphoma, leukemia, colon cancer, ovarian cancer, and prostate cancer	AdaBoostC4.5 is the only one among the all compared classification algorithms that outperform C4.5. Comparing between ensemble methods, Random Forests and AdaBoost C4.5 outperform Bagging C4.5 significantly
	[28]	Bag boosting	50 ransom partition	SRBCT, Brain A, leukemia, colon, prostate, lymphoma	The misclassification error of simple boosting and bagging is continuously reduced by using bag boosting.

8.3 MATERIAL AND METHODS

As the microarray data contain numerous amounts of genetic information but a smaller number of samples, applying the machine learning methods to the microarray data will suffer from one main issue known as the small sample size issue. The microarray data is very hard to tackle but the perfect interpretation of the data is the key concept behind the good diagnosis result. To avoid this issue, the researchers have found the solution as the dimensionality reduction employing which the high dimensional data can be resolved to a considerable dimension. In this result, we have applied the maximum relevance minimum redundancy feature selection method. The reduced data sets are used for training the classifiers such as support vector machines, decision tree, Naïve-Bayes, neural network, logistic regression, and K-nearest neighbor classifier.

8.3.1 Data Set Description

The gene expression data set is collected from the site [36]. The data set description is given in Table 8.2. All the collected data considered for classification are of a binary class. All of the data sets have thousands of properties, while the samples are in the tens and hundreds.

8.3.2 Maximum Relevance Minimum Redundancy (MRMR)

In practice, at each iteration i, a score is computed for each feature to be evaluated (f) in Equation (8.1):

$$score_i(f) = \frac{F(f, target)}{\sum_{s \in features\ selected\ until\ i-1} corr(f, s)|/(i-1)} \tag{8.1}$$

where i is the iteration number, f is the function being assessed, F is the F-statistic, and corr is the Pearson correlation. It's worth noting that the correlation is calculated in absolute value. Whether two features correlate as 0.9 or –0.9 makes no difference: they are highly redundant in both cases.

TABLE 8.2
Data Set Description

Data Set	#Attributes	#Samples	#Class
Lung Cancer	1,628	182	2
Brain Cancer	1,072	29	2
Prostate Cancer	3,406	102	2
Colon Cancer	2,001	62	2

8.3.3 Support Vector Machine

It's a supervised machine learning algorithm that aims to locate a hyperplane in a multidimensional space. The SVM's goal is to find the best hyperplane so that the two groups can be segregated. This ideal hyperplane divides the two groups while also increasing the margin between them. The distance between the hyperplane and the SVs is known as the margin. It is widely used because of its primary benefit, which is that it can be very efficient even in high-dimensional spaces. However, the key flaw in this method is that it does not have probabilistic estimations. High precision can be achieved by fine-tuning hyperparameters such as gamma, coat, and kernel level, but in practice, defining the exact hyperparameters can be difficult, which directly enhances the computational cost and overhead.

The hyperplane optimization can be obtained by Equation (8.2):

$$\text{Minimize } \frac{1}{2}\|w_{(v)}\|^2, \quad \text{where } \|w_{(v)}\|^2 = w_{(v)}^T x \tag{8.2}$$

$$\text{Subject to } y_j(w_{(v)}^T x_j + \mathrm{b}) \geq 1 \text{ where j} = 0, 1$$

$$\Rightarrow 1 - y_j(w_{(v)}^T x_j + \mathrm{b}) \leq 0 \text{ where j} = 1, 2, \ldots$$

The Lagrangian optimization problem is defined in Equation (8.3):

$$\tau = \frac{1}{2}\|w_{(v)}\|^2 + \sum_{j=1}^{n} \alpha_j(1 - y_j(w_{(v)}^T x_j + \mathrm{b})) \tag{8.3}$$

The first derivative of the above equation is taken with respect to $w_{(v)}$ and b, and then we have the following Equation (8.4):

$$w_{(v)} + \sum_{j=1}^{n} \alpha_{\mathrm{j}}(-\mathrm{y_j})\mathrm{x_j} = 0 \tag{8.4}$$

$$\Rightarrow w_{(v)} = \sum_{j=1}^{n} \alpha_{\mathrm{j}}\mathrm{y_j}\mathrm{x_j}$$

$$\Rightarrow \sum_{j=1}^{n} \alpha_{\mathrm{j}}\mathrm{y_j} = 0 \text{ where } \alpha_{\mathrm{j}} \geq 0$$

For the non-linear classification problem, we introduce another dimension to create a bigger dimensional space. Here, ξ_j is introduced to represent the approximated misclassified data samples. So, the classification model is represented as in Equation (8.5):

$$f(x) = \frac{1}{2} w_{(v)}^T w_{(v)} + c\sum_{j=1}^{n} \xi_j \tag{8.5}$$

subject to $y_j(w_{(v)}^T x_j + \mathrm{b}) \geq 1$ Where j = 1, 2, … and $\xi_j \geq 1$

where c represents the trade-off between the margin and training error and c is a constant. We have to minimize the $f(x)$ for a better-optimized hyperplane.

8.3.4 Decision Tree

The decision tree attempts to construct a rule based on classification given a collection of attributes. In a decision tree, the process usually begins with a root and progresses through the data attributes based on the knowledge gain ranking. The root node, test node, and decision node are the three types of nodes found in the decision tree (DT). A DT is being constructed by using some classifiers such as ID3, CART, CHAID, etc., which generally defines a tree automatically. But the main objective of the classification algorithm is to construct an optimized decision tree for the given data set. It makes the utilization of different algorithms to decide whether one node can be divided into two more sub-nodes. The main advantage of a DT is that it requires very little data preprocessing before implementation and is also able to handle both numerical and categorical data. But overfitting is the main disadvantage of this classification technique.

Training set $W = w_1, \ w_2, \ldots \ldots .., w_n$.
With responses $S = s_1, \ s_2, \ldots \ldots \ldots, s_n$.
Bagging repeatedly "E" times.
For $e = 1, 2, \ldots \ldots E$.

The prediction for unseen samples y′, by averaging the prediction from all individual regression tree on y′ as Equation (8.6):

$$\hat{f} = \frac{1}{E} \sum_{e=1}^{E} f_e(y') \tag{8.6}$$

To find out the uncertainty of the prediction using Equation (8.7):

$$\sigma = \frac{\sqrt{\sum_{e=1}^{E} (f_e(y') - \hat{f})^2}}{E - 1} \tag{8.7}$$

8.3.5 Naïve-Bayes

Naïve-Bayes (NB) classification algorithm works on the basis of Bayes' conditional probability theorem. In this, probability means the degree of belief. The conditional probability is being used to classify the data. The most important part of this algorithm is that it works with the assumption that all of the attributes are independent of each other. There are three different kinds of NB-based algorithms present as the Gaussian NB, multinomial NB, and Bernoulli NB. The main advantage present behind this classification is that it requires a very small amount of training data for estimating the conditional parameters but the estimation time depends upon the data set size. If the dimension of the data set is very high, then the NB will be acting as a bad estimator as the estimation time and cost increases concerning the data set.

For each class of (positive, negative)
For each word in (phrase)

$$P(W|C) < num(W|C) \mid num(Class) + num_{total} \tag{8.8}$$

$$P(C) = P(C) * P(W|C) \tag{8.9}$$

Return max {P (+ve), P (−ve)}

$$P(G|S) = \frac{P\ (S|G)\ *\ P(G)}{P(S)} \tag{8.10}$$

$$P\ (G|S)\ = P\ (S_1|G)\ *\ P\ (S_2|G)\ *\ P(S_3|G) \ldots\ldots\ldots *\ P(S_N|G)\ *\ P(G) \tag{8.11}$$

$P\ (G|S)$ –> Posterior probability of class (d, target) given predictor (y, attribute). Defined in Equation (8.10) and (8.11):

$P\ (G)$ –> Class of prior probability

$P\ (S|G)$ –> Likelihood

$P(S)$ –> Predictor as the prior probability

$P(C)$ –> Class probability is defined as Equation (8.9).

8.3.6 Neural Network

The learning interaction that occurs in the human brain inspires neural networks. They have a forgery feature that allows the computer to learn and calibrate itself by investigating new data. Every parameter, also known as a neuron, is a function that generates an output after receiving one or more sources of information. These outputs are then passed on to the next layer of neurons, which incorporate them into their functions and generate additional output. These yields are then passed on to the next layer of neurons, and so on until all of the layers of neurons have been considered and the terminal neurons have received their corresponding output. At that point, the model's result is determined by the terminal neurons.

8.3.7 Logistic Regression

Logistic regression is the regression model that can be used to predict the probability of a given data. Its working depends upon the well-defined model known as the logistic function and also known as the sigmoid function. In this model, the probabilities define the possible outcomes of a single trial tuned by the sigmoid function. The main advantage of this classification model is that it can be easily implemented on independent variables defined in Equation (8.12):

$$F(A) = \frac{1}{1 + e^{-A}} \tag{8.12}$$

$m_{i,j}$ –> Feature vector of length 'N'.

$$j = 1, \ldots\ldots\ldots, N.$$

$$i = 1, \ldots\ldots\ldots, h.$$

$$M = \begin{bmatrix} m_{11}, m_{12}, \ldots m_{1N} \\ m_{21}, m_{22}, \ldots m_{2N} \\ \cdot \\ m_{h1}, m_{h2}, \ldots m_{hN} \end{bmatrix}_{h*N} \tag{8.13}$$

$$R = \begin{bmatrix} r_1 \\ r_2 \\ \cdot \\ \cdot \\ r_h \end{bmatrix} \tag{8.14}$$

$$P(R|M) = \frac{1}{1 + e^{-f(m)}} \text{ (posterior)} \tag{8.15}$$

The posterior is defined as Equation (8.15), where M and R are calculated, applying Equations (8.13) and (8.14).

f(m) Is feature (m_j) is defined in Equations (8.16) and (8.17).

$$f(m) = m_0 + m_1\beta_1 + \ldots\ldots\ldots + m_N\beta_N + \epsilon \tag{8.16}$$

$$m,\ \beta,\ f(m) \in P^N$$

$$\log\left[\frac{P(R|M)}{1 - P(R|M)}\right] = m_0 + m_1\beta_1 + \ldots\ldots\ldots + m_N\beta_N + \epsilon = f(m) \tag{8.17}$$

Maximum likelihood estimation is defined as the following Equation (8.18):

$$argmax\text{: } \log\left\{ \prod_{i=1}^{h} P(R_i|M_i)\, R_i\, (1 - P(R_i|M_i)^{(i-R_i)} \right\} \tag{8.18}$$

8.3.8 KNN

Neighbors-based order is a form of languid learning in that it does not attempt to construct an overall inside model, instead of storing cases of preparation data. A simple part of each K closest neighbors is used to process grouping. The key benefits of this classification algorithm are that it is simple to use and that it is resistant to noise in the training data. The determination of the K value is one of the model's drawbacks, as an incorrect K value will result in poor results.

8.3.9 Proposed Stacking Ensemble Model

The gene expression data is subjected to a feature selection process using the MRMR method to extract the data set's most important features. Science MRMR is a ranking system for feature selection in which a subset of the top-ranked features is chosen, such as 5, 10, 20, 30, 40, and classifiers are trained individually using these relevant features. The stacking model uses the best five classifiers with high classification accuracy, which were trained on a dimensionally reduced data set with suitable features. The proposed structure for the stacking model employs SVM, kNN, NN, DT, and LR as base classifiers. The diversity is preserved in the proposed framework by using a different subset of features for each algorithm. For example, SVM, kNN, NN, LR, and DT are trained on data sets with 5, 10, 20, 30, and 40 features, respectively. Individual classifiers' predictions for class labels for samples in data sets are recorded, and the majority voting procedure is used to find the subsequent class labels for the examples in the data set, with the classification accuracy calculated by comparing the initial class labels of the samples in the data set. Since an odd number of classifiers is needed for majority voting, five classifiers out of six were chosen for model construction based on the performance. In practice, one attempts to integrate as many "diverse" classifiers as possible, hoping to maximize efficiency by using the complementary knowledge contained in the individual classifiers' outputs. Voting methods are based on an independent framework that integrates predictions from classification models that have been independently standardized using several empirical causes. The most simple and intuitive approach is the majority voting rule, which assigns a sample based on the most common class assignment, while the sample is not graded in the event of ties. A tenfold cross-validation technique is used to evaluate the accuracy of individual classifiers. The results of the individual classifiers for each class level are combined using the majority voting technique, and the resulting classification accuracy is determined using the model shown in Figure 8.1.

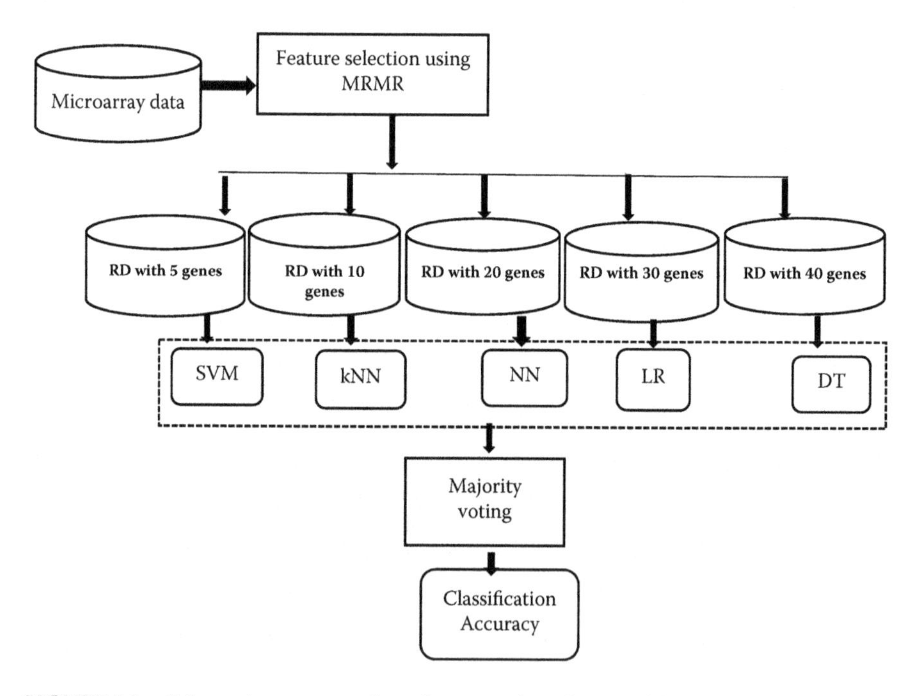

FIGURE 8.1 Schematic representation of proposed stack ensemble model.

ALGORITHM

Input: Microarray data
Output: Classification Accuracy

Step 1. Perform feature selection using MRMR
Step 2. Construct reduced data set RD_i with 5,10,20,30, and 40 features selected in step 2
Step 3. *for* $i = 1$ to 5

for $n = [10,15,25,29,40]$
do
Train Classifier *Ci* with n features
Validate *Ci* with 10-fold cross validation
Record the predicted class labels
end for

Step 4. Use majority voting to determine the class labels
Step 5. Compare the initial class labels with the measured class labels in step 4 to determine the resultant accuracy.

8.4 EXPERIMENTAL RESULTS AND DISCUSSION

The experiment is run on a device with an Intel Core i7 processor and Windows 10 operating system, using Python 3.9.4. This section contains a summary of the data set as well as the experimental findings.

8.4.1 Performance Measure

The following criteria are used to evaluate the classifiers: the accuracy, specificity, and sensitivity are defined in Equations (8.19), (8.20), and (8.21), respectively.

$$Accuracy = \frac{TP + TN}{TP + FP + FN + TN} \tag{8.19}$$

$$Specificity = \frac{TN}{TN + FP} \tag{8.20}$$

$$Sensitivity = \frac{TP}{TP + FN} \tag{8.21}$$

where TP = True Positive, TN = True Negative, FP = False Positive, FN = False Negative.

8.4.2 Results and Discussion

The data from the microarrays are initially normalized using the min-max process. The feature selection is then done using MRMR. Reduced training data sets are created with 5, 10, 20, 30, 40 features, and classification models SVM, KNN, NB, DT, NN, and LR are trained and validated using the tenfold cross-validation process. Table 8.4 shows the classification accuracy of the individual classifier with a different subset of data. The SVM classifier performs best of all in a lung cancer data set with 30 features. With 30 features, KNN outperforms all other models in the brain cancer data set. With 20 characteristics of prostate cancer data, ANN performs better. With 10 and 20 features of colon cancer data, the LR and DT classifiers perform better. Table 8.3 reveals that for the same data set, different classifiers have varying degrees of classification accuracy. We chose the five classifiers for building the stacking model because they display better results for different data sets.

TABLE 8.3
Classification Accuracy of Different Classifiers with 5, 10, 20, and 30 Features Selected by MRMR

Date Set	MRMR	Classification Accuracy with 5, 10, 20, and 30 Features					
	#selected Features	SVM	kNN	NB	DT	ANN	LR
Lung Cancer	5	0.978	0.978	0.977	0.972	0.95	0.955
	10	0.956	0.95	0.951	0.961	0.95	0.945
	20	0.972	0.961	0.962	0.956	0.95	0.934
	30	0.989	0.978	0.979	0.978	0.97	0.973
	40	0.953	0.951	0.95	0.96	0.95	0.963
Brain Cancer	5	0.883	0.82	0.791	0.881	0.905	0.883
	10	0.75	0.679	0.804	0.733	0.833	0.75
	20	0.929	0.893	0.895	0.928	0.938	0.929
	30	0.933	0.964	0.967	0.933	0.941	0.933
	40	0.925	0.923	0.93	0.93	0.936	0.936
Prostate Cancer	5	0.803	0.831	0.911	0.911	0.913	0.911
	10	0.847	0.848	0.764	0.764	0.769	0.765
	20	0.812	0.958	0.824	0.812	0.986	0.812
	30	0.797	0.808	0.901	0.901	0.902	0.901
	40	0.843	0.843	0.824	0.824	0.82	0.82
Colon Cancer	5	0.78	0.79	0.812	0.791	0.693	0.793
	10	0.791	0.839	0.854	0.783	0.854	0.93
	20	0.783	0.709	0.746	0.926	0.774	0.912
	30	0.826	0.774	0.961	0.742	0.87	0.823
	40	0.813	0.756	0.817	0.752	0.743	0.783

TABLE 8.4
Comparison of the Proposed Model to Other State-of-the-Art Ensemble Models in Terms of Performance

Data Set	Ensemble Model	AUC	CA	Specificity	Sensitivity
Lung Cancer	Adaboost	89.9	95.5	95.4	95.5
	Random forest	97.8	98.9	98.9	98.9
	Bagging	96.8	98.3	98.3	98.3
	Proposed stack model	98.6	98.9	98.8	98.9
Brain Cancer	Adaboost	85.7	85.7	85.7	85.7
	Random forest	88	89.2	89.2	89.4
	Bagging	91.8	85.7	85.7	85.7
	Proposed stack model	97.3	99.5	99.5	99.5
Prostate Cancer	Adaboost	79.3	79.4	79.3	79.6
	Random forest	92.3	92.1	92.1	92.1
	Bagging	93.3	85.3	85.3	85.7
	Proposed stack model	94.04	86.3	86.3	86.4
Colon Cancer	Adaboost	78.8	80.6	80.6	80.6
	Random forest	82.7	80.6	80.6	80.6
	Bagging	82	76.8	77.1	77.8
	Proposed stack model	90.1	82.3	82.3	82.8

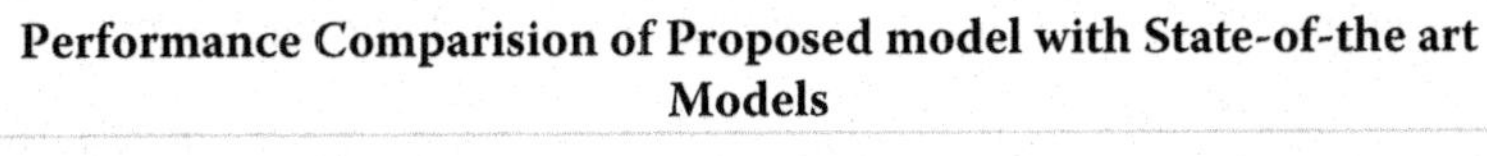

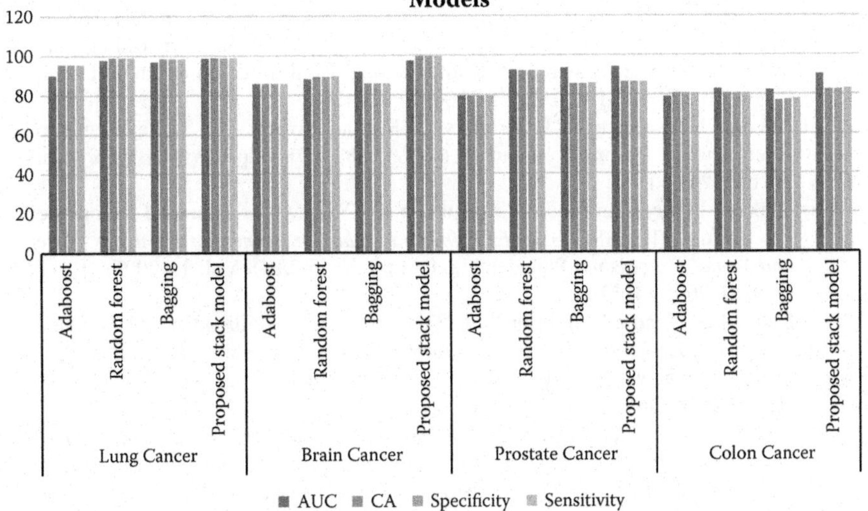

FIGURE 8.2 Study of the proposed model's accuracy in comparison to other ensemble models.

The individual classifier accuracies are combined using the majority voting combination technique, and the resulting classification accuracy is determined. The results of the proposed stacking model, as well as Adaboost, random forest, and bagging, are summarized in Table 8.4. In contrast to Adaboost, random forest, and bagging models, the proposed stacking model performs better for lung cancer, brain cancer, and colon cancer. In contrast to the proposed staking model, the random forest model performed better in the prostate cancer data. Figure 8.2 shows the comparison of performance with other ensemble model performance.

8.5 CONCLUSION

A stacking-based ensemble model for microarray cancer data classification is proposed in this chapter. The proposed model is unique in that it combines the outcomes of individual models using majority voting and incorporates several simple classifiers trained with different reduced data sets. The proposed stacking model is showing better results in comparison to other ensemble methods in the literature. The techniques presented in the current study may encourage similar types of ways to other software development efforts in clinical bioinformatics.

REFERENCES

[1] Baronti F., Micheli A., Passaro A., and Starita A. "Machine learning contribution to solve prognostic medical problems." *Outcome Predict Cancer* (2006): 261.

[2] Rokach L. "Ensemble-based classifiers." *Artificial Intelligence Review* 33, no. 1–2 (2010): 1–39.

[3] Kuncheva L. I., and Whitaker C. J. "Measures of diversity in classifier ensembles and their relationship with the ensemble accuracy." *Machine Learning* 51, no. 2 (2003): 181–207.

[4] 16. Dembczyński K., Cheng W., and Hüllermeier E. "Bayes Optimal Multilabel Classification via Probabilistic Classifier Chains." ICML'10: Proceedings of the 27th International Conference on International Conference on Machine Learning. Pages 279 286, (2010), 10.5555/3104322.3104359

[5] Hoeting J. A., Madigan D., Raftery A. E., and Volinsky C. T. Bayesian Model Averaging: A Tutorial: 14, no. 4 (1999): 382–401 https://www.jstor.org/stable/2676803?seq=1

[6] Sankar A. "Bayesian Model Combination (BAYCOM) for Improved Recognition." Proceedings. (ICASSP '05). *IEEE International Conference on Acoustics, Speech, and Signal Processing*. Philadelphia, PA, pp. I/845–I/848 Vol. 1, (2005), 10.1109/ICASSP.2005.1415246.

[7] Dadhich S., Sandin F. and Bodin U. "Predicting Bucket-Filling Control Actions of a Wheel-Loader Operator Using a Neural Network Ensemble." *International Joint Conference on Neural Networks (IJCNN), Rio de Janeiro*, pp. 1–6, (2018), 10.1109/IJCNN.2018.8489388.

[8] Rodríguez J. J., Kuncheva L., and Alonso C. J. "Rotation forest: A new classifier ensemble method." *IEEE Transactions on Pattern Analysis and Machine Intelligence*: 28, no. 10 (2006): 1619–1630: 10.1109/TPAMI.2006.211

[9] Kourou K., Exarchos T. P., Exarchos K. P., Karamouzis M. V., and Fotiadis D. I. "Machine learning applications in cancer prognosis and prediction." *Computational and Structural Biotechnology Journal* 13 (2015): 8–17.

[10] Polikar R. "Ensemble-based systems in decision making." *IEEE Circuits and Systems Magazine*. 6, no. 3 (2006): 21–45.
[11] Jacobs R. A., Jordan M. I., Nowlan S. J., and Hinton G. E. "Adaptive mixtures of local experts." *Neural Computation*. 3, no. 1 (1991): 79–87.
[12] Dietterich T. G. "Ensemble methods in machine learning." In *Multiple Classifier Systems. Springer*, Berlin, Heidelberg, pp. 1–15, (2000).
[13] Kalousis A., Prados J., and Hilario M. "Stability of feature selection algorithms: a study on high-dimensional spaces." *Journal of Knowledge and Information Systems* 12, no. 1 (2007): 95–116.
[14] Gordon G. J., Jenson R. V., Hsiao L. L., et al. "Translation of microarray data into clinically relevant cancer diagnostic tests using gene expression ratios in lung cancer and mesothelioma." *Journal of Cancer Research*: 62, no. 17 (2002): 4963–4967
[15] Nagi S., and Bhattacharyya D. K. "Classification of microarray cancer data using ensemble approach." *Netw Model Anal Health Inform Bioinformatics*: 2 (2013): 159–173
[16] Hsieh S.-L., Hsieh S.-H., Cheng P.-H., Chen C.-H., Hsu K.-Pi., Lee I-S., Wang Z., and Lai F. "Design ensemble machine learning model for breast cancer diagnosis." *Journal of Medical Systems* 36 (2012): 2841–2847
[17] Livieris, I. E., Kanavos, A., Tampakas, V., and Pintelas, P. "A weighted voting ensemble self-labeled algorithm for the detection of lung abnormalities from X-rays." *Algorithms* 12 (2019): 64.
[18] Gao Y.-C., Zhou X.-H., and Zhang W. "An ensemble strategy to predict prognosis in ovarian cancer based on gene modules." *Frontiers in Genetics*, 24 April 2019, (2019).
[19] Kwon H., Park J., and Lee Y. "Stacking ensemble technique for classifying breast cancer." *Healthcare Informatics Research*, Oct; 25, no. 4 (2019): 283–288.
[20] Adeyemi O. J., Adebayo V. O., Olaniyan O., Olusanya O. O., and Idowu P. A. "A stack ensemble model for the risk of breast cancer recurrence." *International Journal of Research Studies in Computer Science and Engineering (IJRSCSE)* 6, no. 3 (2019): 8–21.
[21] Saha S., Mitra S., and Kant Yadav R. "A stack-based ensemble framework for detecting cancer microRNA biomarkers." *Genomics, Proteomics & Bioinformatics*, 15, no. 6 (2017): 381–388.
[22] Rishika V., and Sowjanya M. "Prediction of breast cancer using stacking ensemble approach." *International Journal of Management, Technology, and Engineering*, volume IX, the issue I, (2019).
[23] Kumar D., and Batra U. "Classification of Invasive Ductal Carcinoma from histopathology breast cancer images using Stacked Generalized Ensemble." *Journal of Intelligent and Fuzzy Systems*, 40, no. 3, (2021): 4919–4934.
[24] Maa B., Menga F., Yana G., Yana H., Chaia B., and Song F. "Diagnostic classification of cancers using extreme gradient boosting algorithm and multi-omics data." *Computers in Biology and Medicine* 121, (2020): 103761
[25] Assiri, A. S., Nazir, S. and Velastin, S. A. "Breast tumor classification using an ensemble machine learning method." *Journal of Imaging*, 6, no. 6 (2020): 39.
[26] Imad Abed S. "Predicting breast cancer using gradient boosting machine." *International Journal of Science and Research (IJSR)* 8, no. 6 (2019): 885–891.
[27] Hu H., Li J., Plank A., Wang H., and Daggard G. "A Comparative Study of Classification Methods for Microarray Data Analysis." *Data Mining and Analytics 2006, Proceedings of the Fifth Australasian Data Mining Conference (AusDM2006)*, Sydney, NSW, Australia, 29–30, (2006).
[28] Dettling M. "BagBoosting for tumor classification with gene expression data." *Bioinformatics* 20, no. 18 (2004): 3583–3593.

[29] Khamparia A., Singh P. K., Rani P., Samanta D., Khanna A., and Bhushan B. "An internet of health things-driven deep learning framework for detection and classification of skin cancer using transfer learning." *Transactions on Emerging Telecommunications Technologies*. pp. 1–11, John Wiley & Sons, (2020).
[30] Sharma N., Bhushan B., Kaushik I., Gautam S., and Khamparia A. Applicability of WSN and Biometric Models in the Field of Healthcare, Chapter 16, pp. 304–329, (2020).
[31] Pattnayak P., and Jena O. P. "Innovation on Machine Learning in Healthcare Services-An Introduction", Chapter 1, *Machine Learning for Healthcare Applications*, pp. 1–14, (2021), Wiley Scrivener Publisher, Beverly.
[32] Jindal M., Gupta J., and Bhushan B. "Machine Learning Methods for IoT and their Future Applications." 2019 International Conference on Computing, Communication, and Intelligent Systems (ICCCIS), (2019).
[33] Kumar S., Bhusan B., Singh D., and Choubey D. K. "Classification of Diabetes using Deep Learning." 2020 International Conference on Communication and Signal Processing (ICCSP).
[34] Panigrahi N., Ayus I. and Jena O. P. "An Expert System-Based Clinical Decision Support System for Hepatitis-B Prediction and Diagnosis", Chapter 4, *Machine Learning for Healthcare Applications*, pp. 57–75, (2021), Wiley Scrivener Publisher, Beverly.
[35] Paramesha K., Gururaj H. L. and Jena O. P. "Applications of Machine Learning in Biomedical Text Processing and Food Industry", Chapter 10, *Machine Learning for Healthcare Applications*, pp. 151–167, (2021), Wiley Scrivener Publisher, Beverly.
[36] https://www.ncbi.nlm.nih.gov/geo/

9 Performance Comparison of Different Machine Learning Techniques towards Prevalence of Cardiovascular Diseases (CVDs)

Sachin Kamley
Department of Computer Applications, Samrat Ashok Technological Institute, Vidisha, Madhya Pradesh, India

CONTENTS

9.1 INTRODUCTION

In the human body, the heart is one of the main body organs and plays an important role in a human body like the brain; it circulates blood to each of the body parts. However, the circulating system is so important because it carries oxygen, blood, or other materials to the different organs of the body [1,2]. For the last couple of years, CVDs or heart

DOI: 10.1201/9781003189053-9

disease have become the most prominent problem in medical science, and the number of people suffering from this problem is increasing day by day. The well-known or common types of heart diseases are hypertensive heart disease, CVDs, pulmonary stenosis, heart murmurs, and heart failure, etc. [3,4]. Every year, approximately 17 million people died of CVDs, specifically strokes and heart attacks reported by the World Health Organization (WHO) [5]. In this way, identifying necessary symptoms and health habits contribute towards CVDs or create heart problems. Table 9.1 shows some of the most common symptoms or factors of heart disease.

There are various issues or symptoms associated with CVDs that make it very complicated to diagnose or detect at the right time (Table 9.1) [7,8]. Therefore, various tests are conducted before diagnosing CVDs i.e. ECG, fasting blood sugar level, blood pressure and cholesterol level, etc. These tests are not suitable for all of the patients because these tests are more time-consuming and expensive. On the

TABLE 9.1
Most Common Symptoms or Factors of Heart Diseases [6,7]

S. No.	Factors	Description	General Symptoms
1	Age	Elderly people suffer more from heart disease	{Chest pain, breath shortness, irregular heartbeat, fainting, fatigue, swollen feet}
2	Sex	Males have greater chances of heart attack than females	
3	Smoking	Smokers have highly risk of heart disease than non-smokers	
4	Family History	Probability of heart disease is high if relatives or family have heart diseases	
5	Poor Diet	For development of heart, dieting is essential	
6	Cholesterol Level	High blood cholesterol level increases formation of plaque	
7	Blood-Pressure (BP)	BP can thicken the blood vessels and narrow and harden arteries	
8	Diabetes	Increases sugar level in body	
9	Obesity	Overweight people have more chances of heart disease	
10	Stress	Damage arteries	
11	Poor Hygiene	Increases heart disease	
12	Physical Inactivity	Physical activity helps the heart function properly	

other hand, patients' health condition is also an important factor during these tests [9,10]. The prioritization of these tests is very important if the patient's condition is critical and he/she needs immediate treatment [11,12].

Due to the advent of digital technology and the growing size of data, there is a huge amount of data collected by the healthcare industry throughout the year in their databases [13,14]. However, the data stored in the databases is very complicated and very challenging to analyze. For effective decision-making and to find useful patterns, it needs to be mined rigorously.

Data mining and machine learning techniques have utilized by academicians and researchers to retrieve useful patterns and knowledge from data sets. It would help medical professionals or healthcare people in the diagnosis of heart diseases or CVDs. Today, machine learning and data mining is an emerging field that is extensively used due to the growing size of the data [15]. To gain information or knowledge from a vast data set, traditional statistical methods and software are not suitable. In this direction, data mining tools and techniques can retrieve hidden patterns, knowledge, and relationships from large databases while machine learning techniques can train large data sets and gain insights from these data sets that is impossible for human eyes [16].

In this study, performance comparison of different machine learning techniques like logistic regression (LR), Bayesian regularization neural network (BRNN), Naïve-Bayes (NB), and support vector machine (SVM) are made on the heart disease data set. However, their performances are compared based on accuracy measures like a confusion matrix. Finally, the highest performance accuracy is recorded by the BRNN method i.e. 96.39% among other existing approaches as well as we have also classified the data based on class label attribute disease which can be detected easily that a particular patient has heart disease or not. To prevalence of heart disease or deaths in the hospitals, medical professionals can utilize these tools and techniques and can design better policy from results. Hence, patient will be diagnosed at right time by implementing these tools and techniques [17].

The primary focus of this study is to highlight the role of prediction techniques in healthcare centers where these techniques will be helpful for enhancing the quality of services in healthcare centers as well as automatic diagnosis of the CVDs. To save the life of the people, it would be very helpful for doctors, clinicians, and specialists to make the correct decision on time.

Some eminent researchers' work is focused in Section 9.2, followed by a data pre-processing process in Section 9.3. After that, proposed methodologies is focused on in Section 9.4. Section 9.5 focuses on experimental results and Section 9.6 focuses on the conclusion and future scopes of the study.

9.2 LITERATURE REVIEW

Prediction plays a very important role to diagnose and detect heart disease accurately and efficiently. For many years, prominent researchers have designed various machine learning algorithms to contribute in the medical science field. Some eminent researchers' works are discussed here in brief.

Jackins et al. (2021) [18] have used different kinds of patient data like diabetes, cancer, heart disease, etc. to help the doctor to diagnose the particular patient health conditions. For this purpose, they have utilized artificial intelligence (AI) techniques like random forest (RF) and Naïve-Bayes (NB) to classify the data set and check the patient has a disease or not disease. Therefore, they had applied performance evaluation criteria to the data set and found that the RF method outperformed NB in terms of results.

Goyal et al. (2021) [19] have suggested wearable healthcare systems with inter-association allowed medical gadgets and their combinations to enhance the healthcare system quality in a broader scale network. However, they have also addressed various issues like security, privacy, and scalability and utilized various technologies such as cloud computing, big data, and augmented reality and patients' health-related issues are also generated by the system.

Aldahiri et al. (2021) [20] have discussed the comprehensive study of various supervised and unsupervised machine learning algorithms like Gradient Boosted Decision Tree (GBDT), random forest (RF), K-nearest neighbor (KNN), support vector machine (SVM), decision tree (DT), and Naïve-Bayes (NB) as well as their applications on IoT medical data. In their study, they have addressed the positive and negative points of the proposed algorithms based on the training data set size, number of parameters, time, sensitivity, etc. and finally they stated that the SVM method had secured excellent performance over other approaches.

Nahar et al. (2013) [21] have analyzed the performance of heart disease data sets using data mining techniques like Apriori, Tertius, and Predictive Apriori. They have identified some risk factors like rest_ECG (normal, hyper) are common in man and woman both. Based on the findings they have concluded that the possibility of heart disease in women is less than in men and only in hyper form, rest_ECG is considered a risk factor in men as well as this parameter could be also be selected as a primary factor for heart disease prediction in women. Finally, experimental results stated that the precision of Apriori was recorded at 90% which is higher than others.

Rajeshwari et al. (2012) [22] have recorded the performance of the neural network (NN) algorithm with the feature selection method for the ischemic heart disease problem. A total of 12 parameters was considered for their research work. The experimental results stated that the precision rate in training and testing mode recorded 89.4% and 82.4%, respectively, when all the features (parameters) are considered. Moreover, they have concluded that the reduction of any features or parameters also decreases the precision rate in both training and testing modes.

Shah et al. (2020) [23] have considered a heart disease data set from the UCI repository consisting of 76 attributes and 303 samples. For study purposes, only 14 attributes are selected for testing purposes out of these 76 attributes. For heart disease prediction, they have adopted various machine learning techniques like Naïve-Bayes, K-nearest neighbor (K-NN), random forest, and decision tree. Finally, the best performance was recorded by the K-NN method.

Walker et al. (2014) [24] have stated that the heart is the main cause of death in Texas, America. In their research study, the cluster analysis approach considered the analysis of different areas of Texas. Their experimental results had shown that poor hygiene and economic deprivation or other conditions are responsible for heart disease problems.

Ahmad et al. (2013) [25] have designed a machine learning classifier system using random forest (RF) and support vector machine (SVM) methods. To classify the data set, the liver, cancer, and heart disease data with different kernel parameters are considered. The liver, cancer, and heart disease data with varying kernel parameters are considered. Finally, the SVM method had excellent performance over others shown by experimental results.

Kara et al. (2006) [26] have adopted the artificial neural network (ANN) approach for the diagnosis of optic nerve disease with pattern electrifying signals. Therefore, Levenberg Marquardt (LM) backpropagation algorithm is used to train the multilayer perceptron (MLP) network. Finally, experimental results have shown that the proposed method performs excellent and the results are classified in two categories i.e. disease or healthy.

Masetic et al. (2016) [27] have presented a random forest (RF) classification approach with tenfold cross-validation to improve accuracy. For this purpose, different accuracy measures are used by them such as receiver operating characteristics (ROC) curve and F-measure, etc. Finally, the proposed method gives better accuracy than others.

Olaniyi and Oyedotun (2015) [28] have designed artificial neural network (ANN) model with three phases to diagnose heart disease in angina. The 88.89% classification accuracy was recorded. The main benefit of their system is that it can be easily incorporated into healthcare centers.

Jabbar et al. (2013) [29] have designed a machine learning classifier system to diagnose heart disease. They have adopted a backpropagation method with a feature selection algorithm for the research study. Finally, the proposed system received excellent performance accuracy shown by experimental results.

Taneja (2013) [30] selected various supervised machine learning classification techniques like J48, multilayer perceptron (MLP), and Naïve-Bayes (NB) for study purposes. The data mining tool WEKA is adopted for analysis purposes. The J48 method with tenfold cross-validation outperformed others concluded by the research study.

Dewedi (2017) [31] has selected various machine learning classification methods with tenfold cross-validation techniques for analyzing the CVDs' data set. However, the algorithms used for performance evaluations are Naïve-Bayes (NB), decision tree (DT), artificial neural network (ANN), logistic regression (LR), K-nearest neighbor (K-NN), and support vector machine (SVM). The proposed algorithms had achieved 83%, 77%, 84%, 85%, 82%, and 80% accuracy, respectively. Finally, they have concluded that LR provides better accuracy than others.

Chourasia et al. (2014) [32] have utilized various machine learning techniques for the detection of heart disease problems. The data set is downloaded from the UCI repository and contains only 11 attributes. Therefore, data mining techniques used for prediction are J48, Naïve-Bayes (NB), and bagging. Finally, the highest classification rate was secured by bagging, i.e. 85.03%.

Shafique et al. (2015) [33] compared the performances of the three most prominent machine learning classification techniques, neural network (NN), Naïve-Bayes (NB), and decision tree (DT), to gain insights from the heart disease data set. The NB method secured excellent performance over other methods.

Sundar et al. (2012) [34] developed a prototype based on data mining techniques like weighted associative classifier (WAC) and Naïve-Bayes (NB). Therefore, these techniques found hidden relationships, patterns, and knowledge from the heart disease data sets. Moreover, the proposed model could be successfully implemented in hospitals for the diagnosis of heart patients. For model validation, a confusion matrix measure is used.

This study is augmented by using various machine learning techniques like logistic regression (LR), Naïve-Bayes (NB), support vector machine (SVM), and Bayesian regularization neural network (BRNN) for the heart disease data set.

9.3 DATA PRE-PROCESSING

The healthcare industry collects a vast amount of data every year that is incomplete, inconsistent, and fuzzy. It is very difficult to make predictions from such kinds of data. The data pre-processing is an important step that embodies the treatment of missing values [35]. The data set obtained from the Kaggle data source contains more errors, missing values, and repeated attributes. Finally, data is not suitable for prediction tasks and can't directly apply any prediction methods. To remove inconsistency and missing values from the data set, a data pre-processing process is utilized. However, the process prepares the data for the prediction task and reduces risk level [35,36]. The data set contains 305 samples and consists of 14 attributes like age, sex, resting blood pressure (RBP), fasting blood sugar (FBS), old peak (OP), slope of peak exercise (SPE), number of major vassals (NME), etc. [37]. The attribute description is shown in more detail in Table 9.2.

Here, we are showing only a sample of the data set due to the large size. A sample of the data set is shown in Table 9.3.

9.4 PROPOSED METHODOLOGIES

9.4.1 Support Vector Machine (SVM)

Cortes and Vapnik proposed the SVM model first in 1995 [38]. The model follows the concept of structure risk minimization and statistical learning theory. In 1998, Vapnik modified the model further [38,39]. In N-dimensional space, the SVM model classifies the data sets in positive or negative decision boundaries. Moreover, the data points are separated in such a way that some points reside on one side of the plane and the other resides on another side of the plane. However, support vectors are those points that are closest to the hyperplane. The largest distance analysis is used to identify the classes and error minimization w.r.t. data separation based on the largest margin classifier is performed by using a hyperplane [39,40]. Figure 9.1 shows a simple representation of the SVM model.

It is clearly shown by Figure 9.1 that the hyperplane divides the data points into two decision boundaries i.e. positive or negative class, respectively, which is shown by blue and red colors. Figure 9.2 states the flow chart of the SVM model.

TABLE 9.2
Description of Attributes for Heart Disease Data Set [37]

S. No.	Attribute	Value {Min–Max}	Description
1	Age	{29–77}	Person Age
2	Sex	{0–1}	Sex (Male -1, Female -0)
3	CPT	{1–4}	Chest Pain Type{Typ_Angina-1, Atyp_Angina-2, Non_Anginal-3, Asympt-4}
4	RBP	{94–200}	Resting Blood Pressure in mm/hg
5	FBS	{0–1}	Fasting Blood Sugar {0-No, 1-Yes}
6	OP	{0–6.2}	Old Peak (ST Depression Induced by Exercise)
7	SPE	{1–3}	Slope of Peak Exercise{Up-Sloping-1, Flat-2, Down-Sloping-3}
8	NME	{0–3}	No. of Major Vassals
9	Thal	{3–7}	Thalassemia {Norma-3, Fixed Defect-6, Reversable Defect-7}
10	MHR	{71–202}	Maximum Heart Rate
11	ECG	{0–2}	Electro Cardio Gram {Normal-0, StTWave_Abnormality-1, LeftVent_Hyper-2}
12	SC	{126–564}	Serum Cholesterol
13	EIA	{0–1}	Exercise Included Angina {1-Yes, 0-No}
14	Disease (Class)	{0–1}	{Present-1, Absent-0}

TABLE 9.3
Sample of Heart Disease Data Set [37]

S. No.	Age	CPT	RBP	FBS	ECG	MHR	EIA	SPE	NMV
1	60	3	170	0	0	135	1	2	3
2	55	2	140	0	0	170	1	2	0
3	52	1	160	1	0	125	0	1	0
4	42	2	150	0	0	143	0	2	1
5	41	3	130	0	0	140	0	1	1
6	38	4	140	0	0	135	0	1	0
7	52	1	170	1	2	122	1	2	1
8	54	2	190	0	0	125	1	2	1
9	59	4	130	0	0	125	0	3	2
10	56	1	150	0	1	122	1	3	3
11	52	1	150	0	1	170	0	3	0
12	60	3	120	0	0	125	0	1	0
13	55	4	140	1	0	143	1	1	0
14	57	1	130	1	0	140	0	2	2
15	38	2	140	0	0	166	0	1	1
16	60	1	160	0	2	135	0	2	0
17	55	1	170	0	0	150	0	2	2

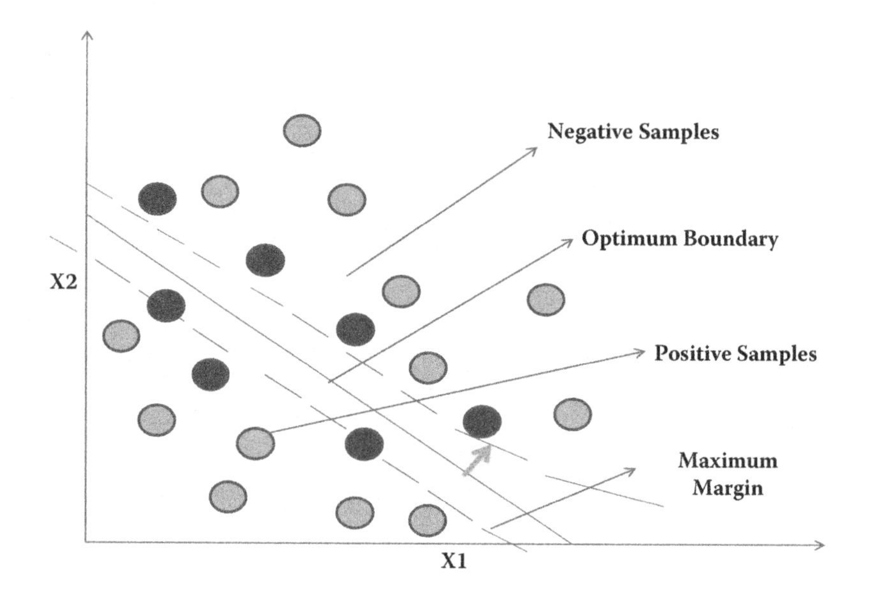

FIGURE 9.1 SVM model representation [40].

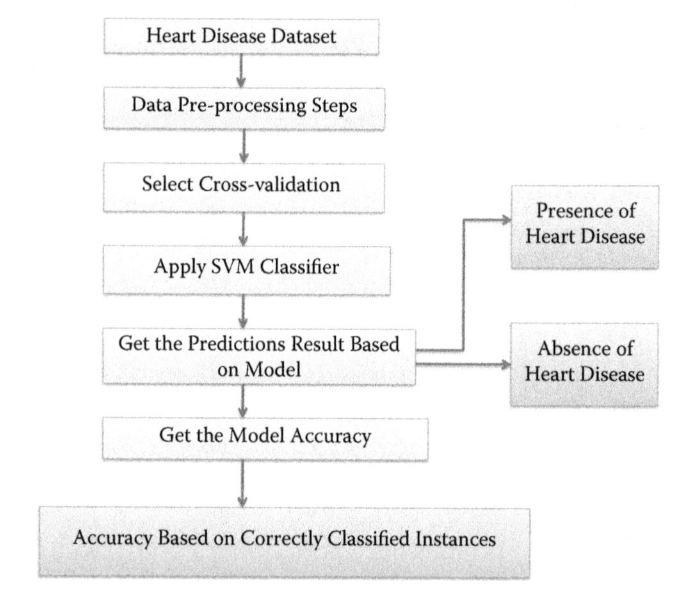

FIGURE 9.2 Flow chart of the SVM model [41].

9.4.2 Naïve-Bayes (NB)

Naïve-Bayes (NB) is the most prominent and effective machine learning algorithm in the classification family that is based on the principle of Bayes' theorem. Therefore, the algorithm states that occurrences of particular features of a class are independent of the presence or absence of other features [35] [42]. It is a powerful classification algorithm that is being extensively used for heart disease prediction. As with conditional probability, in NB, the posterior probability of each class is calculated for classifying the data. The class label of attribute is predicted by using the NB formula that is shown by equation (9.1).

(9.1)

where C = class label for instance,

Y = instances for prediction.

Figure 9.3 shows the flow chart of the NB model.

9.4.3 Logistic Regression (LR)

One major drawback of linear regression is that it is used to predict continuous variables like size. Therefore, logistic regression is very similar to linear regression and predicts discrete variables i.e. something like true or false [42,43]. However, LR is used to solve classification problems (binary and multi-class) not regression problems. One major strength of LR is a sigmoid function that is used to convert the independent variable into an expression of probability concerning for 0 to 1 (dependent variable). The formula for the sigmoid function is as follows:

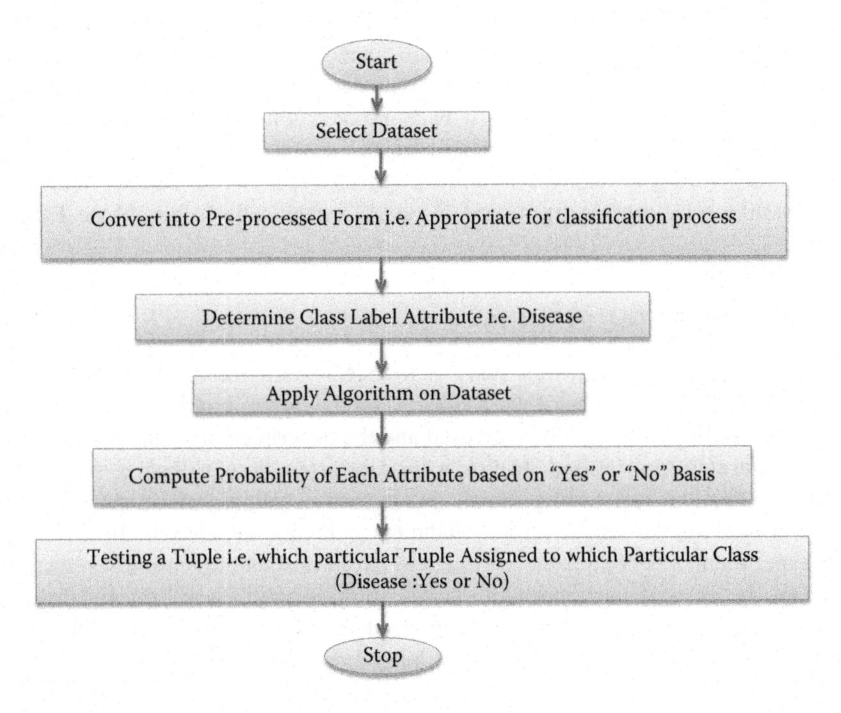

FIGURE 9.3 Flow chart of the NB model [41,42].

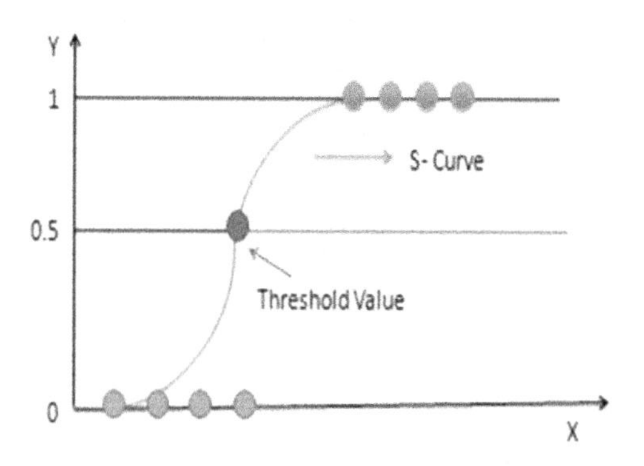

FIGURE 9.4 Logistic regression representation [35,41].

(9.2)

where Z = steepness parameter

LR fits a data in an S-shaped curve instead of fitting data to a line, which is shown in Figure 9.4.

9.4.4 Bayesian Regularization Neural Network (BRNN)

In the artificial neural network (ANN) family, Bayesian regularization (BR) is one of the well-known and popular algorithms. However, the method is more robust i.e. high level of functionality and eliminating the need for the lengthy cross-validation process as compared to the standard back propagation neural network (BPNN) method [42–44]. One major advantage of BRNN is that it adopted a mathematical process that is used to map the non-linear regression into well-defined statistical problems like ridge regression [44,45]. Figure 9.5 states a flow chart of the BRNN model.

9.5 EXPERIMENTAL RESULTS

The main focus of this research study is to select the optimum classification algorithm as well as predict heart disease based on that algorithm. However, the four different classification algorithms are used and the experimental purpose MATLAB machine learning tool is used. In this way, data separation is done in two parts: training (70%) and rest testing (30%). For effective training and testing performance, a well-known tenfold cross-validation technique is selected. In this way, each experiment was conducted ten times to avoid unstable operation results, and based on the comparison, optimum classification accuracy was achieved finally. Figure 9.6 shows the performance comparison of predicted disease vs. observed disease for the support vector machine (SVM) model.

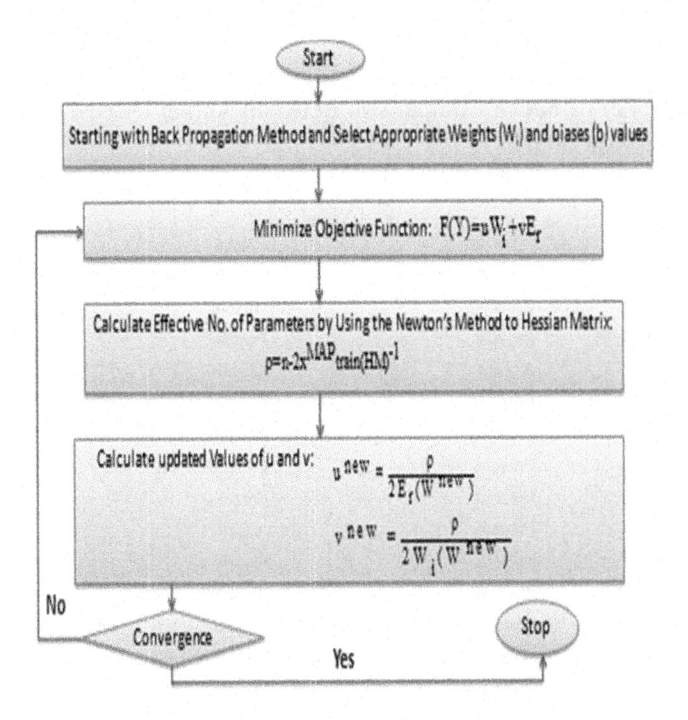

FIGURE 9.5 Flow chart of the BRNN model [45,46].

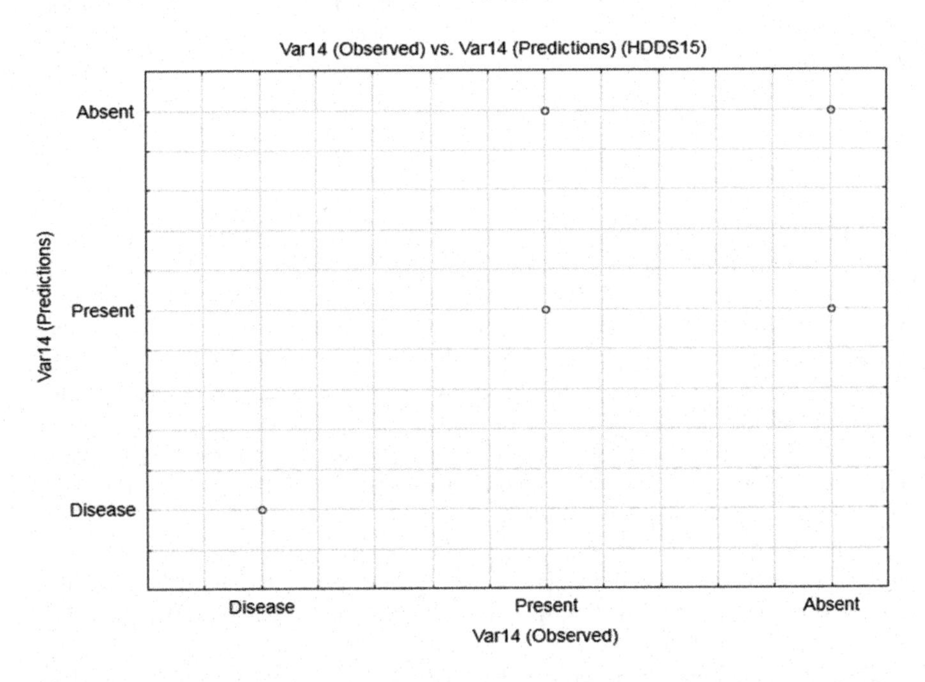

FIGURE 9.6 Performance comparison of predicted disease vs. observed disease for the SVM model.

TABLE 9.4
SVM Model: Performance Comparison between Actual Disease (AD) vs. Predicted Disease (PD)

S.No.	AD	PD	Accuracy
1	Present	Present	Correct
2	Absent	Absent	Correct
3	Present	Absent	Incorrect
4	Present	Present	Correct
5	Absent	Absent	Correct
6	Present	Present	Correct
7	Present	Present	Correct
8	Present	Present	Correct
9	Present	Present	Correct
10	Present	Absent	Incorrect
11	Present	Present	Correct
12	Present	Present	Correct
13	Absent	Absent	Correct
14	Present	Present	Correct
15	Present	Present	Correct
16	Absent	Present	Incorrect
17	Present	Present	Correct
18	Present	Present	Correct
19	Absent	Absent	Correct
20	Absent	Absent	Correct
21	Present	Present	Correct
22	Absent	Absent	Correct
23	Absent	Absent	Correct

Performance prediction between actual and predicted disease (blue circle) is shown by Figure 9.6. Performance comparison between actual disease (AD) and predicted disease (PD) for the SVM model is shown in Table 9.4.

Figure 9.7 shows a histogram diagram of accuracy (predicted disease) against number of observations.

A histogram diagram of performance accuracy (correct vs. incorrect) is shown in Figure 9.7. Figure 9.8 shows the performance of the Naïve-Bayes (NB) model for actual output against predicted output.

Figure 9.8 clearly states that the model is perfectly fitted by a yellow circle (actual values) and blue circle (predicted values) under the line. Performance comparison between actual disease (AD) and predicted disease (PD) for the NB model is shown in Table 9.5.

Receiver operating characteristic (ROC) curve of the logistic regression (LR) model is shown in Figure 9.9.

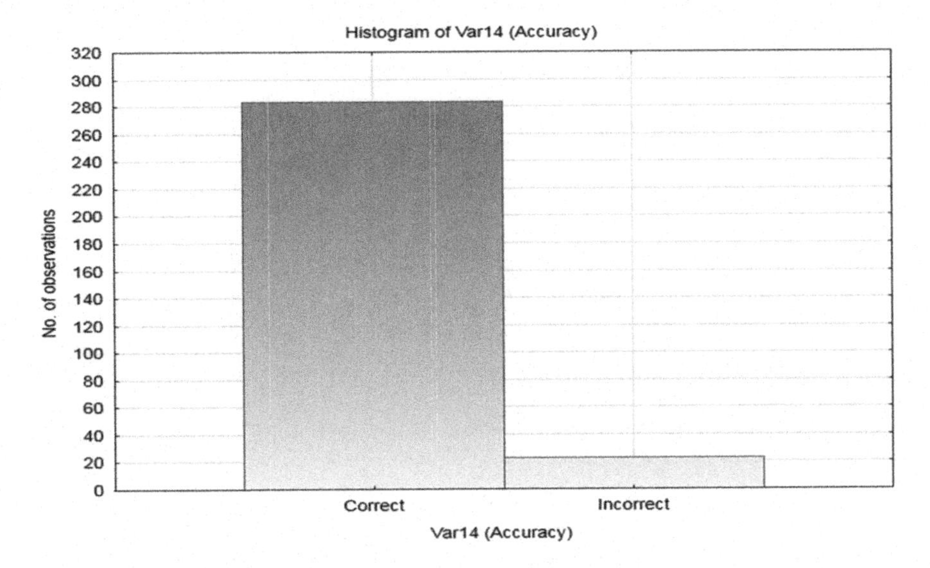

FIGURE 9.7 Histogram diagram of accuracy (predicted disease) against number of observations.

Here, the area under curve (AUC) value of 0.90 indicates the high prediction rate, i.e. model has recorded good performance accuracy. Performance comparison between actual disease (AD) and predicted disease (PD) for the logistic regression (LR) model is shown in Table 9.6.

Figure 9.10 shows the training state of the Bayesian regularization (BR) model.

In Figure 9.10, we have a sum of squared error, gradient value, and mutation values are 4.111, 0.011077, and 0.5, respectively, at epoch number 1,000. Figure 9.11 shows a regression plot between actual vs. predicted output.

Figure 9.11 clearly states the regression plot between actual and predicted output and best regression fit line for training and testing are achieved at 0.91 and 0.63, respectively. Figure 9.12 states the actual vs. predicted output comparison based on error histogram.

Figure 9.12 shows the error histogram for training and testing errors, respectively. Here, training and testing errors are shown by blue and red color, respectively. We also have a zero error, which is shown by a yellow line. A confusion matrix is used to predict the performances of the proposed algorithms, which are shown in Table 9.7.

Table 9.8 depicts the classification accuracy of the proposed algorithms.

Table 9.7 and Table 9.8 show confusion metrics and classification accuracy of the proposed algorithms respectively. Based on experimental results, we can state that the BR algorithm has outstanding classification accuracy, i.e. 96.39% than other algorithms. The second- and third-highest classification accuracy was recorded by SVM and LR algorithms, i.e. 92.45% and 83.27%, respectively. The lowest classification accuracy is recorded by NB algorithm, i.e. 77.21%.

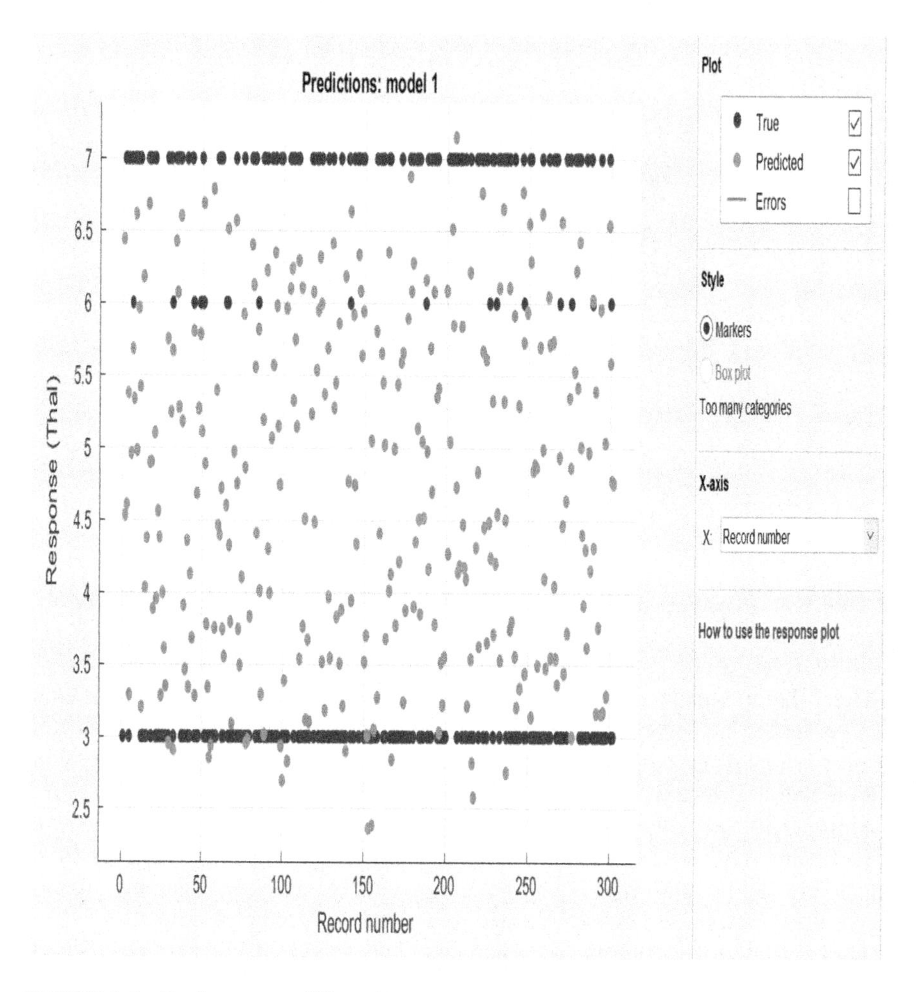

FIGURE 9.8 Performance of Naïve-Bayes (NB) model for actual output against predicted output.

9.6 CONCLUSION AND FUTURE SCOPES OF THE STUDY

In developing countries, heart disease has become the most common problem today. If proper treatment is not provided for the patient on time then it might lead to death. In the medical science field, machine learning techniques and software have widely been used by the researchers due to increasing heart patients worldwide. The main concern of this research study is to predict the occurrence of heart disease as well as compare the performance of different machine learning techniques. The Kaggle data source obtained for study purposes was completely pre-processed and used for testing purposes. Based on the findings, we have concluded that for small data set size, machine learning

TABLE 9.5
NB Model: Performance Comparison between Actual Disease (AD) vs. Predicted Disease (PD)

S. No.	AD	PD	Accuracy
1	Present	Absent	Incorrect
2	Absent	Absent	Correct
3	Present	Absent	Incorrect
4	Present	Present	Correct
5	Absent	Present	Incorrect
6	Present	Present	Correct
7	Present	Present	Correct
8	Present	Present	Correct
9	Present	Present	Correct
10	Present	Absent	Incorrect
11	Present	Present	Correct
12	Present	Present	Correct
13	Absent	Absent	Correct
14	Present	Present	Correct
15	Present	Present	Correct
16	Absent	Present	Incorrect
17	Present	Present	Correct
18	Present	Present	Correct
19	Absent	Absent	Correct
20	Absent	Present	Incorrect

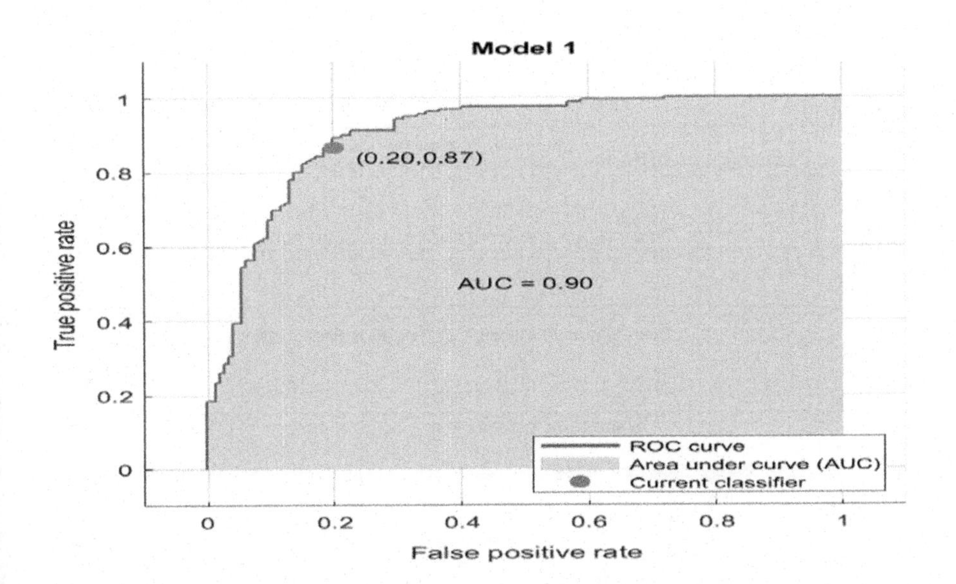

FIGURE 9.9 Logistic regression (LR) model: ROC curve representation.

TABLE 9.6
Logistic Regression (LR) Model: Performance Comparison between Actual Disease (AD) vs. Predicted Disease (PD)

S. No.	AD	PD	Accuracy
1	Absent	Absent	Correct
2	Absent	Absent	Correct
3	Absent	Absent	Correct
4	Absent	Present	Incorrect
5	Absent	Absent	Correct
6	Absent	Absent	Correct
7	Absent	Absent	Correct
8	Present	Absent	Incorrect
9	Absent	Present	Incorrect
10	Present	Absent	Incorrect
11	Absent	Absent	Correct
12	Absent	Absent	Correct
13	Present	Present	Correct
14	Present	Present	Correct
15	Present	Present	Correct
16	Present	Present	Correct
17	Present	Absent	Incorrect
18	Absent	Absent	Correct
19	Absent	Absent	Correct
20	Absent	Present	Incorrect

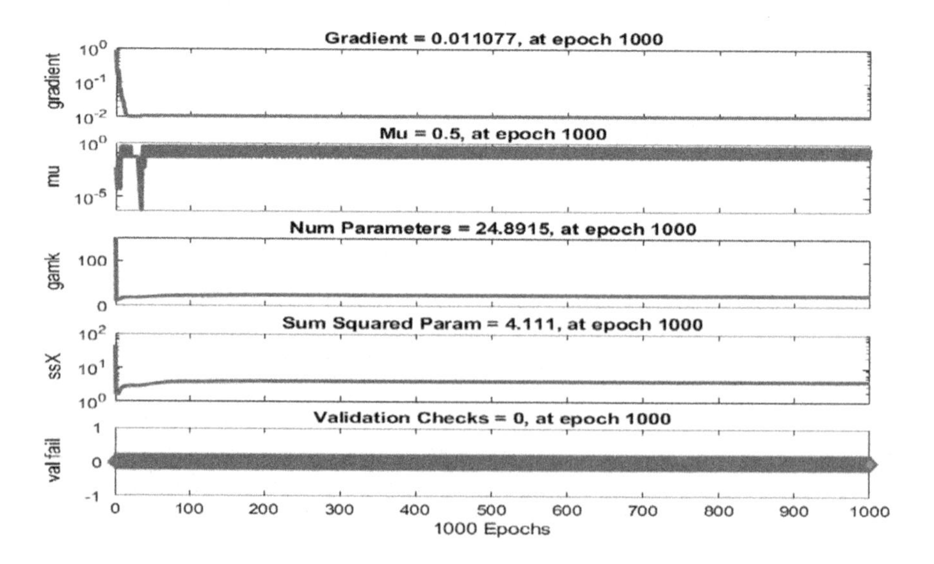

FIGURE 9.10 Training state of the Bayesian regularization (BR) model.

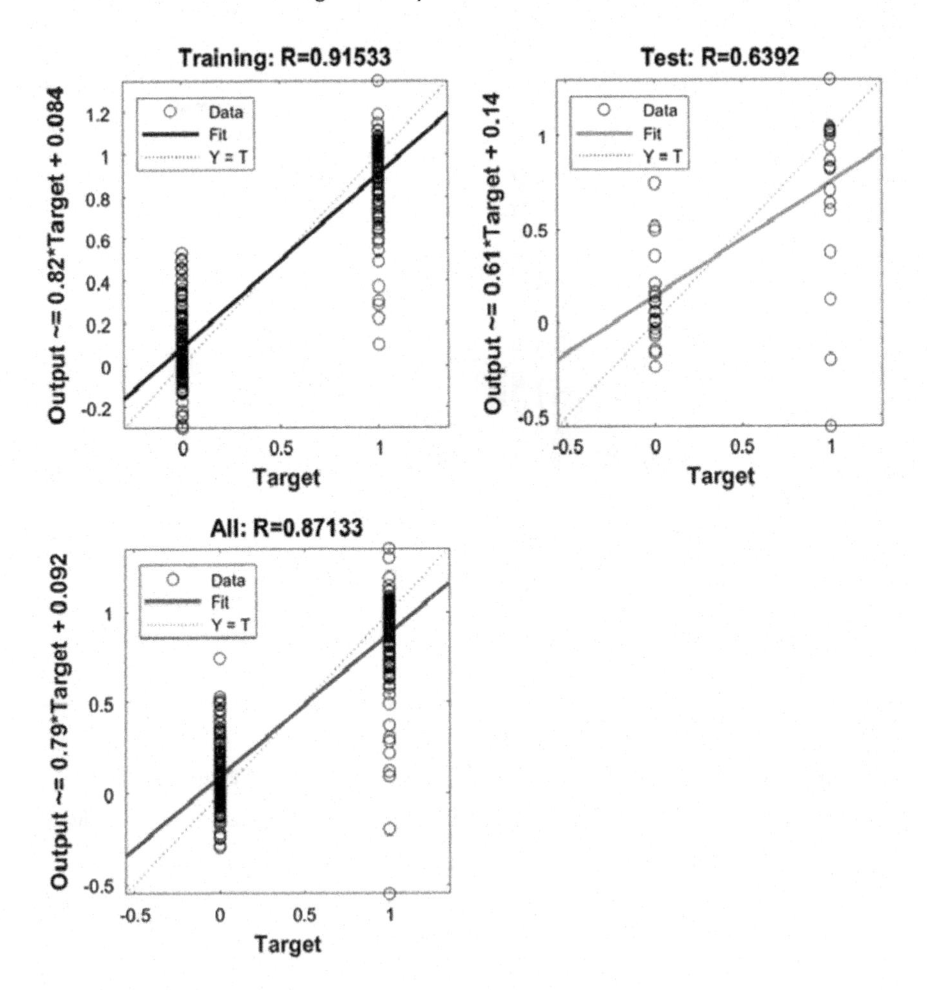

FIGURE 9.11 Regression plot: actual vs. predicted output.

techniques Bayesian regularization (BR) and support vector machine (SVM) outperform, while Naïve-Bayes (NB) and logistic regression (LR) recorded the lowest performance accuracy, i.e. below 90%. Moreover, the model is more appropriate for prediction than existing methods and has great learning ability, i.e. simultaneously learn the multiple records. The accuracy of the system is recorded up to 96.39%, which is acceptable. The proposed models would be helpful for medical professionals to diagnose heart disease on time.

In the future, optimization and hybrid machine learning techniques, such as genetic-fuzzy, neuro-fuzzy, and fuzzy-clustering, etc., will be adopted to improve the accuracy of proposed algorithms and patient feedback will be considered a top priority to update the database records. Additionally, more data variables, such as smoking habit, obesity, patient history, etc., would be considered in the future for improving prediction performance.

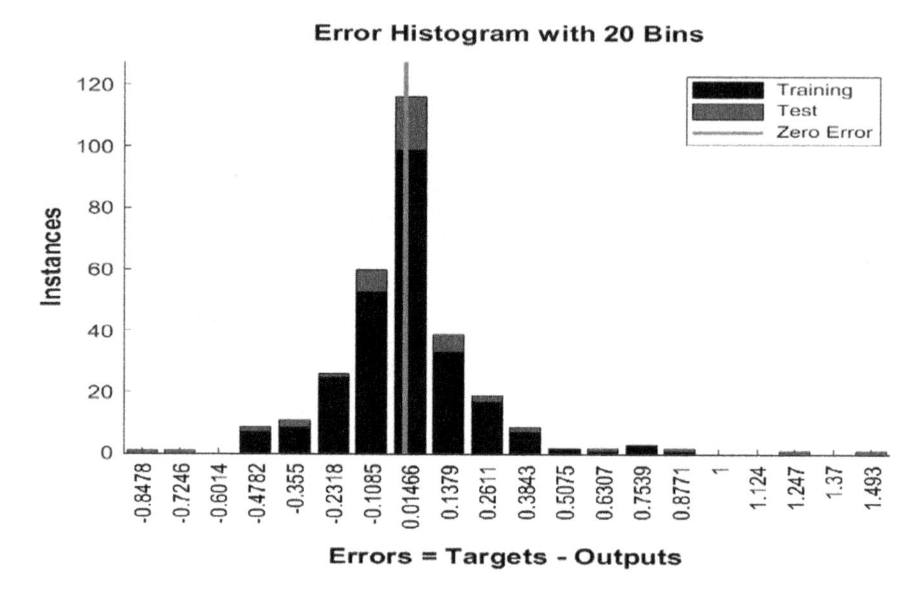

FIGURE 9.12 Actual vs. predicted output comparison based on error histogram.

TABLE 9.7
Confusion Matrices: Performance Prediction of the Proposed Algorithms

Algorithm	Class Observed	Present	Absent
Support Vector Machine (SVM)	Present	130	16
	Absent	7	152
Naïve-Bayes (NB)	Present	114	29
	Absent	41	121
Logistic Regression (LR)	Present	137	21
	Absent	30	117
Bayesian Regularization (BR)	Present	167	23
	Absent	19	127

TABLE 9.8
Classification Accuracy of the Proposed Algorithms

Algorithm	Correctly Classified	Misclassified	Accuracy (%)
Support Vector Machine (SVM)	282	23	92.45%
Naïve-Bayes (NB)	235	70	77.21%
Logistic Regression (LR)	274	31	83.27%
Bayesian Regularization (BR)	294	42	96.39%

REFERENCES

[1] Soni, J., Ansari, U., Sharma, D., and Soni, S. "Predictive Data Mining for Medical Diagnosis: An Overview of Heart Disease Prediction". *International Journal of Computer Applications* 17, no. 8 (2011): 43–48.

[2] Rhoads, J. M., and Stoudemire, A. "Cardiac Screening with Electrocardiography, Stress Echocardiography or Myocardial Perfusion Imaging: Advice for High-value Care from the American College of Physicianscardiac Screening in Low-risk Adults". *Annals of Internal Medicine* 162, no. 6 (2015): 438–447.

[3] Birje, M. N. and Hanji, S. S. "Internet of Things based Distributed Healthcare Systems: A Review". *Journal of Data, Information and Management* 2, (2020): 149–165.

[4] Kumari, M. and Godara, S. "Comparative Study of Data Mining Classification Methods in Cardiovascular Disease Prediction". *International Journal of Computer Science and Technology* 6, (2011): 304–308.

[5] Parthiban, L., and Subramanian, R. "Intelligent Heart Disease Prediction System Using CANFIS and Genetic Algorithm". *International Journal of Biological and Life Science* 15, (2007): 157–160.

[6] Han, J. and Kamber, M. Data Mining: Concepts and Techniques. Second edition, Morgan Kaufmann Publishers, San Francisco, (2006).

[7] Tantimongcolwat, T., and Naenna, T. "Identification of Ischemic Heart Disease via Machine Learning Analysis on Magneto-cardiograms". *Computers in Biology and Medicine*, Elsevier 38, (2008): 817–825.

[8] Yan, H., and Zheng, J. "Development of a Decision Support System for Heart Disease Diagnosis Using Multilayer Perceptron". *Proceedings of the international Symposium on Circuits and Systems* 5, (2003): 709–712.

[9] Hashi, E. K., Zaman, M. S. U., and Hasan, M. R. "An Expert Clinical Decision Support System to Predict Disease Using Classification Techniques". *International Conference on Electrical, Computer and Communication Engineering (ECCE)*, pp. 396–400, (2017).

[10] Hazra, A., Mukherjee, A., Gupta, A., & Mukherjee, A. "Heart Disease Diagnosis and Prediction Using Machine Learning and Data Mining Techniques: A Review". *Research Gate Publications* 10, no. 7 (2017): 2137–2159.

[11] Pattnayak, P., and Jena, O. P. "Innovation on Machine Learning in Health Care Services-An Introduction". *Machine Learning for Healthcare Applications* 1, (2021): 3–16, 10.1002/9781119792611.ch1.

[12] Dey, A., Singh, J., and Singh, N. "Analysis of Supervised Machine Learning Algorithms for Heart Disease Prediction with Reduced Number of Attributes using Principal Component Analysis". *Analysis* 140, no. 2 (2016): 27–31.

[13] Duggani. K., and Nath M. K. "A Technical Review Report on Deep Learning Approach for Skin Cancer Detection and Segmentation". *Lecture Notes on Data Engineering and Communications Technologies book series (LNDECT)* 54, (2021).

[14] Weng, W. H. "Machine Learning for Clinical Predictive Analytics". *Leveraging Data Science for Global Health* (2020): 199–217. 10.1007/978-3-030-47994-7_12

[15] Paramesha, K., Gururaj, H. L., and Jena, O. P. "Application of Machine Learning in Biomedical Text Processing and Food Industry". *Machine Learning for Healthcare Applications* (2021): 151–168. 10.1002/9781119792611.ch10.

[16] Moloud. A., Sharareh, R. N. K., Tole, S., and Imam, M. I. S., "Goli. A Comparing Performance of Data Mining Algorithms in Prediction Heart Diseases". *International Journal of Electrical and Computer Engineering (IJECE)* 5, no. 6 (2015): 1569–1576.

[17] Otoom, A. F., Abdallah, E. E., Kilani, Y., Kefaye, A., and Ashour, M. "Effective Diagnosis and Monitoring of Heart Disease". *International Journal of Software Engineering and Its Applications* 9, no. 1 (2015) 143–156.

[18] Jackins, V., Vimal, S., Kaliappan M. and Lee Young M. "AI based Smart Prediction of Clinical Disease Using Random Forest Classifier and Naïve Bays". *The Journal of Super Computing* 77, (2021): 5198–5219.

[19] Goyal, S., Sharma, N., Bhushan, B., Shankar, A. and Sagayam, M. "IoT Enabled Technology in Secured Healthcare: Applications, Challenges and Future Directions". *Cognitive Internet of Medical Things for Smart Healthcare* 311, (2020): 25–48.

[20] Aldahiri, A., Alrashed, B. and Hussain W. Trends in Using IoT with Machine Learning in Health Prediction System. *Forecasting* 3, (2021): 181–206.

[21] Nahar, J., Tasadduq, I., Kevin, S. T., and Yi-Ping Ph, Ch. "Association Rule Mining to Detect Factors Which Contribute to Heart Disease in Males and Females". *Expert Systems with Application* 40, no. 4 (2013): 1086–1093.

[22] Rajeswari, K., Vaithiyanathan, V., and Neelakantan, T. R. "Feature Selection in Ischemic Heart Disease Identification using Feed Forward Neural Networks". *International Symposium on Robotics and Intelligent Sensors*, Procedia Engineering 41, (2012): 1818–1823.

[23] Shah, D., Patel, S. and Bharti S. K. "Heart Disease Prediction using Machine Learning Techniques". *SN Computer Science, Spring Nature* 1, no. 345 (2020): 1–6.

[24] Walker, K. E. and Crotty, S. M. "Classifying High-prevalence Neighborhoods for Cardiovascular Disease in Texas". *Applied Geography* 57, (2014): 22–31.

[25] Ahmed, A., Sultan, K. A., and Hussain Syed, N. "Comparative Prediction Performance with Support Vector Machine and Random Forest Classification Techniques". *International Journal of Computer Applications* 69, no. 11 (2013): 12–16.

[26] Kara, S., Guvenb, A., and OztUrk, O., "Ayse. Utilization of Artificial Neural Networks in the Diagnosis of Optic Nerve Diseases". *Elsevier Publication, Computers in Biology and Medicine* 36, (2006): 428–437.

[27] Masetic, Z., and Subasi, A. "Congestive Heart Failure Detection Using Random Forest Classifier". *Computer Methods and Programs in Biomedicine* 130, (2016): 54–64.

[28] Olaniyi, E. O., and Oyedotun, O. K. "Heart Diseases Diagnosis Using Neural Networks Arbitration". *International Journal of Intelligent Systems and Applications* 7, no. 12 (2015): 75–82.

[29] Jabbar, M. A., Deekshatulu, B. L., and Chandra, P. "Classification of Heart Disease Using Artificial Neural Network and Feature Subset Selection". *Global Journal of Computer Science and Technology Neural & Artificial Intelligence* 13, no. 11 (2013): 456–462.

[30] Taneja, A. "Heart Disease Prediction System Using Data Mining Techniques". *Oriental Journal of Computer Science and Technology* 6, no. 4 (2013): 457–466.

[31] Dwivedi, A. K., "Analysis of Computational Intelligence Techniques for Diabetes Mellitus Prediction". *Neural Computing & Applications* 13, no. 3 (2017): 1–9.

[32] Chaurasia, V., and Pal, S. "Data Mining Approach to Detect Heart Diseases". *International Journal of Advanced Computer Science and Information Technology* 2, no. 4 (2014): 56–66.

[33] Shafique, U., Majeed, F., Qaiser, H., and Mustafa, U. I. I. "Data Mining in Healthcare for Heart Diseases". *International Journal of Innovation and Applied Studies* 10, (2015): 1312–1322.

[34] Sundar, A. N., Latha, P. P., and Chandra R. M. "Performance Analysis of classification Data Mining Techniques over Heart Disease Database". *International Journal of Engineering Science & Advance Technology* 4, (2012): 470–478.

[35] Pujari, A. K. Data Mining Techniques. Universites (India) Press Private Limited, 10th Edition, Hyderabad (A.P.), (2006).
[36] Han, J. & Kamber, M. Data Mining: Concepts and Techniques, 2nd Edition, Morgan Kaufmann Publishers, San Francisco, (2006).
[37] "Heart Diseases Dataset Downloaded from" (2020). http://www.kaggle.com.
[38] Cortes, C. and Vapnik, V. N. The Natural of Statistical Learning Theory. Springer, New York (U.S.A.), (1995).
[39] Vapnik, V. N. Statistical Learning Theory. Wiley, New York (U.S.A.), (1998).
[40] Bonaccorso, G. Mastering Machine Learning Algorithms: Expert techniques to implement popular machine learning algorithms and fine-tune your models. Packt Publishing Ltd., 1st Edition, Birmingham, U.K., (2018).
[41] Sultana, M., and Haider A. "Heart Disease Prediction Using WEKA Tool and 10-Fold Cross-validation". *The Institute of Electrical and Electronics Engineers* 9, no. 4 (2017): 6766–6773.
[42] Shahi, M., and Gurm, R. K. "Heart Disease Prediction System Using Data Mining Techniques". *Orient J. Computer Science Technology* 6, (2017): 457–466.
[43] Beyene, C., and Kamat, P. "Survey on Prediction and Analysis the Occurrence of Heart Disease Using Data Mining Techniques". *International Journal of Pure and Applied Mathematics* 118, no. 8 (2018): 165–173.
[44] Gomathi, K. and Shanmuga, Priyaa. "Multi Disease Prediction Using Data Mining Techniques". *International Journal of System and Software Engineering* 4, no. 2 (2016): 12–14.
[45] Mann, D. L., Zipes, D. P., Libby, P., and Bonow R. O. "Braunwald's Heart Disease: A Textbook of Cardiovascular Medicine". *Elsevier Health Sciences* 2, (2014).
[46] Das, R., Turkoglu, I., and Sengur, A. "Effective Diagnosis of Heart Disease through Neural Networks Ensembles". *Expert Systems with Applications* 36, no. 4 (2009): 7675–7680.

10 Deep Neural Networks in Healthcare Systems

Biswajit R Bhowmik, Shrinidhi Anil Varna, Adarsh Kumar, and Rahul Kumar
National Institute of Technology Karnataka, Mangalore, Karnataka, India

CONTENTS

DOI: 10.1201/9781003189053-10

10.1 INTRODUCTION

The novel coronavirus disease (COVID) is first identified in Wuhan, Hubei, China, in December 2019 and rapidly spread globally [1]. The World Health Organization (WHO) assesses the COVID 2019 (COVID-19), which has already affected global public health. Later, the organization has declared a global pandemic caused by this virus spill on the March 11, 2020 [2]. An estimation shows there are 45,677,613 COVID cases/patients found till October 30, 2020. This estimation increases to 104,471,838 till early February 2021. But people get affected in different ways depending on their immunity strength. The virus, a new but crucial member in the family of viruses, cause infection and, consequently, illness, ranging from the common cold to severe respiratory syndrome or diseases, e.g., Middle East respiratory syndrome (MERS), severe acute respiratory syndrome (SARS), etc. [3,4]. Most infected people are capable of developing a mild to moderate illness and recover without hospitalization. However, this virus more likely targets people with medical complications like diabetes, cardiovascular, or chronic respiratory diseases. As seen, the virus is highly infectious and, at extreme conditions, can cause respiratory distress or multiple organ failure. It is vital to control and prevent this pandemic by maintaining social distance, timely quarantine, medical treatment, etc., in the absence of any vaccine. In all cases, it is mandatory to detect the virus in terms of the COVID patients as the number of COVID-19 patients increases worldwide. On the other hand, a limited number of available detection kits or medical facilities pose difficulty identifying disease on a large scale. Therefore, researchers and medical practitioners look for an alternative technique, e.g., computer-aided medical diagnosis, to cope with the situation.

Medical image–based analysis of the chest X-rays and CT scans of a COVID-19 patient has proved to be an essential alternative test for detecting the virus. Multiple reasons make the X-ray images and CT scans a frequently used imaging modality. One reason is wide availability, and another reason is a low-cost resource. In this detection method, accuracy might depend on the experience in radiology. However, a diagnosis recommendation system can help clinicians verify patients' pulmonary imaging and reduce the need for a diagnosis doctor. Analysis of the input images on a large scale by a diagnosis recommendation system needs to have different image clusters. Fortunately, deep neural networks have proven to be very successful in classifying medical images from low to high quality. Subsequently, multiple deep learning techniques have achieved state-of-the-art performances in this system. Some sufficient models are highly trained and tested for medial image classification, such as ImageNet, EfficientNet, etc., at different use cases. Complex architectures like these models effectively help in detecting COVID-19 using CT scans and X-ray images taken on the chest.

This chapter critically situates the deep neural networks concerning the healthcare systems concerning current COVID emergence and evolution from the historical, socio-cultural, pedagogical, economic, policy, etc. perspectives. This chapter introduces AI in the healthcare systems and develops a solution to fight against the COVID-19 explosion. It meets various issues like challenges in data collection and visualization of trends of COVID-19. This chapter also presents many forecasting and data-driven analytical models that may help address the diseases. Finally, this work identifies significant challenges and open issues in healthcare systems based on deep neural networks. The work also guides to different forthcoming results. Overall, this chapter elucidates some of the salient problems, interests, and issues around these broad themes.

The rest of this chapter is organized as follows. Section 10.2 describes the COVID-19 evolution and emergence. Section 10.3 explores the detection and measurement history on COVID-19. Section 10.4 shows the importance of AI in COVID-19 disease. Section 10.5 applies AI in fighting against COVID-19. Section 10.6 defines various metrics used in the deep learning–based analysis. Section 10.7 covers different COVID-19 detection techniques. Section 10.8 discusses the forecasting models. Section 10.9 describes data-driven analytical models for COVID-19. Section 10.10 visualizes and predicts the trends of COVID-19. Section 10.11 states multiple challenges in data collection. Section 10.12 concludes this chapter, including its plausible future directions.

10.2 COVID-19 EVOLUTION AND EMERGENCE

In late December 2019, the novel coronavirus is first reported in the Wuhan Province of China [1]. A large outbreak of the virus is immediately observed in many cities in China and later rapidly spread worldwide, including Thailand, Japan, Korea, USA, UK, and one of the largest democratic country Bharat. It is the latest threat to global public health [3].

10.2.1 COVID-19 Situation Worldwide

Health is one of the actual states in human life. In all aspects, one must be mentally and physically fit [5]. But the novel coronavirus is highly infectious, and extreme conditions can cause SARS or multiple organ failure. So far, most frequent manifestation is pneumonia. But significant complications, such as acute respiratory distress syndrome (ARDS) [6], contribute to COVID-19's high mortality rate [3]. Officially, the WHO named the disease caused by the novel coronavirus as

Coronavirus Disease 2019 (COVID-19) [2,7]. The new coronavirus confirms human-to-human transmission. In early 2020, the number of COVID-19 infected people is significantly less. Still, the number dramatically increased every day around the world due to the massive transportation and considerable population mobility, impact of weather [1,8]. Because of the rapid growth of the infected people, the WHO assessed on March 11, 2020, and declared COVID-19 as a pandemic. Another estimation reported that the virus had already infected beyond 1,436,000 people in nearly 200 countries and territories as of April 9, 2020 [1]. As of October 30, 2020, 45,677,613 affected cases were reported worldwide. Figure 10.1 shows an early trend of the COVID-19 instances worldwide. Table 10.1 [9] shows the current number of reported cases worldwide and the top five countries till early November 2020. Several measurements and guidelines have been taken and revised from time to time for detecting COVID-19 at early and later stages. It is essential to deliver proper healthcare supports and services to the COVID-19 patients and protect the rest of the population that is luckily unaffected.

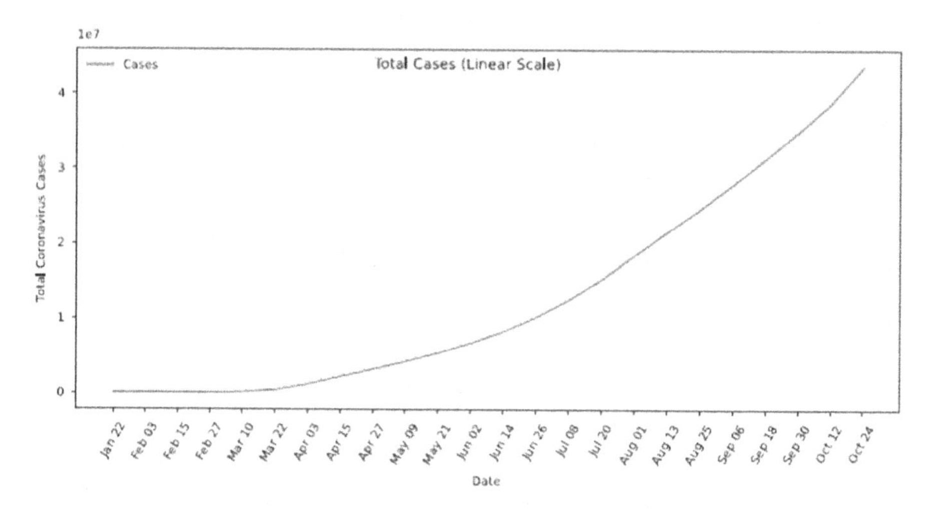

FIGURE 10.1 Early trend of worldwide COVID-19 cases.

TABLE 10.1
Top 5 Countries with Reported COVID-19 Cases

Country	Confirmed	Active Cases	Recovered	Deceased
World	4,88,37,746	1,27,18,189	3,48,83,274	12,36,283
USA	98,51,936	33,06,434	63,05,153	2,40,349
Bharat	84,09,626	5,20,832	77,63,799	1,24,995
Brazil	55,95,081	3,69,468	50,64,344	1,61,269
Russia	17,12,858	4,04,180	12,79,169	29,509
France	16,01,367	14,38,052	1,24,278	39,037

10.2.2 COVID-Situation in Bharat

After the declaration of the coronavirus situation as a pandemic on March 11, 2020, WHO reiterated immediate actions to be by the countries and scale up the response to treat, detect and reduce transmission to save people's lives. Bharat is the second-largest population country. Naturally, detection of the disease at the early stage is essential. According to the MoHFW Bharat report, a total of 909 COVID-19 cases are found till March 28, 2020. Among them, 862 Bharatiya (Indians) are from 27 states/union territories, and 47 are Foreign Nationals. Also, the report says 80 people are cured or discharged already, and 19 deaths. Because of the exponential growth of the virus, Prime Minister Shri Narendra Modi exercises his powers under section 6(2)(i), Disaster Management Act, 2005, and prescribes a full lockdown for containment of the epidemic throughout the country for 21 days with effect from March 25, 2020. The 'whole government' approach and response to the pandemic are pre-emptive, pro-active, and graded with high-level commitment. As a result, the spreading of the disease gets prevented effectively. As of March 2, 2021, there are 11,124,527 confirmed cases in the country. Active cases per million are 7,940, and a total of 157,248 unfortunate deaths are reported. Figure 10.2 [10] gives a trend of a rapidly growing disease while Figure 10.3 provides the current situation of COVID-19 cases [11].

Millions of tests have been conducted throughout the country so far, out of which around 6–7% are detected to be positive. This detection is bound to some degree of error. Considering the cases tested positive (including erroneous ones), they are hardly anything in front of the total number of tests conducted. The reasons stated for this can be many. The patient might have got cured of the disease. The symptoms of other conditions might be in common with that of COVID-19. The need for aggressive testing might have considered many patients who might have never contacted the potential carriers of the disease. A very crucial thing to know in this is that those who have tested negative are overwhelmingly huge in number. The

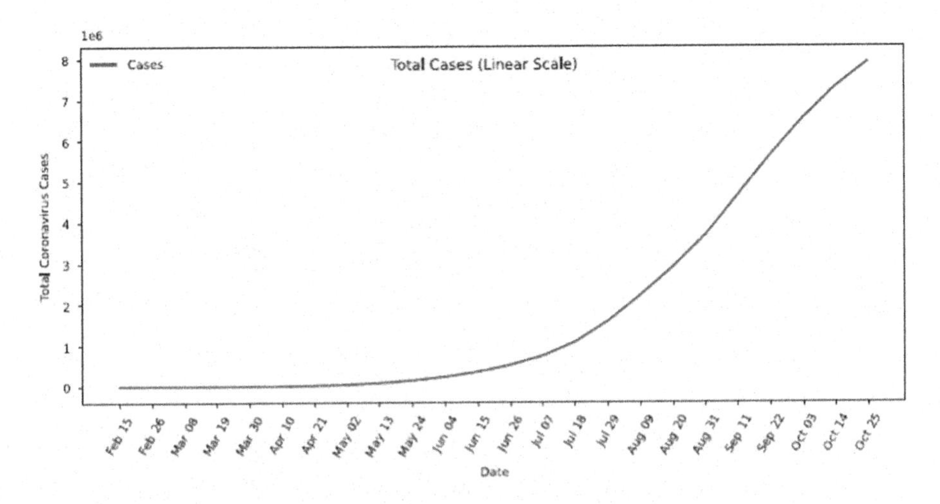

FIGURE 10.2 Early trend of COVID-19 cases in Bharat.

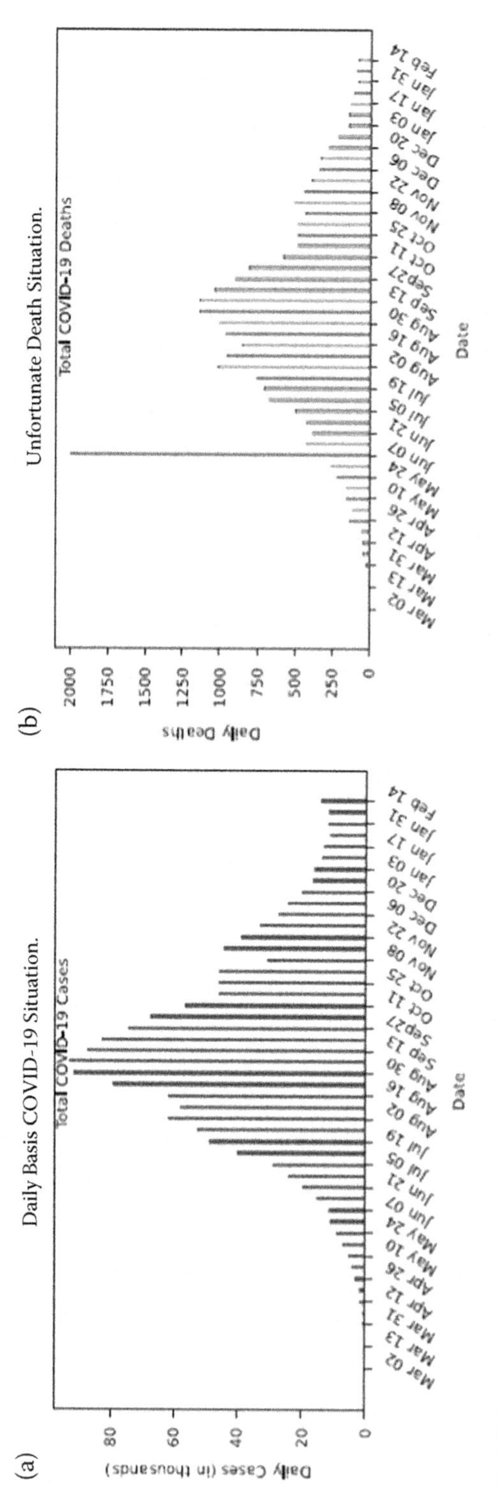

FIGURE 10.3 Current COVID-19 situation in Bharat.

TABLE 10.2
Top 5 States with Reported COVID-19 Cases

State	Confirmed	Active Cases	Recovered	Deceased
Bharat	84,11,034	5,19,508	77,64,763	1,25,029
Maharashtra	17,03,444	1,06,519	15,51,282	44,804
Karnataka	8,38,929	33,095	7,94,503	11,312
Andhra Pradesh	8,35,953	21,878	8,07,318	6,757
Tamil Nadu	7,36,777	19,061	7,06,444	11,272
Uttar Pradesh	4,91,354	23,150	4,61,073	7,131

handful of positive cases are the ones that will help the deep learning models learn about the characteristics of this disease.

To get more such cases to study, one should conduct a test for a sufficiently colossal number. The number that is worrying is falsely detected cases. False negatives constitute the most dangerous part of the patients who get tested for COVID-19. They are potential carriers without their knowledge. One way of overcoming this could be conducting multiple tests over a few days. Such a false negative increases the chance of reaching closer to the fact or ground truth. The goal is to minimize falsely detected cases, keeping in mind the community transmission that has already taken place with medical machinery working at its highest capacity. Table 10.2 [12] shows the number of reported cases in the country and its five states that are badly affected by this disease till November 6, 2020.

10.3 COVID-19 DETECTION AND MEASUREMENT HISTORY

There seems to be no sign that the infections and fatalities will decline, and the situation is regulated. The study states that the cumulative number of cases is still massive, with about 3.4% (as of November 31, 2020) of mortality, with about 4,60,15,562 deaths and 11,94,906 deaths per day. The WHO has lifted COVID-19's risk assessment to the highest degree and deemed it a global pandemic, leading to its terrible state as COVID-19. With this enormous impact of COVID-19 globally, many steps resolve the COVID-19 epidemic. The policymakers in nearly all impacted countries have prioritized isolating infected citizens as soon as possible. This pandemic would be prevented primarily by the government, for example, the closure of infection-reducing areas, the medical system's reaction to the outbreak, a series of crisis steps to minimize the national economy's effect, and the implementation of adaptive policies based on the situation in COVID-19. Simultaneously, following specific recommendations, such as wearing masks in public places, frequent hand washing, maintaining social isolation policies, and communicating the latest news on symptoms to regional health centers, encourage people to keep fit and protect others. Following this pandemic, the cure for the disease is a priority for the researchers, facilitating the slowdown of viral transmission and disease containment. In addition to attempts to develop effective COVID-19 coronavirus vaccines and drug treatments by medical practitioners and scientists globally, computer researchers have also made initial efforts to combat COVID-19 and enhance them.

Scientific experts suggest that developing a vaccine can defeat the COVID-19 and guarantee herd immunity in the people, especially the young generations because the vaccine is less effective in older people [13]. Many complications, such as acute respiratory distress syndrome (ARDS), contribute to the high mortality rate of COVID-19, despite the syndrome present shortly after the onset of symptoms. Various methods for the detection and monitoring of these respiratory manifestations play a significant role. For example, chest X-rays (CXR), antibody tests, and chest computed tomography (CT) scans are commonly used methods. In some cases, CT scans have shown abnormal findings in patients [3]. If it becomes the gold standard for diagnosis, make sure that COVID-19 X-ray cases are time-consuming. The suspected patient's obstacles can arise as quickly as possible from both a high false-negative rate and low sensitivity. The patient's general signs of COVID-19 are flu-like, such as fever, cough, shortness of breath, viral issues with coughing, and pneumonia [14]. But these signs alone have little meaning. Individuals do not show any symptoms in 41 cases, but their chest CT scan and pathogenicity scans are positive for COVID-19. Thus, to detect illness, positive pathogen tests and positive CT chest X-rays/photographs use the symptoms.

The chest X-ray of a COVID-19 patient has proved a definitive test for the diagnosis of COVID-19 cases because of increased sensitivity. Even as the number of patients is immense, X-ray diagnosis accuracy depends heavily on expertise with radiology. A device that will help doctors monitor lung pictures is the diagnostic recommender. For patients and physicians, such a system would minimize the difficulty of diagnosis. Software for deep learning is an artificial neural network. Similar to neurons in the human nervous system, each layer has many functioning neurons. A convolutional neural network (CNN) [2,15] is a deep learning network technique proven to be successful and reliable in medical image recognition. Many researchers use the CNN to detect pneumonia and other X-ray-based illnesses. Research to classify variations in lung disease has been suggested based on the structure of CNN. About 100,000 X-ray photographs of chest X-ray data are used for developing CNN diagnostic models of 14 diseases. It forecasts pneumonia by CNN. A suggestion method may help identify the contaminated region on the CT picture by radiologists. Real-time PCR is used as a standard testing technique for pathological studies [14]. The COVID-19 expansion research facilities include testing the medical systems around the world. The assessments would increasingly contribute to the detection and isolation of infected individuals. However, reliability cannot be assured by availability. At this point, the government's key concern is false-negative test outcomes – negative or hostile contaminated persons are the test product. Without knowing it, such a person will spread the virus to other individuals, so infection and panic are spreading quickly. Another reason is publishing and believing in incorrect research findings or false claims. Erroneous research findings hurt attempts to prevent proliferation from happening. There is no precise or reliable information on the results of these test characteristics regarding this issue's effect on insecure health and public employees' welfare. The sensitivity of these experiments is uncertain.

10.4 AI IN COVID-19 DISEASE

Currently, the world is fighting with a shortage of specialists trained enough to diagnose COVID-19. A concerted move adopts AI where deep learning–based methods are particularly used for the pandemic diagnosis and prognosis. Recently, Deep learning is being treated as the core technology of the rising AI. Well-annotated data on these methods always plays a critical role. For example, an essential diagnostic accuracy is reported in medical imaging for automatic lung disease detection using a deep learning method [1,3,16,17]. This section briefly explains the AI and its areas used to detect COVID-19. This section also describes various AI components and describes how this technology helps develop a solution for COVID-19 detection.

10.4.1 Artificial Intelligence

In multiple intelligent systems, artificial intelligence is a highly advanced technology in various fields, such as automobile, medical diagnostics, healthcare systems, network monitoring, image recognition, finance banking, computer vision, natural language processing, or image processing and so on. In many aspects of machine learning (ML), artificial intelligence (AI), and deep learning (DL) there are two fundamental approaches. Machine learning usually offers insight into understanding and identifying functional patterns from data. The performance of algorithms and systems based on machine learning is mainly dependent on representative functions. At the same time, through a clear voice, one can master a deep learning model. According to Ian et al. [18], deep learning has two primary characteristics that allow the learning of proper representation. It shows a deep learning feature, and deep learning helps the machine understand the data in depth, using several layers to learn increasingly meaningful representations. AI is used to diagnose pathogens of infections such as COVID-19 that have taken remarkable strides. According to the studies cited, it is essential to review and consider the problems related to AI's possibilities and infections to use modern AI approaches successfully.

10.4.2 Supervised Learning

Supervised learning is a part of machine learning that deals with features and labels. The features and labels are given to the machine learning model, which creates some patterns out of the given data and predicts the input-output. Supervised learning can provide an ingenious step in mastering the observation and prediction of COVID-19. It is also possible to create a nervous system to eliminate this disease's visual reflections, which will help control and legally treat those affected. A depth-based CNN method, e.g., Xception model [19], involves layers recognizable by convolution. It starts with two convolution layers. Then deeply separable convolution layers, a fully connected layer, and four convolution layers follow them. With its powerful functions and effective results, it can be a valuable tool against COVID-19.

10.4.3 Unsupervised Learning

Unsupervised learning is also called training the machine using the relevant information that is neither classified nor labeled. It permits the algorithm to take action on that information without any guidance. Unlike the training mentioned previously using verified data, this training technique does not use information signals and does not use names. This technique generally finds the coverage structure of a given piece of data and breaks it down into neighboring collections. In the medical world, one of the best-known professions of this learning technique is identifying oddities. This calculation forces the client to determine the generated k-cluster number. The primary purpose is to distinguish noise from PD signals [20]. A little consideration is paid to such subcategories and disturbance congregations that may exist within PD. One can apply this idea to CT scans, including COVID-19 and other various medical applications under the umbrella of the Internet of medical things (IoMT) [21].

10.4.4 Reinforcement Learning

Reinforcement learning (RL) is a machine learning field connected to how virtual agents can behave to optimize accumulated rewards in the environment. This learning technique is neither of the two approaches above but a progressive hybridization method. There is a reserve or sole authority in this technology, which has acceptable behavioral significance in certain circumstances. The ultimate goal is for them to strive to increase their vast bonus or total score. Practitioners will learn the best way to map a state to a movement without understanding the natural data. It differs from the usual supervised learning strategy, which generally relies on an instantaneous, deep, and supervised signal. It uses inspection, evaluation, and deferred entries to address ongoing dynamic issues. These peculiarities carry out the RL method as a logical choice for development of breakthrough devices in various fields of human medicine. In these fields, diagnostic or treatment options are usually the delayed and continuous strategies.

10.5 AI APPLICATIONS IN FIGHTING AGAINST COVID-19

This section introduces AI applications in fighting against COVID-19 and its use in controlling the spread of the disease, panic, and allowing proper dissemination of information related to COVID-19.

10.5.1 Detection and Diagnosis of COVID-19

Currently, the standard method for detecting the COVID-19 virus is reverse transcription-polymerase chain reaction (RT-PCR). Some dedicated plans improve this technique. Due to the unavailability of sufficient testing kits or time and cost constraints, this method faces difficulties in reaching the rapid testing process. A simple and low-cost solution to this problem is to make use of AI frameworks. AI frameworks are cost-efficient, fast computing abilities, and in abundance due to cloud space and the Internet's availability to many people. Since COVID-19 has

TABLE 10.3
Comparison of AI Detection Techniques

Study	Images	Metric Used	Value
Wang et al. [b17]	13,975	Accuracy	93.30%
Chagani et al. [b94]	668	POO	97%
Tang et al. [b95]	176	Sensitivity	93.30%

to do with the respiratory tract, some patients underwent X-ray and computed tomography (CT) scans. The X-ray images and CT scans act as an input set for a deep learning model built in [22]. The output, as expected, is infected with something other than COVID-19. The deep learning model then does a three-class classification of the input image. This method is highly efficient and uses transfer learning for computational complexity and achieves higher accuracy [23], image augmentation, ResNet model, and other efficient models. The process got an accuracy of over 90%. Hyper-parameter tuning of a deep neural network can improve the accuracy further. The limitation of using this approach is the quality and quantity of images available. Table 10.3 refers to a comparative study done using ML/DL and AI techniques so far. The missing values in the table are due to the unavailability of the exact values.

10.5.2 Identifying, Tracking, and Predicting the Outbreak

The susceptible infected removed (SIR) model is a traditional scheme that predicts infectious disease. The following non-linear differential equations express this SIR model, where I, R, and S represent infected, removed, and susceptible individuals, respectively. The β, γ denotes the transmission rate, and recovering rate, respectively [24–26].

$$\frac{dS}{dt} = -\beta SI \tag{10.1}$$

$$\frac{dI}{dt} = \beta SI - \gamma I \tag{10.2}$$

$$\frac{dR}{dt} = -\gamma I \tag{10.3}$$

The tracking method helps raise the alarm to push towards lockdowns in the city and take other prevention methods. The earlier few months in 2020 had confusion going on where doctors and the WHO didn't have conclusive evidence to prove whether a mask was a preventive measure or not. After collecting enough data, various institutions and research teams in the world verified these data. They suggested that wearing masks could significantly reduce the exposure and spread of the virus. Later, various governments worldwide rolled out an advisory to enforce wearing masks while traveling. Further research has already predicted how this pandemic shaped over the coming months and year. The present data is used and updated daily to predict the future course of the pandemic. The prediction of the outbreak is essential because if a prediction is made early, the governments can plan to reduce/increase movement restrictions and estimate the restored normalcy. The shape of the curve would give an idea in which stage a town/state/country arrived in containing the virus. The steps are per the situation of the outbreak. The studies are done using various machine learning or deep learning models in [27–29]. These models were applied in the U.S. infected cases due to enough data and the highest quality of research teams available during April 2020, when not many countries had started testing rapidly. Later on, other countries followed the same testing strategy and made predictions on their national data collected.

10.5.3 AI for Infodemiology and Infoveillance

When an outbreak hits the world, everybody is well informed regarding the situation outside due to the digital and social medium, unlike previous years. This success is purely possible due to technologies and AI. During this pandemic, the two most important things related to circulated data on COVID-19 are integrity and availability. The integrity of any information needs to be checked. The power of deciding the integrity of data is under the hands of WHO and Health Ministries of respective countries. Any fake news that is making the rounds needs to be shut down. All of this is possible using AI. Since social media has many users, it is nearly impossible for an organization to keep checking what information is disseminated anytime by anyone. AI can help by deploying bots that keep checking if any wrong or fake news is getting spread. This is of utmost importance because the health ministry cannot afford the public to get panicked or ill-informed by any means that can hamper the progress made so far in recovering from this outbreak. The social media websites such as Facebook, Instagram, Twitter, YouTube, and so on have taken this conscious step to keep the information in check to prevent incorrect data circulation. The reach of data with integrity is of utmost importance, and hence social media websites are coming in handy.

10.5.4 AI for Biomedicine and Pharmacotherapy

When clinically verified drugs aren't available, it becomes essential to discover new medicines and use existing drugs more to treat this coronavirus. This has both economic and scientific benefits, especially using AI. AI can make the process faster and cheaper. Deep learning extracts features from the given data that is difficult to do manually. More reasons why AI may benefit biomedical research, and why AI is essential are discussed in [30]. The provision of critical biomedical data has prompted the use of the AI industry in biomedicine and pharmaceuticals. Biomedical data such as transcriptomic and proteomics involve a lot of high-dimensional, unstructured data with non-linear relationships. Deep neural networks can handle complex scenarios, as mentioned previously. Due to the seriousness of the pandemic, AI recently identified medical applications to restrict coronavirus dissemination, primarily focusing on predicting protein structure, drug discoveries, and drug repositioning.

10.6 METRICS FOR DEEP LEARNING–BASED ANALYSIS

In the last decade, deep learning applications have expanded to a wide range of areas [2], especially in the healthcare systems, e.g., medical image processing (MIP) comprising disease diagnosis [31], organ segmentation [32], etc. Figure 10.4 gives a framework for diagnosis of COVID-19 using DL. CNN [15] is one of the leading classic deep learning technologies used in the above applications. While applying this technology, it keeps in mind to evaluate a series of metrics during its performance exhibitions. The metrics are confusion matrix, true/false positive, precision, recall, sensing, specificity, etc., [18,33] defined below.

Definition 1: ***Confusion Matrix*** is the table when the model predictions versus the ground-truth labels is visualized in a tabular format. It is generally not treated as a metric, but essential to know! It is four types based on the combinations True/False and Positive/Negative parameters.

- True Positive (TP): When both ground truth and the prediction are true.
- True Negative (TN): When both ground truth and the prediction are negative.
- False Positive (FP): When the ground truth is false, but the prediction is true.
- False Negative (FN): When the ground truth is true, but the prediction is false.

For example, the simple truth is that the patient has the disorder, but the forecast tells us what the classification/model tells the patient that the illness is contracted on a data basis.

Definition 2: ***Classification Accuracy*** is the number of accurate forecasts divided by the total number of projections. It is an example of how similar the predictions of the fundamental truth are.

Definition 3: ***Precision*** is the fraction of the appropriate instances of the samples obtained (also referred to as the positive predictive value).

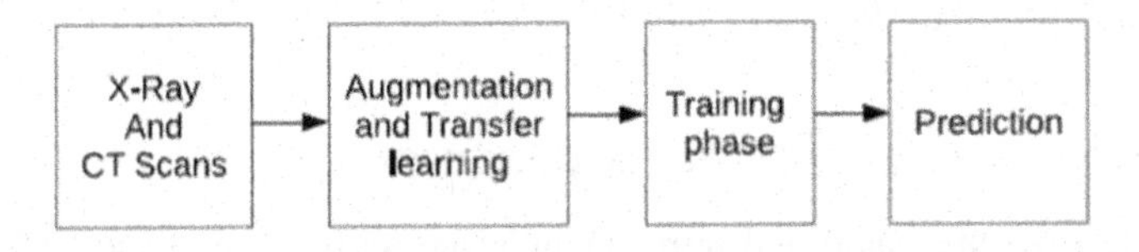

FIGURE 10.4 A framework for diagnosis of COVID-19 using DL.

Definition 4: ***Recall (or sensitivity)*** is a proportion of the total number of instances currently detected. The metric is equated in Equation 10.4 below.

$$Recall = \frac{TP}{TP + FN} \tag{10.4}$$

Definition 5: ***F1 Score*** demonstrates the combination of accuracy and recall. The maximum value of an F-score is 1, which means complete accuracy and reminder, and the lowest possible value is 0. Hence, the name is F1 score. This metric is equated in Equation 10.5.

$$F1\ Score = \frac{2 \times Recall \times Precision}{Recall + Precision} \tag{10.5}$$

Definition 6: ***Sensitivity*** is the metric to determine the potential of a model for predicting the true positive attributes of each group available. The sensitivity is measured in the same way as that of the recall.

$$Sensitivity = Recall = \frac{TP}{TP + FN} \tag{10.6}$$

Definition 7: ***Specificity*** is the approach that tests a model's capacity to predict actual negatives of each type accessible. This metric is reverse of the sensitivity or recall and equated in Equation 10.7.

$$Specificity \frac{True\ Negative}{True\ Negative + False\ Positive} \tag{10.7}$$

Definition 8: According to the receivers' cut-off threshold, a graph showing the output of a binary classifier is the practical characteristic curve. This graph is the ***receiver operating characteristic curve*** (ROC). It displays the true positive rate (TPR) for specific threshold values against the false positive rate (FPR). The curve plots TP vs. FP rate at different classification thresholds. Figure 10.5 shows a typical ROC curve.

Definition 9: ***AUC*** is the area under ROC curve. It represents an aggregated estimate of a binary classifier's output on any possible threshold level (and is thus an invariant threshold). Figure 10.6 represents an AUC. The AUC value ranges from 0 to 1. If a model's predictions are 100% wrong or correct, it has an AUC of 0.0 or 1.0, respectively.

10.7 COVID-19 DETECTION TECHNIQUES

Since the last decade, rapid and tremendous progress has been observed on deep learning–based solutions in healthcare systems, ranging from computer vision to

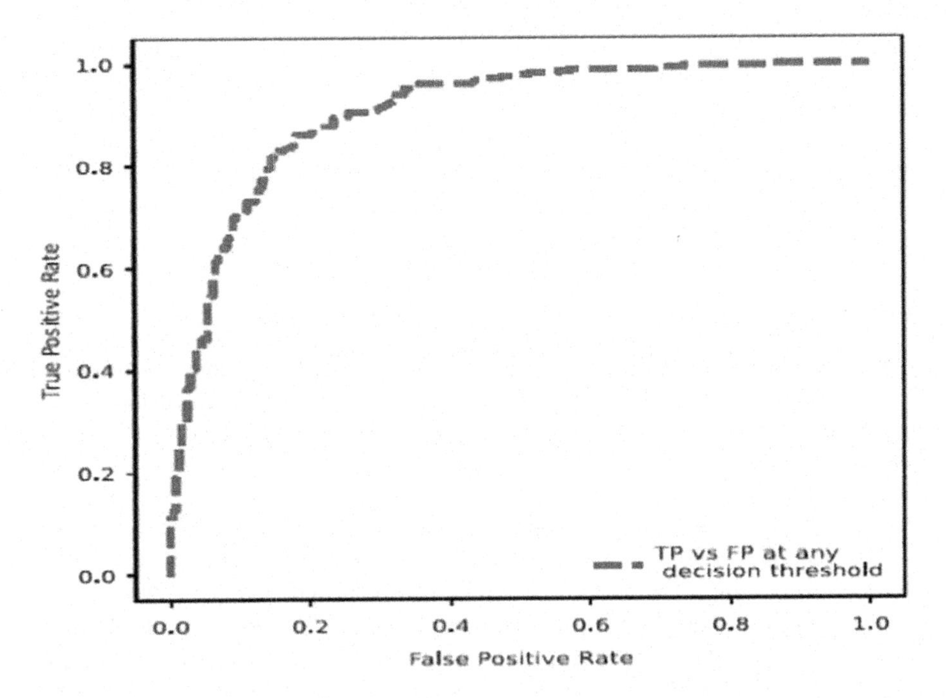

FIGURE 10.5 Typical ROC curve.

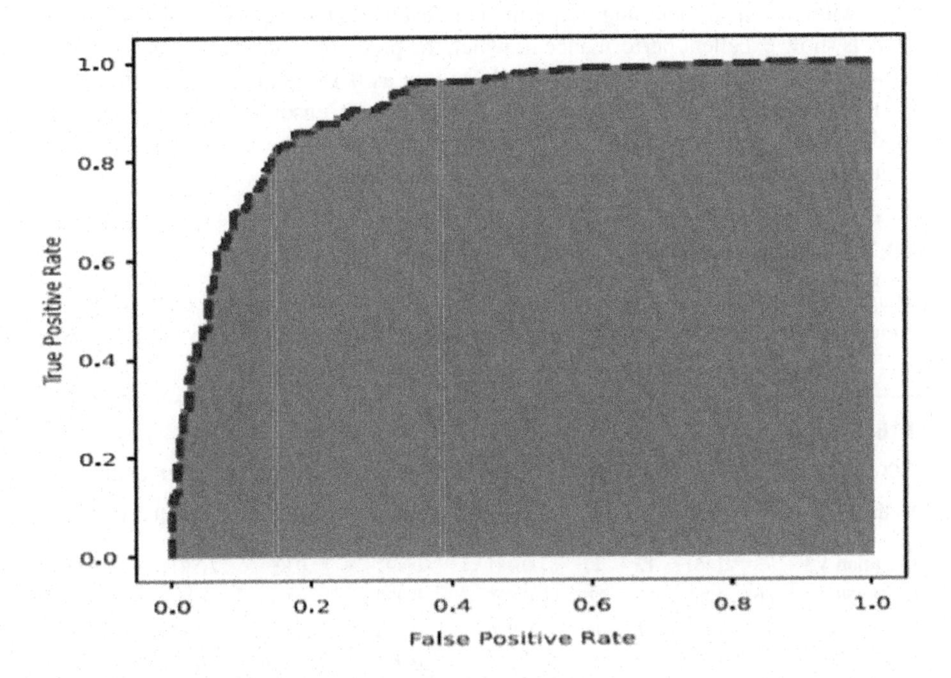

FIGURE 10.6 Area under the ROC curve.

annotated large-scale data sets, including the most recent image-based COVID-19 detection and diagnosis and classification of diabetes [34]. Compared to ancient and traditional shallow methodologies, different deep learning techniques used to detect COVID-19 offer improved quantitative performances in detection, recognition, and segmentation. One reason may be the previous methods built upon hand-crafted image features [31]. This section discusses different AI techniques that can fight against the COVID-19 explosion.

10.7.1 Use of Chest X-rays and CT Images for COVID-19

A regression model is used to find COVID-19 cases on the exploitation of chest X-rays and CT images. The central idea is to use a transformation function that relates linear or non-linear predictors to the mean response. Further, the procedure ensures that the mean is within a satisfactory scope. These are recommended features because the constituent data is a vector of some integral parts with associated information. In other words, the image is scalable.

For example, a Dirichlet censored linear regression (DCLR) model is based on displacement scaling. The response variable is a component variable related to the shape, scale, and position parameters of the corresponding displacement scaling Dirichlet distribution. To get these parameters, one can use the maximum likelihood estimation method techniques followed by using the gradient climb to update the parameters during the prediction in real time. Various ways like Inception V3, ResNet50, MobileNet, and Xception [19,35] are standard models in a neural network without transfer learning. Experimental results on the implementation of these models show excellent performance in which the prediction accuracy is as good and is nearly 97%. The time for an update is as low as 0.15 seconds [36]. Table 10.4 [14] provides the experimental results. These results ensure that the regression model might be more efficient and powerful than a set of the latest corresponding technologies.

10.7.2 Image-Based Diagnosis of COVID-19 Using ML

Image moments are another popular technique used for diagnosing COVID-19 in which one defines projection of images based on polynomials. These moments are

TABLE 10.4
Accuracy Result Using Different Neural Network without Transfer Learning

Method	FN	TN	TP	FP	Precision	Accuracy	Specificity	Recall	F1 Score
Inception V3	73	1461	12	17	0.981	0.992	0.859	0.811	0.834
ResNet50	86	1203	4	270	0.825	0.997	0.956	0.242	0.386
MobileNet	79	1462	11	11	0.986	0.993	0.878	0.878	0.878
Xception	56	1466	7	34	0.974	0.995	0.889	0.622	0.732

the extraction of low-level and high-level features from these images. Using fractional orthogonal polynomials to project the digital frames produced fractional orthogonal moments could extract the digitally provided image's coarse low-level and derived functions. These moments give high precision [37] on deriving from the fractional order of a new orthogonal exponential moment and each COVID-19 input image. Such a method diagnoses COVID-19 cases in the chest X-ray pictures visually. The proposal uses fractional moments to draw functions from COVID-19 X-ray images. A simplified version of manta foraging optimization (OFDM) can be implemented as a function collection tool, followed by using the differential evolution (DE) to adjust it and boost OFDM's ability to identify specific features extracted from the functions. A K-nearest neighbors (KNN) classifier used in the manta-ray foraging optimization and differential evolution (MRFODE) feature selection process decides if a given chest X-ray image is COVID-19 or normal. Compared to the famous CNN architecture MobileNet model, this approach shows similar accuracy indicators, recall, and accuracy rating with the minor features and functionality while tested on two separate data sets. By selecting the essential functions, the method thus achieves both performance and high resource consumption.

10.7.3 X-Ray Images Utilizing Transfer Learning with CNN

Transfer learning is an approach in which information extracted by CNN from considering data is transferred to resolve distinct but relevant tasks, which involve new data, which one is generally a tiny population that forms a CNN start from scratch. This role requires initial CNN training for basic tasks such as classification in deep learning, using an extensive range of data sets. Data availability for initial training is the most important consideration for training for practical work in CNN. CNN can learn and retrieve data from an image to extract essential features. In the next step, CNN can enable a new collection of pictures of various types and extract features based on CNN's feature extraction information during the initial training. Two widely used techniques exist to take advantage of the capacities of pre-trained CNNs. The first approach extracts the function, which is why it is often called extraction of the transfer learning method, which allows a methodology in which the pre-training model maintains both its original architecture and any weights acquired. The second approach in which particular improvements to the pre-trained model produce the best outcomes refers to this technique as a more nuanced process. These changes can involve modifications to the device configuration and parameter adjustments. Only some necessary information gained from the previous tasks is retained in this direction. The most common transfer learning practice in medical activities is CNN applications, which participated in and stood out in the large-scale ImageNet visual recognition competition, which tested algorithms for object identification and large-scale image classification. Data improvement is an important method that can enhance the network's training collection and is primarily employed when only a limited number of samples are used in the testing data set. These are rapid, reproducible, and effective approaches. Effectively, increasing

TABLE 10.5
Accuracy Result Using Different Neural Networks with Transfer Learning

Network	Accuracy 2-Class (%)	Accuracy 3-Class (%)
VGG19	98.75	93.48
MobileNet v2	97.4	92.85
Inception	86.13	92.85
Xception	85.57	92.85
Inception ResNet v2	84.38	92.85

the volume of data will increase CNN training and testing accuracy, minimize losses, and improve the network's robustness. The experiment's results are shown in Table 10.5 [38,39].

10.7.4 Computer Vision and Radiology for COVID-19 Detection

Although a lot of research is ongoing to improve methods for the rapid identification of COVID-19 and to use artificial intelligence to develop its cures, there is still no apparent process that the medications used to diagnose COVID-19 can perform best the information box test of the author. The residual network (ResNet) is better than the previous classification network (such as CNN) to classify the image type of tasks. However, these deep neural networks require large amounts of information to train the model and get the most advanced performance. Adding specific parameters such as hyperparameter learning rate and dropout rate can improve the model's successful outcome. This model typically plays a crucial role in delivering the best results in a shorter period and alleviating overfitting problems [39]. Using X-ray scans to detect the COVID-19 virus, we have implemented a new approach. It is also possible to differentiate between pneumonia patients and COVID-19 because they share the same symptoms and the two patients are also confused by the procedure adopted. Using X-rays to detect COVID-19 is much simpler than COVID-19 medical test kits and as quick as new thermal imaging technology. One can use this technology for the initial scanning of airports, hotels, and shopping malls. Table 10.6 shows a few findings from its trial.

TABLE 10.6
Accuracy Results Using Different ResNet Models

Model	Accuracy	Error Rate
ResNet-34	66.67%	33.33%
ResNet-50	72.38%	27.62%

10.8 FORECASTING MODELS

Different methods and various input sources can do the forecasting. Various forecasting models discussed below are helpful in terms of the detection of COVID-19 diseases.

10.8.1 Big Data

Big data is a large quantity of organized or unstructured data sets. A broad range of fields use big data, including biomedical applications, electronic medical reports (EMRs), intelligent computational means (ICMs) to support patient facilities. Various formats of data, e.g., text or video, are generated from multiple channels, including online media networks, mobile devices, IoT devices, or public data. Inside healthcare systems, machine learning methods for IoT, data mining, and big data technologies are beneficial [40–44]. The big data model also uses its data aggregation capacities to use high volumes of data for early identification to exploit the potential predictability of the COVID-19 outbreak. Colossal data collection, including contaminated patients, from various sources, will lead to large-scale research on COVID-19, which produces detailed and accurate care plans. Data analysis is centered on this analysis, and big data analysis is how several data classes are gathered and processed to find hidden useful trends and other information (such as COVID-19 data discovery).

10.8.2 Social Media Data/Other Communication Media Data

Social networking and Internet searches are the most available channels in this digital era to supply more information on COVID-19. Social networking and web searches are linked to the number of chronic cases of COVID-19. With that in mind, certain researchers have been using data sets from Google, Baidu search engines [45,46], mobile phones [46,47], newspapers [48], and numerous websites [49,50] such as Github [51] for a certain amount of time. These data sets are evaluated using various techniques, i.e., machine learning techniques or mathematical/theoretical stochastic equations based on the parameters discussed previously. Zhu et al. [47] presents a pandemic spatial model for estimating the number of deaths. This analysis aims to construct a statistical model that will evaluate the development of the virus for March, taking into account the current dynamics of COVID-19. The analysis has three separate scenarios: (a) it comprises people who have a history of travel in Wuhan and local people impacted; (b) the degradation rate has also been included in the report to assess various cities' efforts to reduce disease spread; (c) the phone gathers data from town residents who returned from Wuhan, and from the town model, the latest images were used and tested in new cases as early as by February 11, 2020. In the three previous scenarios, to forecast issues before March 13, 2020, the report had predicted a combination of 72,172, 54,285, and 149,675 accidents, respectively. The possible outcome of the analysis is a spatial model. Its projections would undoubtedly increase the distribution of resources in each region over the following month when a pandemic evolves into a severe condition.

10.8.3 Stochastic Theory/Mathematical Models

The standard mathematical and random theory method is used in previous epidemics to estimate human loss and forecast the total number of deaths up to a specific time or end of an epidemic. This conventional approach is very successful and projects better. Then the researchers in [52–57] employed the same traditional procedure for determining the number of deaths and the distribution of COVID in the present epidemiological situation of COVID-19. This strategy has also estimated the overall death rate until the conclusion of the outbreak. Databases from registered or search engines, smartphone data, and media accounts are analyzed. Using mathematical models, Sameni [58] has generated a pattern for the virus. This analysis used a model from the famous segmented model family called the contaminated recovery model. Research has shown that country-specific behaviors impact the mortality rate positively. The infrastructure set up to handle the infections has indeed done a lot to avoid the epidemic outbreak. But this mathematical model has precise drawbacks due to its design for a strained data collection. The study on Boltzmann function by Yuan et al. [59] has shown that vision correction is more straightforward and helps determine the condition's seriousness and respond accordingly—the effect of gender and age on the number of deaths by statistical means. Dowd et al. [60] has shown that this virus affects more older people. The age framework of a nation now plays a vital role in this situation. The threat for countries with similar age systems to Italy, South Korea, is rising more strongly in Italy; 23% of the population is over 65. Policies such as social distancing and quarantine will also help slow the virus's propagation and discourage it. Mathematical simulations in this infection and studying the transmission rate revealed the impact of presymptomatic transmission on mortality. The rate is normally deduced from observation. Transmission peaked on symptoms or before they happened. And before the first signs are physically evident, 44% of propagation is seen. Therefore, while reducing the disease's dissemination, specialists in disease control need to consider the presymptomatic transmission. Some works worth mentioning are [61–66]. Gianakias et al. [61] developed the stochastic principle online health assessment method. The effect of underlying disorders such as heart disease and diabetes on mortality has been shown by Banerjee et al. [62]. Note that Alexander et al. [63], Chen et al. [64], Ma et al. [65], and Shi et al. [66] have introduced the mobility of COVID-19.

10.8.4 Data Science and ML Techniques

Machine learning (ML) techniques are nowadays applied globally. Applications range from household to healthcare, domestic to enterprise, and agriculture to military. In other way, ML-based applications encompass all walks of life [67–69]. In the current scenario, to find the infection rates in China and Italy, Kumar and Himbram [70] introduced a model that is based on the logistics equation, the Weibull equation, and the Hill equation. This research work evaluates data to clarify the effect due to the accuracy of the forecasts. However, there are various difficulties in using machine learning techniques because very few details are usable.

The problems involved in model training are (a) the required parameter collection and (b) prediction selection of the right model for ML. The researchers in [71–75] have used the best ML models in conjunction with the data set given by Kumar and Hembram [70], a model based on the logistic equation, the Weibull equation, and the Hill equation to figure out the rates of Chinese and Italian diseases. Data analysis during this study explains the effect on the COVID-19 distribution of environmental factors. The data analyses took place in four Chinese cities: Beijing, Chongqing, Shanghai, and Wuhan, and four Italian cities, namely Bergamo, Cremona, Lodi, and Milan, where people were more infected. Three environmental variables, namely maximum air temperature, relative humidity, and wind speed, are specifically discussed in this report. The statistics were from the WHO's survey in China and Italy. The findings indicate that moisture and wind speed have no relationship to COVID-19 propagation.

More temperatures have a "slight to moderate effect" on virus dissemination. However, there is no indicator that the weather has a direct impact on the virus. Based on the data collection, however, findings can differ. A model that uses regression, driven grading trees, and a hybrid model that uses Medicare data is suggested by DiCaprio et al. [7]. These models' outcomes help to initiate management techniques and take corrective steps to control their time distribution. It is clear from the literary analysis that both studies took data from structured data sources. However, no acquisition organization or its partner organizations have yet structured the data sets. These experiments have neglected to handle spatial and statistical deviations into account. However, these may be helpful for improved forecasting. The literature discusses the effect on the distribution of COVID-19 of environmental and mobility variables. The various stages of the COVID-19 epidemic are well illustrated [48], as it will help to minimize the rate of spread by understanding the steps of an outbreak. Different models of machine learning in literature are studied. Deep learning models [48] may therefore be utilized to achieve improved forecasts and more accuracy. Moreover, predictions can be rendered more precisely by using active learning models on these crowded, interactive data [76] instead of a single projected form.

10.9 DATA-DRIVEN ANALYTICAL MODELS OF COVID-19

Although hospitals, charities, governments, and organizations worldwide have been publicizing several databases and studies, full literature review and data compilation are missing. They are not complete from an empirical point of view to segmented data analysis at the first level of the COVID-19 study. This study is conferred, for example, an early March 2020 prediction model. The virus evolves rapidly, resulting in an incorrect measurement of pathogens. This section covers the most current data sets and sample projections.

10.9.1 Exponential Model

The number of infectious patients would escalate rapidly over time without successful responses (such as in the early stages of a pandemic). Equation 10.8 determines the diagnostic data sequence of pathogens.

$$I(t) = I(0) \times e^{rt} \tag{10.8}$$

I(t) is the number of infections diagnosed over time and r is the rate of growth that is obtainable from the observed data when the model runs. The authors analyzed the exponential model, but the forecast does not have credible figures because of the active government reactions.

10.9.2 Logistic Model

Compared to the exponential model, the logistic growth model functions almost exponentially at the beginning. In contrast, the growth is almost unregulated as you reach the upper end of the form, called the load power, and the rate decreases. Equation 10.9 gives growth in the logistic model [77].

$$I(t) = \frac{N}{1 + e^{b-c(t-t_0)}} \tag{10.9}$$

Where I (t) is the total number of confirmed cases, N is the maximum predicted number of confirmed cases (population carrier capacity), b and c are the coefficients of modifications obtainable from the current data collection, t_0 is the time when the first outbreak was detected, and t is the number of days following the first case. The disease patterns have been forecast by related regression and logistic production models in [6,28,78–82]. The researchers in these works suggested, for example, a sectoral model of Poisson, which has incorporated a force law and an exponential law to determine shooting. However, the model reliably forecasts the last pandemic scale based on the recent COVID-19 developments worldwide.

10.9.3 SIR Model

The susceptible and susceptible contagious recovered (SIR) model [6] explains infectious diseases' movement among persons in five states: susceptible, infectious, and recovered that can be distributed as follows [79].

$$\frac{dS(t)}{d(t)} = -\frac{\beta}{N} \times S \times I \tag{10.10}$$

$$\frac{dI(t)}{d(t)} = \left(\frac{\beta}{N} \times S - \gamma\right) \times I \tag{10.11}$$

$$\frac{dR(t)}{d(t)} = \gamma \times I \tag{10.12}$$

Where β, γ are the transmission and recovery rate, respectively. The expression N = S + I + R is a constant. Thus, the primary reproduction number R_0 in the SIR model is below.

$$R_0 = \frac{\beta}{\gamma}\left(1 - \frac{I_0}{N}\right) \tag{10.13}$$

The SIR model has many variations in literature as a standard model for predicting COVID-19. An updated epidemiological approach [83], for example, the susceptible exposed removed (SEIR) model, was seen in the Chinese New Year in respect of the mass inhabitants of Wuhan by incorporating motion-in, moving-out, in(t), and out(t). A stochastic SIR (SSIR) model [84] brings randomness into the forecast.

10.9.4 MetaWards

Authors in [85] have modified the existing stochastic disease propagation model metabolism to forecast the possible timing of the COVID-19 increase in England and Wales. The population of this model is split into elections. The authors believed the persons contributing at night and during the day to the contagion of the "domestic" pavilion. A fixed transmission rate for a variable transmission rate over time is substituted to predict the possible low transmission rate over the summer months. Equalization transmission rate r is defined in Equation 10.14.

$$r = \beta \times \left(1 - \frac{m}{2} \times \left(1 - cos\frac{2\pi t}{365}\right)\right) \tag{10.14}$$

Where m denotes the seasonal transmission variation varies from 0 (non-seasonal) to 1 (extreme seasonality without summer transmission). However, the MetaWards model didn't take COVID-19 strategies into account, along with seasonal variables, which resulted in significant infection patterns.

10.9.5 SIDARTHE

The work in [86] suggests a more detailed model called the SIDARTHE model, which takes into account several phases of S-sensitive (uninfected) infection; D: diagnosed (asymptomatic infected, undetected); A: ailing (infected symptoms, undetected); R: recognized (infected symptoms, detected); T: endangered (infecting with life-threatening symptoms, detected); H: healed (recovered); E: extinguished (dead) [6]. Figure 10.7 shows SIDARTHE's stage transitions. It consists precisely of eight ordinary differential equations, which model population evolution at each point. The population at each stage and Greek letters as parameters are positive figures. The rate of transmission is between S and I, D, A, and R is α, β, γ, and δ. The probabilities of asymptomatic and symptomatic instances of and θ are, respectively, detectable. An infected subject's degree of likelihood is not aware of and learns of infection is ζ and η. The μ and v show the chances of unrecognized and

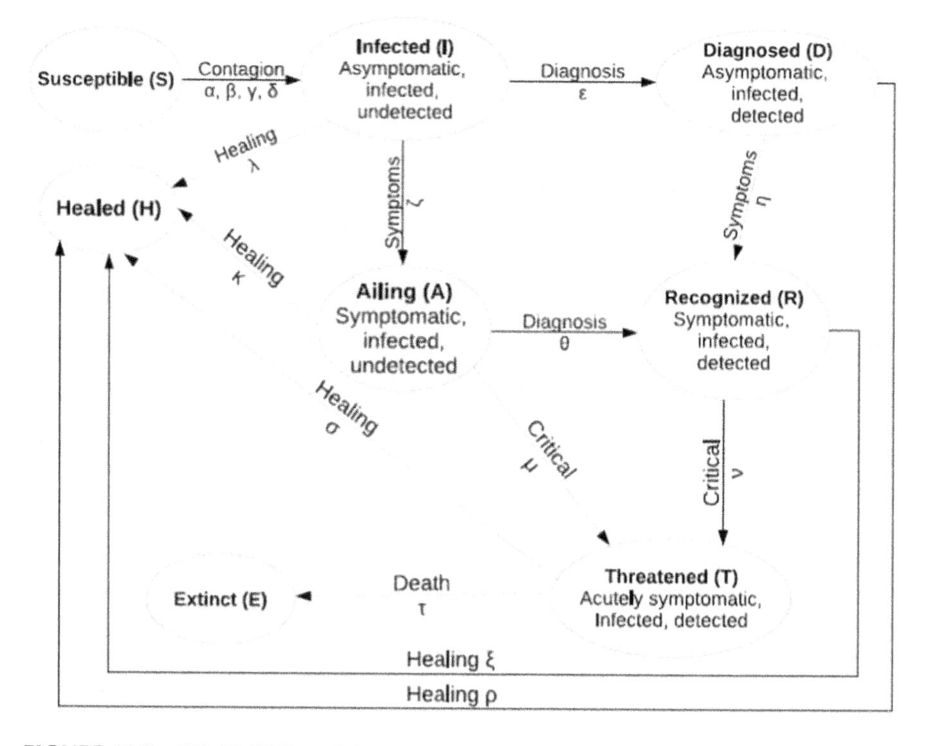

FIGURE 10.7 SIDARTHE model as an SIR model.

observed compromised participants having extreme symptoms. The death rate is τ. The survival rate of patients in five groups (S, I, D, A, and R) is λ, κ, ξ, ρ, and σ. Figure 10.7 refers to a pictorial representation of the SIR model.

10.10 VISUALIZING TRENDS OF COVID-19

When the outbreak was in its nascent stage, anything was difficult to predict. A few days' or weeks' assessments can capture any particular trend—the pattern studies concerns the virus's spread in different weather and geographical locations. The directions were quite interesting across age groups. The death rate increased with an increase in age, and patients with comorbidities were more vulnerable. The death rate plays a crucial role in visualized data. There are several ways one could imagine this trend. Data visualization helps in making complicated things look simpler to both professionals and the public. The professionals include data scientists, physicians, chemists, etc. The trend dictates the movement of people in their town. There have been several heatmaps made in various levels, including city, district, state, country, and international levels. The heat map shows the areas affected by the virus. They give an idea about to what extent the infection can spread in a locality. Several such graphs and maps have made the public understand a simple way to spread the disease. The crowd, in general, can now understand the various forms of analyzing the data visualized by statisticians as they have gotten used to it.

10.11 CHALLENGES IN DATA COLLECTION

Artificial intelligence has gained great potential in the global fight against the current pandemic. The challenges will continue to be addressing solutions in the future, in addition to the apparent benefits. Furthermore, many challenges are there in data collection, as learned, and provide study groups and experts with some recommendations.

10.11.1 Regulation

Different approaches are introduced to contain the disease, such as confinement, social segregation, detection, and large-scale testing, with the epidemic's outbreak and the tremendous rise in reported cases every day. In this way, regulators play a crucial role in defining policies that facilitate individuals, scientists and researchers, companies, giant technologies, and major corporations and coordinate different entities' execution to eradicate hurdles and obstacles. As far as this challenge is concerned, from the first confirmed COVID-19 case to the current scenario, many attempts have been made. South Korea's quarantine policy is one example, which will take effect on April 1, 2020. In particular, all passengers entering South Korea must be put under quarantine at their registered address or assigned address facility for 14 days. Besides, all passengers must carry out a self-test twice a day and send information on their cell phones using the self-test program that is enabled. The Seoul metropolitan government launched a calling device for artificial intelligence tracking to automatically check people's health who do not have a mobile phone or have not installed self-diagnosis software. Zhejiang's provincial government and the Alibaba DAMO Academy jointly developed an artificial intelligence platform for automatic COVID-19 study and research groups.

10.11.2 Data Inefficiency

The lack of standard data sets has created considerable difficulties in finding a stable response against the COVID-19 virus for AI and big data systems and applications. Several artificial intelligence algorithms and big data platforms are not tested against the same data set mentioned in the preceding sections. For example, it has been observed that the algorithms in [6,87] achieved 82.90–98.27% precision, 80.50–97.60% specificity, and 84–98.93% sensitivity, respectively. However, two data sets with different sample sizes cannot decide which algorithm is more suitable for virus detection. Furthermore, most of the data sets found in the literature are generated by personal efforts. Most data sets are collected on the Internet, for example, and then consolidated to construct their own data sets and test using the algorithms developed already. Governments, giant corporations, and healthcare institutions (such as the WHO and CDC) have played a crucial role in solving this problem so they can collaborate to access massive high-quality data sets. These agencies may generate various data points, such as hospital X-rays and CT scans, satellite data, personal records, and self-diagnostic application notes. For instance, Georgetown Security Center and other partners (such as the All AI Institute, the Chen Zuckerberg Project, Microsoft Research, and the National Institutes of Health) maintain the COVID-19 data set. Furthermore, the Alibaba DAMO Academy has partnered with many hospitals in China to set up an AI initiative to classify COVID-19 infected cases. Among them, the Alibaba DAMO Academy is responsible for developing the AI algorithm, and the hospital supports over 5,000 confirmed CT scans for coronavirus 2019 viral disease cases. The machine has recently been used by more than 20 hospitals in China because of its outstanding performance, hitting 96% accuracy in just 20 seconds. A shared data set of medical images of COVID-19 can be maintained as a personal initiative, and a global database of COVID-19–based open access projects can be accessed at [88].

10.11.3 Privacy

Today, the important thing is to keep people healthy and control the situation as soon as possible. However, how to protect the security and privacy of personal data is still needed. The Zoom video conferencing app security and privacy scandal is one manifestation of this challenge. Authorities may encourage their workers to share their data in a pandemic, such as the location of GPS, CT scans, medical history, routes of transport, and daily routines so that the situation gets controlled, followed by establishing new policies and decisions for emergency action. Data is a requirement for any artificial intelligence and big data platform to be efficient. However, where there is no statutory requirement, persons do not necessarily wish their confidential information to be exchanged. There are privacy/security and efficiency trade-offs.

10.12 CONCLUSION AND FUTURE SCOPE

Studying this chapter aims to reduce the testing time and increase the model's accuracy to minimize the false negative and false positive cases, making it easier for the middlemen and experts to conduct tests and make it automated. The extended goal must build a custom neural network architecture inspired by existing great neural network complex architectures. Since AI and cloud computing are on the rise, there is a considerable scope of improvement in this outbreak. The data is available in significant amounts to study the trend and visualize it using various techniques. But as one explores the data available for patients who underwent any of the two COVID-19 tests and X-ray/CT scans, the tested patients' composition is noticed. A few challenges faced so far by different researchers working in this domain are noted down: (1) The number of negative cases (both false negatives and true negatives) is overwhelming, more than the number of positive cases (true positives and true negatives); (2) another challenge that exists is a fewer number of images in the public domain. Due to massive data set's unavailability, it becomes difficult to train a model to have good testing accuracy. Some authors have trained a data set having 13,975 images and had an accuracy of 93.3%. This accuracy can certainly increase using a better neural network design; (3) a patient who has the disease but tested negative can cause huge problems. A false positive case is mainly tolerated, but they form a tiny percentage of the total data combined with the false negatives. The area of improvement is surely bringing down the number of falsely detected cases. However, this will bring out only a marginal increase in the overall accuracy. But the crucial part of this improvement is the decrease of falsely detected cases. This can be done by making use of custom neural network architecture. An architecture built using transfer learning techniques and complex and sophisticated neural networks designed for computer vision problems with very high accuracy, hyper-parameter tuning, etc., can learn the classification problem much more efficiently and accurately. A newly designed method may help reduce the chaos that false detections and predictions of the disease can cause. What motivates us to take up this problem is its relevance and promising result, and to tackle this disease a little more wisely in the future.

REFERENCES

[1] X. Wang, X. Deng, Q. Fu, Q. Zhou, J. Feng, H. Ma, W. Liu, and C. Zheng, "A weakly-supervised framework for COVID-19 classification and lesion localization from chest ct," *IEEE Transactions on Medical Imaging* 39, no. 8 (2020): 2615–2625.

[2] X. Ouyang, J. Huo, L. Xia, F. Shan, J. Liu, Z. Mo, F. Yan, Z. Ding, Q. Yang, B. Song, F. Shi, H. Yuan, Y. Wei, X. Cao, Y. Gao, D. Wu, Q. Wang, and D. Shen, "Dual-sampling attention network for diagnosis of COVID-19 from community acquired pneumonia," *IEEE Transactions on Medical Imaging* 39, no. 8 (2020): 2595–2605.

[3] Y. Peng, Y. Tang, S. Lee, Y. Zhu, R. M. Summers, and Z. Lu, "Covid-19-ct-cxr: A freely accessible and weakly labeled chest x-ray and ct image collection on COVID-19 from biomedical literature," *IEEE Transactions on Big Data* 7, no. 1 (2021): 3–12.

[4] G. Jain, D. Mittal, D. Thakur, and M. K. Mittal, "A deep learning approach to detect COVID-19 coronavirus with x-ray images," *Biocybernetics and Biomedical Engineering* 40, no. 4 (2020): 1391–1405.

[5] N. Sharma, S. G. Ila Kaushik, B. Bhushan, and A. Khamparia, "Applicability of wsn and biometric models in the field of healthcare," in *Deep Learning Strategies for Security Enhancement in Wireless Sensor Networks* (A. D. A. K. Martin Sagayam, B. Bhushan and V. H. C. de Albuquerque, eds.), ch. 6, pp. 304–329, Hershey, PA: IGI Global, (2020).

[6] Y. Mao, S. Jiang, and D. Nametz^, "Data-driven analytical models of covid-2019 for epidemic prediction, clinical diagnosis, policy effectiveness and contact tracing: A survey," (2020). 10.36227/techrxiv.12613355.

[7] W. H. Organization et al., "Who director-general's remarks at the media briefing on 2019-ncov on 11 february 2020," (2020).

[8] K. Singh and A. Agarwal, "Impact of weather indicators on the COVID-19 outbreak: A multi-state study in india," (2020). 10.1101/2020.06.

[9] "Reported cases and deaths by country, territory, or conveyance". Available at: https://www.worldometers.info/coronavirus.

[10] "Reported cases and deaths in Bharat by coronavirus". Available at: https://www.worldometers.info/coronavirus/country/Bharat/.

[11] "Current COVID-19 cases in Bharat". Available at: https://cdn.who.int/media/docs/default-source/wrindia/situation-report/india-situation-report-57.pdf?sfvrsn= ee392ca6_4.

[12] "Reported cases and deaths by bharat". Available at: https://www.covid19india.org/.

[13] R. F. Sear, N. Vel´asquez, R. Leahy, N. J. Restrepo, S. E. Oud, N. Gabriel, Y. Lupu, and N. F. Johnson, "Quantifying COVID-19 content in the online health opinion war using machine learning," *IEEE Access*, 8 (2020): 91886–91893.

[14] R. Sethi, M. Mehrotra, and D. Sethi, "Deep learning based diagnosis recommendation for covid19 using chest x-rays images," in 2020 Second International Conference on Inventive Research in Computing Applications (ICIRCA), pp. 1–4, (2020).

[15] Y. LeCun, B. Boser, J. S. Denker, D. Henderson, R. E. Howard, W. Hubbard, and L. D. Jackel, "Backpropagation applied to handwritten zip code recognition," *Neural Computation*, 1, no. 4 (1989): 541–551.

[16] F. Shi, J. Wang, J. Shi, Z. Wu, Q. Wang, Z. Tang, K. He, Y. Shi, and D. Shen, "Review of artificial intelligence techniques in imaging data acquisition, segmentation, and diagnosis for COVID-19," *IEEE Reviews in Biomedical Engineering* 14 (2021): 4–15.

[17] K. Suzuki, "Overview of deep learning in medical imaging," *Radiological Physics and Technology* 10, no. 3 (2017): 257–273.

[18] I. Goodfellow, Y. Bengio, A. Courville, and Y. Bengio, *Deep Learning*, vol. 1. MIT press, Cambridge, (2016).

[19] A. E. Eltoukhy, I. A. Shaban, F. T. Chan, and M. A. Abdel-Aal, "Data analytics for predicting COVID-19 cases in top affected countries: Observations and recommendations," *International Journal of Environmental Research and Public Health* 17, no. 19 (2020), p. 7080.

[20] A. A. Hussain, O. Bouachir, F. Al-Turjman, and M. Aloqaily, "Ai techniques for COVID-19," *IEEE Access* 8 (2020): 128776–128795.

[21] A. Khamparia, D. Gupta, K. Shankar, A. Slowik and A. E. Hassanien, *Cognitive Internet of Medical Things for Smart Healthcare. Springer Nature Switzerland AG*: Springer International Publishing, Switzerland, (2021).

[22] D. Shen, G. Wu, and H.-I. Suk, "Deep learning in medical image analysis," *Annual Review of Biomedical Engineering* 19 (2017): 221–248.

[23] A. Khamparia, P. K. Singh, P. Rani, D. Samanta, A. Khanna and B. Bhushan, "An internet of health things-driven deep learning framework for detection and classification of skin cancer using transfer learning," *Transactions on Emerging Telecommunications Technologies* 1 (2020): 1–11.

[24] L. Wang, Z. Q. Lin, and A. Wong, "Covid-net: A tailored deep convolutional neural network design for detection of COVID-19 cases from chest x-ray images," *Scientific Reports* 10, no. 1 (2020): 1–12.

[25] S. Chaganti, A. Balachandran, G. Chabin, S. Cohen, T. Flohr, B. Georgescu, P. Grenier, S. Grbic, S. Liu, F. Mellot, et al., "Quantification of tomographic patterns associated with COVID-19 from chest ct," *arXiv preprint arXiv:2004.01279*, (2020).

[26] Z. Tang, W. Zhao, X. Xie, Z. Zhong, F. Shi, J. Liu, and D. Shen, "Severity assessment of coronavirus disease 2019 (COVID-19) using quantitative features from chest ct images," *arXiv preprint arXiv:2003.11988*, (2020).

[27] X. Zhong, F. Deng, and H. Ouyang, "Sharp threshold for the dynamics of a sirs epidemic model with general awareness-induced incidence and four independent brownian motions," *IEEE Access* 8 (2020): 29648–29657.

[28] X. Zhou, X. Ma, N. Hong, L. Su, Y. Ma, J. He, H. Jiang, C. Liu, G. Shan, W. Zhu, et al., "Forecasting the worldwide spread of COVID-19 based on logistic model and seir model," *MedRxiv*, (2020).

[29] C. Bayes, L. Valdivieso, et al., "Modelling death rates due to COVID-19: A bayesian approach," *arXiv preprint arXiv:2004.02386*, (2020).
[30] M. Magdon-Ismail, "Machine learning the phenomenology of COVID-19 from early infection dynamics," *arXiv preprint arXiv:2003.07602*, (2020).
[31] X. Wang, Y. Peng, L. Lu, Z. Lu, M. Bagheri, and R. M. Summers, "Chestx-ray8: Hospital-scale chest x-ray database and benchmarks on weakly-supervised classification and localization of common thorax diseases," in 2017 IEEE Conference on Computer Vision and Pattern Recognition (CVPR), pp. 3462–3471, (2017).
[32] O. Ronneberger, P. Fischer, and T. Brox, "U-net: Convolutional networks for biomedical image segmentation," in International Conference on Medical image computing and computer-assisted intervention, pp. 234–241, Springer, Sarıyer - İstanbul/Turkey, (2015).
[33] X. Zhang, L. Yao, D. Zhang, X. Wang, Q. Z. Sheng, and T. Gu, "Multi-person brain activity recognition via comprehensive eeg signal analysis," in Proceedings of the 14th EAI International Conference on Mobile and Ubiquitous Systems: Computing, Networking and Services, MobiQuitous 2017, (New York, NY, USA), p. 28–37, Association for Computing Machinery, (2017).
[34] S. Kumar, B. Bhusan, D. Singh, and D. k. Choubey, "Classification of diabetes using deep learning," in 2020 International Conference on Communication and Signal Processing (ICCSP), pp. 0651–0655, (2020).
[35] T. Pham, "A Comprehensive Study on Classification of COVID-19 on Computed Tomography with Pretrained Convolutional Neural Networks," *Scientific Reports* 5 (2020): 16942 https://doi.org/10.1038/s41598-020-74164-z
[36] N. Zamzami, P. Koochemeshkian, and N. Bouguila, "A distribution-based regression for real-time COVID-19 cases detection from chest x-ray and ct images," in 2020 IEEE 21st International Conference on Information Reuse and Integration for Data Science (IRI), pp. 104–111, IEEE, (2020).
[37] M. A. Elaziz, K. M. Hosny, A. Salah, M. M. Darwish, S. Lu, and A. T. Sahlol, "New machine learning method for image-based diagnosis of COVID-19," *Plos One* 15, no. 6 (2020), p. e0235187.
[38] I. D. Apostolopoulos and T. A. Mpesiana, "Covid-19: automatic detection from x-ray images utilizing transfer learning with convolutional neural networks," *Physical and Engineering Sciences in Medicine* 43, no. 2 (2020): 635–640.
[39] R. Punia, L. Kumar, M. Mujahid, and R. Rohilla, "Computer vision and radiology for COVID-19 detection," in 2020 International Conference for Emerging Technology (INCET), pp. 1–5, (2020).
[40] C. Bhatt, N. Dey, and A. S. Ashour, "Internet of things and big data technologies for next generation healthcare," Springer, Cham, (2017).
[41] A. E. Hassanien, N. Dey, and S. Borra, *Medical Big Data and internet of medical things: Advances, challenges and applications*. CRC Press, (2018).
[42] K. Lan, D.-t. Wang, S. Fong, L.-s. Liu, K. K. Wong, and N. Dey, "A survey of data mining and deep learning in bioinformatics," *Journal of Medical Systems* 42, no. 8 (2018): 1–20.
[43] A. Jain and V. Bhatnagar, "Concoction of ambient intelligence and big data for better patient ministration services," *International Journal of Ambient Computing and Intelligence (IJACI)* 8, no. 4 (2017): 19–30.
[44] M. Jindal, J. Gupta, and B. Bhushan, "Machine learning methods for iot and their future applications," in *2019 International Conference on Computing, Communication, and Intelligent Systems (ICCCIS)*, pp. 430–434, (2019).
[45] L. Li, Z. Yang, Z. Dang, C. Meng, J. Huang, H. Meng, D. Wang, G. Chen, J. Zhang, H. Peng, et al., "Propagation analysis and prediction of the COVID-19," *Infectious Disease Modelling* 5 (2020): 282–292.

[46] S. Lai, I. I. Bogoch, N. W. Ruktanonchai, A. Watts, X. Lu, W. Yang, H. Yu, K. Khan, and A. J. Tatem, "Assessing spread risk of wuhan novel coronavirus within and beyond china, january-april 2020: a travel network-based modelling study," *MedRxiv*, (2020).

[47] X. Zhu, A. Zhang, S. Xu, P. Jia, X. Tan, J. Tian, T. Wei, Z. Quan, and J. Yu, "Spatially explicit modeling of 2019-ncov epidemic trend based on mobile phone data in mainland china," *MedRxiv*, (2020).

[48] D. Giuliani, M. M. Dickson, G. Espa, and F. Santi, "Modelling and predicting the spread of coronavirus (COVID-19) infection in nuts-3 italian regions," *arXiv preprint arXiv:2003.06664*, (2020).

[49] C. Anastassopoulou, L. Russo, A. Tsakris, and C. Siettos, "Data-based analysis, modelling and forecasting of the COVID-19 outbreak," *PloS One* 15, no. 3 (2020) p. e0230405.

[50] C. Li, L. J. Chen, X. Chen, M. Zhang, C. P. Pang, and H. Chen, "Retrospective analysis of the possibility of predicting the COVID-19 outbreak from internet searches and social media data, china, 2020," *Eurosurveillance* 25, no. 10 (2020), p. 2000199.

[51] J. Bayham and E. P. Fenichel, "The impact of school closure for COVID-19 on the us healthcare workforce and the net mortality effects". *Lancet Public Health* 5, (2020): e271–e278. 10.1016/S2468-2667(20)30082-7

[52] P. Magal and G. Webb, "Predicting the number of reported and unreported cases for the COVID-19 epidemic in south korea, italy, france and germany," *Italy, France and Germany* (March 19, 2020), 2020.

[53] A. Victor, "Mathematical predictions for COVID-19 as a global pandemic," Available at SSRN 3555879, (2020).

[54] H. Wang, Y. Zhang, S. Lu, and S. Wang, "Tracking and forecasting milepost moments of the epidemic in the early-outbreak: framework and applications to the COVID-19," *F1000Research* 9 (2020).

[55] A. E. Botha and W. Dednam, "A simple iterative map forecast of the COVID-19 pandemic," *arXiv preprint arXiv:2003.10532*, (2020).

[56] F. C. Coelho, R. M. Lana, O. G. Cruz, C. T. Codeco, D. Villela, L. S. Bastos, A. P. y Piontti, J. T. Davis, A. Vespignani, and M. F. Gomes, "Assessing the potential impacts of COVID-19 in brasil: mobility, morbidity and impact to the health system," *medRxiv*, (2020).

[57] A. Weber, F. Ianelli, and S. Goncalves, "Trend analysis of the COVID-19 pandemic in china and the rest of the world," *arXiv preprint arXiv:2003.09032*, (2020).

[58] R. Sameni, "Mathematical modeling of epidemic diseases; a case study of the COVID-19 coronavirus," *arXiv preprint arXiv:2003.11371*, (2020).

[59] Y. Gao, Z. Zhang, W. Yao, Q. Ying, C. Long, and X. Fu, "Forecasting the cumulative number of COVID-19 deaths in china: a boltzmann function-based modeling study," *Infection Control & Hospital Epidemiology* 41, no. 7 (2020): 841–843.

[60] J. B. Dowd, L. Andriano, D. M. Brazel, V. Rotondi, P. Block, X. Ding, Y. Liu, and M. C. Mills, "Demographic science aids in understanding the spread and fatality rates of COVID-19," *Proceedings of the National Academy of Sciences* 117, no. 18 (2020): 9696–9698.

[61] V. Giannakeas, D. Bhatia, M. T. Warkentin, I. Bogoch, and N. M. Stall, "Estimating the maximum daily number of incident COVID-19 cases manageable by a healthcare system," *MedRxiv*, (2020).

[62] A. Banerjee, L. Pasea, S. Harris, A. Gonzalez-Izquierdo, A. Torralbo, L. Shallcross, M. Noursadeghi, D. Pillay, C. Pagel, W. K. Wong, et al., "Estimating excess 1-year mortality from COVID-19 according to underlying conditions and age in england: a rapid analysis using nhs health records in 3.8 million adults," *MedRxiv*, (2020).

[63] A. F. Siegenfeld and Y. Bar-Yam, "Eliminating COVID-19: A community-based analysis," *arXiv preprint arXiv:2003.10086*, (2020).
[64] B. Chen, H. Liang, X. Yuan, Y. Hu, M. Xu, Y. Zhao, B. Zhang, F. Tian, and X. Zhu, "Roles of meteorological conditions in COVID-19 transmission on a worldwide scale," *MedRxiv*, (2020).
[65] Y. Ma, Y. Zhao, J. Liu, X. He, B. Wang, S. Fu, J. Yan, J. Niu, J. Zhou, and B. Luo, "Effects of temperature variation and humidity on the death of COVID-19 in wuhan, china," *Science of the Total Environment* 724 (2020) p. 138226.
[66] P. Shi, Y. Dong, H. Yan, X. Li, C. Zhao, W. Liu, M. He, S. Tang, and S. Xi, "The impact of temperature and absolute humidity on the coronavirus disease 2019 (COVID-19) outbreak-evidence from china," *MedRxiv*, (2020).
[67] P. Pattnayak and O. P. Jena, *Innovation on Machine Learning in Healthcare Services–An Introduction*, ch. 1, pp. 1–15. John Wiley & Sons Ltd., (2021).
[68] K. Paramesha, H. Gururaj, and O. P. Jena, *Applications of Machine Learning in Biomedical Text Processing and Food Industry*, ch. 10, pp. 151–167. John Wiley & Sons, Ltd, (2021).
[69] N. Panigrahi, I. Ayus, and O. P. Jena, *An Expert System-Based Clinical Decision Support System for Hepatitis-B Prediction & Diagnosis*, ch. 4, pp. 57–75. John Wiley & Sons, Ltd, (2021).
[70] J. Kumar and K. Hembram, "Epidemiological study of novel coronavirus (COVID-19)," *arXiv preprint arXiv:2003.11376*, (2020).
[71] S. James Fong, E. Herrera Viedma, et al., "Finding an accurate early forecasting model from small data set: A case of 2019-ncov novel coronavirus outbreak," (2020).
[72] M. Batista, "Estimation of the final size of the second phase of the coronavirus COVID-19 epidemic by the logistic model," (2020).
[73] H. Z, "Evaluating the effect of public health intervention on the global-wide spread trajectory of covid19," (2020).
[74] L. Jia, K. Li, Y. Jiang, X. Guo, et al., "Prediction and analysis of coronavirus disease 2019," *arXiv preprint arXiv:2003.05447*, (2020).
[75] D. DeCaprio, J. Gartner, T. Burgess, S. Kothari, and S. Sayed, "Building a COVID-19 vulnerability index," *arXiv preprint arXiv:2003.07347*, (2020).
[76] K. Santosh, "Ai-driven tools for coronavirus outbreak: need of active learning and cross-population train/test models on multitudinal/multimodal data," *Journal of Medical Systems* 44, no. 5 (2020): 1–5.
[77] L. Jia, K. Li, Y. Jiang, X. Guo, et al., "Prediction and analysis of coronavirus disease 2019," arXiv preprint arXiv:2003.05447, (2020).
[78] K. Wu, D. Darcet, Q. Wang, and D. Sornette, "Generalized logistic growth modeling of the COVID-19 outbreak: comparing the dynamics in the 29 provinces in china and in the rest of the world," *Nonlinear Dynamics* 101, no. 3 (2020): 1561–1581.
[79] D. T´atrai and Z. V´arallyay, "Covid-19 epidemic outcome predictions based on logistic fitting and estimation of its reliability," *arXiv preprint arXiv:2003.14160*, (2020).
[80] L. Kriston and L. Kriston, "Projection of cumulative coronavirus disease 2019 (COVID-19) case growth with a hierarchical logistic model," *Bull World Health Organ*, (2020).
[81] R. Huang, M. Liu, and Y. Ding, "Spatial-temporal distribution of COVID-19 in china and its prediction: A data-driven modeling analysis," *The Journal of Infection in Developing Countries* 14, no. 03 (2020): 246–253.
[82] X. Zhang, R. Ma, and L. Wang, "Predicting turning point, duration and attack rate of COVID-19 outbreaks in major western countries," *Chaos, Solitons & Fractals* 135 (2020) p. 109829.

[83] Z. Yang, Z. Zeng, K. Wang, S.-S. Wong, W. Liang, M. Zanin, P. Liu, X. Cao, Z. Gao, Z. Mai, et al., "Modified seir and ai prediction of the epidemics trend of COVID-19 in china under public health interventions," *Journal of Thoracic Disease* 12, no. 3 (2020) p. 165.

[84] A. Simha, R. V. Prasad, and S. Narayana, "A simple stochastic sir model for covid 19 infection dynamics for karnataka: Learning from europe," *arXiv preprint arXiv:2003.11920*, (2020).

[85] L. Danon, T. House, and M. J. Keeling, "The role of routine versus random movements on the spread of disease in great britain," *Epidemics* 1, no. 4 (2009): 250–258.

[86] G. Giordano, F. Blanchini, R. Bruno, P. Colaneri, A. Di Filippo, A. Di Matteo, and M. Colaneri, "Modelling the COVID-19 epidemic and implementation of population-wide interventions in italy," *Nature Medicine* 26, no. 6 (2020): 855–860.

[87] S. Wang, B. Kang, J. Ma, X. Zeng, M. Xiao, J. Guo, M. Cai, J. Yang, Y. Li, X. Meng, et al., "A deep learning algorithm using ct images to screen for corona virus disease (COVID-19)," *MedRxiv*, (2020).

[88] F. Hu, J. Jiang, and P. Yin, "Prediction of potential commercially inhibitors against sars-cov-2 by multi-task deep model," *arXiv preprint arXiv:2003.00728*, (2020).

11 Deep Learning and Multimodal Artificial Neural Network Architectures for Disease Diagnosis and Clinical Applications

Jeena Thomas and Ebin Deni Raj
Indian Institute of Information Technology, Kottayam, Valavoor, Kerala, India

CONTENTS

DOI: 10.1201/9781003189053-11

11.1 INTRODUCTION

Different technologies were introduced and adopted in the medical field, thereby resulting in expanded automation. Artificial intelligence (AI), or machine intelligence, has been identified as the most important technology for medical diagnosis and clinical applications [1]. It can solve various medical challenges at different levels of difficulty in complex medical operations. Checking for anomalies and suggesting proper medical intervention is one of the benefits of AI in clinical applications. AI presents rapid innovations in clinical areas and evaluates information and clinical reports. If a digital database is used to store patients' data, it can be utilized for further diagnosis, and an appropriate software can be developed to automate the various operations in a hospital. It facilitates more informed decisions regarding the patient and also provides excellent services accordingly.

AI provides digital automation with rapid and steady outcomes. It also aids in virtual interaction with doctors; thereby, the healthcare industry becomes efficient in solving various challenging tasks. For a complicated surgery, AI systems can provide accurate and fast responses despite the hectic schedules of medical practitioners. It can check, organize, and observe strategies with improved effectiveness and minimum risk of errors. AI performs a prominent role in scanning technologies like X-rays, magnetic resonance imaging (MRI), and computed tomography (CT) [1]. Medical imaging, automatic electrocardiogram (ECG), medical laboratory evaluation, respiratory tracking, and anesthesia are the other significant application areas of AI in medical diagnosis. A variety of large data sets are generated in the medical field, and accurate processing of this information is essential.

The introduction of technologies in the medical field has resulted in the digitization of patients' health records as electronic health records (EHRs) [2]. Earlier, a clinical resolution aiding system was developed on the rule-based approach for illness prediction and diagnosis. The emergence of smartphone apps, biometric models [3], and Internet of Things (IoT) devices [4] that can monitor the human body is one of the greatest innovations of AI. Nowadays, wearable sensors can track physiological parameters of the human body over a longer period of time [5]. Image-based medical diagnosis is one of the successful domains of artificial intelligence application in the healthcare sector, and most of the medical disciplines rely on the same. Medical image computing, a domain of scientific computing mainly used for image-based diagnosis, predominantly works on a mathematical model that uses the techniques of artificial intelligence such as machine learning and deep learning.

The motivation of this chapter is to furnish a comprehensive and exhaustive summary of prominent technologies existing in the domain of disease diagnosis as well as clinical applications. This chapter provides an intuition to the popular technologies used in healthcare for ailment analysis and prediction. This study is an exploration of all the prevailing and latest technological applications in healthcare using artificial intelligence, machine learning, deep learning, and deep neural network architectures. Our aim is to suggest a framework capable of experimental evaluation, which can be used for disease prediction and labeling. We have contributed a hybrid model involving restricted Boltzmann machine (RBM) and long short term memory (LSTM) for effective disease prediction and semantic labeling. The proposed model will help healthcare practitioners ease labeling of medical images and reduce their workload.

The remaining part of the chapter is structured as follows: Section 11.2 specifies the various technologies used in the healthcare sector. Section 11.3 gives an overview of the various applications of artificial intelligence and emphasizes its key applications in healthcare. Section 11.4 discusses different algorithms of machine learning which are mainly used in clinical applications. Section 11.5 considers the deep learning approach for diagnosing diseases in various medical disciplines. Section 11.6 explains the various deep neural network architectures in the medical field and clinical diagnosis. Section 11.7 illustrates the hybrid models of machine learning and deep learning in the medical field, while also specifying its experimental results. Section 11.8 explains the proposed mathematical model for disease prediction and labeling using the integrated approach of RBM and LSTM. Section 11.9 concludes the study.

11.2 TECHNOLOGIES IN HEALTHCARE SECTOR

The digitization flow of the global medical system predicts that the processed medical services' facts are expected to generate large exabytes of fresh data in 2020 [2]. A huge amount of this healthcare data and lack of insights from these big data is one major problem in the current scenario. The central and current technologies that solve the problems of the medical field and clinical applications are: a) artificial intelligence, b) machine learning, c) deep learning, and d) deep neural networks.

An efficient diagnostic system based on artificial intelligence techniques is required for processing big data in medical diagnosis and clinical applications. In order to efficiently discover the knowledge from big data generated from the healthcare sector, we require some algorithms and mechanisms of deep learning and machine learning. An overview of various technologies used in the healthcare sector is illustrated in Figure 11.1. This chapter discusses AI's application in the healthcare industry and various machine learning techniques for implementing artificially intelligent systems in the medical field. It also provides the basic understanding and latest applications of deep learning and various deep neural network architectures in medical diagnosis and clinical operations.

11.3 APPLICATIONS OF ARTIFICIAL INTELLIGENCE IN HEALTHCARE

Game playing, heuristics, expert systems, natural language processing (NLP), and machine learning are the main application areas of AI. Expert systems work on

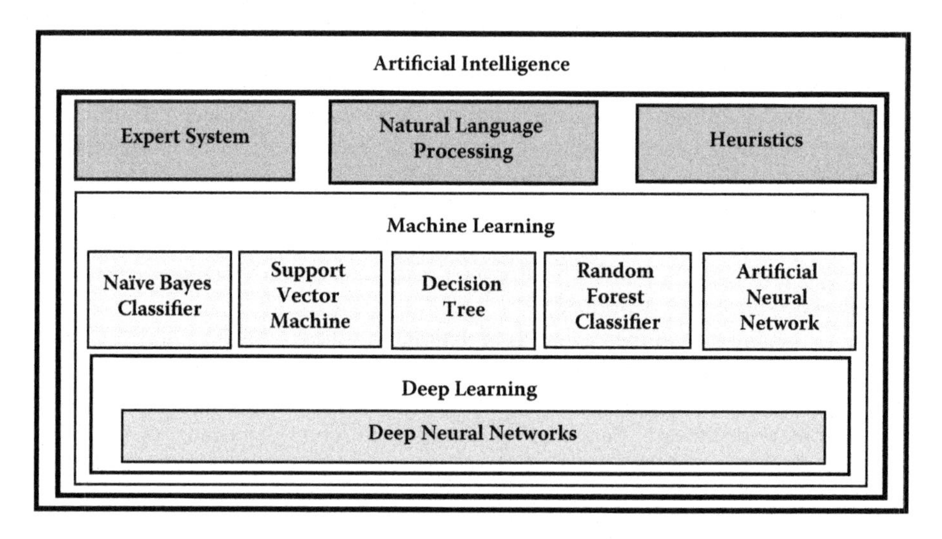

FIGURE 11.1 Overview of technologies in the healthcare sector.

domain specific knowledge, which combines problem recognition and a group of heuristic problem fixing regulations. To develop such systems, knowledge should be gained from a human domain expert, and the AI specialist is responsible for imposing this aptitude in a program. Mycin is an expert system that uses expert clinical knowledge to determine bacterial disease of the blood and spinal meningitis. Artificial intelligence helps doctors achieve efficient healthcare tasks like disease diagnosis, drug development, surgery, radiology, hospital administration, and medical records. The various benefits of artificial intelligence in disease diagnosis and clinical applications are represented in Figure 11.2.

Guo et al. proposed a novel artificial intelligent system, which helps the clinical establishments to procure trusted clinical-assisted prognosis models, thereby

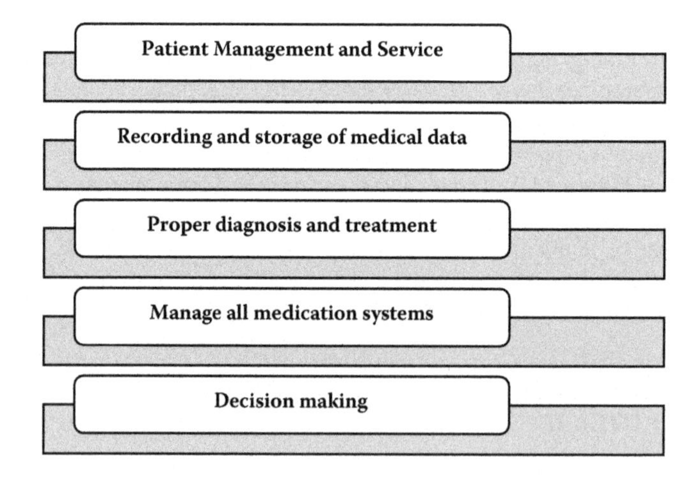

FIGURE 11.2 AI in healthcare.

minimizing the task of doctors and improving the efficiency of medical organizations [6]. AI can be used within the area of radiology for the automated functions of image acquisition, assessment of image quality, image interpretation, reporting, and management. The various applications of AI in medical imaging are clearly explained by Chassagnon et al. in the field of chest radiography for thoracic imaging, such as lung nodule evaluation, quantification of diffuse lung diseases, tuberculosis, and pneumonia detection [7]. As reported by the Global Burden of Disease (GBD) in 2016, stroke is identified as one of the major reasons for global mortality. Ma et al. made a detailed study about the recent and current advances of AI in the sphere of strokes with AI-established examination, forecasting, decision making, medication, and recovery [8].

Barricelli et al. narrated a novel technology called digital twin (DT), its application in the medical field, like hospital management and precision medicine, and also analyzed its state-of-the-art definitions [9]. Bouletreau et al. investigated AI applications in orthognathic surgery, especially in maxillofacial imagery, treatment planning, custom orthodontic and surgical appliances, and treatment follow-up [10].

11.4 MACHINE LEARNING TECHNIQUES IN THE HEALTHCARE SECTOR

Machine learning (ML) is an approach of AI that models the computer system to carry out unique projects without specific instructions and instead depends on patterns and reasoning. Learning can be of three types: supervised, unsupervised, and reinforcement learning. In supervised learning, the machine learns with guidance and uses labeled data to notify the input and output. A target output is present and it is tested with the obtained output. Regression and classification problems come under supervised learning. For predicting a continuous quantity, regression is used, whereas classification problems are mainly used to predict a label for a class. Discovering the patterns is the primary element related with the unsupervised approach. Here, the input is provided, which is then explored for the hidden patterns to find the output. The data is not labeled and there is no target output. Unsupervised learning mainly deals with association and clustering problems. Consequently it discovers the patterns in data and co-occurrence. In clustering, the data will be grouped based on similarity. Reinforcement learning follows the hit and trial concept. There is an agent and it is put in an unknown environment. This agent has to explore the environment by taking actions and making transitions from one state to another to get maximum rewards.

Artificial intelligence and machine learning have progressed in the healthcare industry. They play an essential role in the healthcare industry, especially in medical image processing, segmentation, interpretation, recapture, inspection, image fusion, and computer-aided analysis. Machine learning systems extract information from images and represents the information effectively and competently. AI and ML techniques can assist doctors so that they can predict diseases faster and more accurately [11–13]. Machine learning techniques involve conventional algorithms like Naïve-Bayes classifier, support vector machine, decision trees, random forest classifier, and artificial neural networks. The healthcare industry is generating massive amounts of data that need to be mined to discover the hidden patterns that can be used for effective prediction, classification, and decision making.

11.4.1 Naïve-Bayes Classifier

Naïve-Bayes classifiers are statistical classifiers that can anticipate probabilities of class membership that a given pattern belongs to a specific case. Classification based on this method depends on the Bayes' theorem. One advantage is that it needs very little information for categorization. Using Bayes' theorem, the target class's posterior probability can be calculated as

$$P(H|F) = \frac{P(F|H)P(H)}{P(F)} \tag{11.1}$$

It is proportional to $P(F|H)$, predictor class's probability, where $P(H)$ is class H's probability of being true and $P(F)$ is the predictor's prior probability.

The Naïve-Bayesian approach is used for breast cancer prediction, where it classifies patients as benign and malignant. Non-cancerous patients are marked benign and cancerous patients fall under the malignant group. Orphanou et al. developed a Naïve-Bayes classification model incorporated with temporal association rules for the prognosis of cardiovascular disease [14]. A hybrid model consisting of Naïve-Bayes classifier and K-nearest neighbour algorithms was implemented to recognize epileptic seizures against EEG signals. To predict the function of an obscure protein, Sinha et al. used the Naïve-Bayes classifier for the evaluation of the *Leishmania donovani* parasite that causes a deadly sickness, Visceral Leishmaniasis, in humans [15].

11.4.2 Support Vector Machines

A support vector machine (SVM) is used to segregate linear as well as non-linear data, and a hyperplane may partition the data from different classes. A SVM finds the hyperplane using support vectors and margins. This technique is significantly less prone to overfitting when compared to other ML techniques and can be used for prediction and classification. For constructing an optimal hyperplane and to minimize error, a SVM performs iterative training algorithm. For a binary categorization task *{a, b}* where *a* indicates data points and *b* as corresponding labels separated by hyperplane is represented in equation (11.2).

$$W^T a + c = 0 \tag{11.2}$$

where W is coefficient vector which is normal to hyperplane and c is offset from the origin.

Timely forecasting of liver afflictions is remarkable because the proper functioning of the liver is crucial for optimum health. It plays a vital role in metabolism, including some critical functions like the decomposition of red blood cells.

Joloudari et al. proposed a computer assisted resolution making system for the diagnosis of liver disorder using particle swarm optimization (PSO) integrated with a SVM by selecting significant features [16]. Breast cancer is considered as an exponentially rising malady among women in developing nations. A report by the National Cancer Registry says that this disease is significantly prevalent in the urban communities of India such as Delhi, Mumbai, Ahmadabad, and Chennai. Vijayarajeswari et al. explored the early detection of breast cancer with the Hough transform and SVM classifier [17]. The Hough transform is employed for feature identification in mammogram images and the latter is utilized for classification. An efficient system for classifying medical data using SVM and fruit fly optimization algorithm (FOA) was proposed and evaluated on the Parkinson data set, the Pima Indians diabetes data set, breast carcinoma data set, and the thyroid disease data set. Tuberculosis (TB) is another substantial problem in many developing countries due to socioeconomic factors. In accordance with the World Health Organization's (WHO) Global Tuberculosis Report, TB is the ninth main cause of demise worldwide. For the effective treatment of TB, a SVM is used as a classification algorithm. A novel multi-classified system was developed for disease diagnosis with sequential minimal optimization (SMO), a variation of a SVM, which acts as a base classifier along with elephant herding optimization (EHO) that considers the parameters like cost and tolerance.

11.4.3 Decision Trees

Tree-based learning algorithms are acknowledged as one of the greatest supervised learning methods. Decision tree is an algorithm that contains only conditional control statements where internal node represents test on attributes and leaf nodes represent class labels. The route from root to leaf nodes indicates the classification rule. The procedure of dividing into two or more subnodes is known as splitting. The process to reverse splitting is called pruning. Using the parameters, information gain and entropy with an approach of divide and conquer, a decision tree is constructed. The purity and impurity of data instances can be measured with a parameter known as entropy. Entropy for a given set of examples S, containing negative and positive instances of a target output can be measured as:

$$H(S) = \sum_{j=1}^{a} P_j \log_2 P_j \tag{11.3}$$

where H indicates entropy, P_j represents the probabilistic frequency of occurrence of class j, which could be positive or negative. In the medical field, decision trees are used with prioritization of emergency for patients' treatment. It builds a predictive model considering diverse aspects like age, gender, the severity of pain, and location. The most commonly used decision trees are ID3, C4.5, C5.0, and CART. The ID3 algorithm designs decision tree occupies information gain, whereas C4.5 is based on gain ratio.

Complication during pregnancy has turned out to be another complicated problem for women. During gestation, women might undergo various psychological changes and severe health problems, which sometimes lead to the death of the mother and the fetus. Pregnant women should be protected from these complications. A C4.5 classifier is effectively used for predicting the respective risks related to pregnancy. A hybrid model was developed to predict type 2 diabetes; J48 decision tree is used for classification and K-means clustering algorithm is used for data reduction and tested on Pima Indians Diabetes data set. A hierarchical decision tree was induced in a standard single nucleotide polymorphism (SNP) database, which reduces communication overhead and scales well with data volume and dimension. Zhang et al. devised a Gaussian-based decision tree (GDT) for effective classification and representation of biosignals of sample sizes that are extremely small [18].

11.4.4 Random Forest Classifier

Random forest classifier uses numerous decision trees during the training phase and generates the mean prediction of individual trees. It is a supervised learning technique that uses collective learning algorithms for improving performance. Random forest classifier creates forests with an arbitrary volume of trees that reveal the root node and subdivide the features randomly. Consider the input set M and corresponding output set N; the random forest tries to determine the correlation between M and N that requires a learning data set of $L=\{(M_1, N_1), (M_2, N_2), \ldots, (M_n, N_n)\}$. To discover the finest split of the set, the data is broken up into different subsets during training of each node on a splitting criterion, α which is moved to the child nodes a and b. The information gain that is used to estimate the best split over a set of samples S_n can be calculated by equation (11.4):

$$Information\ Gain(\alpha) = R(S_n) \sum_{i=a}^{b} \frac{|S_i(\alpha)|}{|S_n|} R(S_i(\alpha)) \tag{11.4}$$

where R evaluates randomness of sample S.

Brain computer interface (BCI) is one of the prominent disciplines in recent years which allows communication between the brain and external devices. BCI reads different signals from the brain and recognizes the various mental states. Random forest classifier is used to construct a BCI model to foresee mental conditions like meditation and concentration. Since diabetes is considered to be one of the deadliest diseases affecting humans, and it may also create severe complications in pregnant women, early detection is the only preventive remedy. Three different ML classification algorithms, such as Naïve-Bayes, decision tree, and SVM, have been applied to predict diabetes in patients. Zabihi et al. used random forest classifier to detect atrial fibrillation (AF), which leads to irregular heartbeats that may result in blood clots and stroke, by monitoring ECG [19]. A combined approach of discrete state Markov model and random forest classifier was used for the detection of AF in sole lead electrocardiogram, and the tested results showed the highest sensitivity value.

11.4.5 Artificial Neural Networks

Artificial neural network (ANN) mimics the functionality of the human brain, which contains multiple neurons and mathematically formalizes the computation of the brain. The human brain processes information through billions of interconnected neurons. The first neural network, McCulloch Pitts (MP) neuron, was introduced in 1943. It is primarily used to implement logic gates and also used to solve linearly separable problems. The key characteristics of this neural network is that there exists no training algorithm in order to calculate the output. The weights and thresholds are analytically determined. Perceptron, another variant of neural network introduced by Rosenblatt in 1958, solves only linear separable problems. Multi-layer perceptron (MLP) has been introduced to solve many non-linear and complex problems to overcome this difficulty. It includes three distinct layers such as input, hidden, and output layers. To train these neural networks, many epochs are usually performed with a new input sample by adjusting weights and bias.

The major mathematical concept related to ANN is: a set of inputs x_i, weight vector W_i, net input net_{in}, activation function f and output y. Consider input x as $\{x_1, x_2, \ldots, x_n\}$, weight vector w as $\{w_1, w_2, \ldots, w_n\}$ and bias parameter b, the net input net_{in} can be calculated as

$$net_{in} = \sum_{i=1}^{n} x_i w_i + b \tag{11.5}$$

The output for the neural network is computed by applying the activation function over net input.

$$y = f\,(net_{in}) \tag{11.6}$$

An artificial neural network system based on MLP model was developed by aiding security for medical chips that have the ability to classify between genuine and fake glucose measurement. An efficient machine learning system was developed with the combined approach of grasshopper optimization algorithm (GOA) and multi layer perceptrons (GOAMLP) and applied over the data sets of patients of orthopaedic disorders, coronary heart disease, Parkinson's disease, diabetes, and breast cancer. An adaptive MLP framework was used for effective noise removal in X-ray medical images based on a principal component decomposition algorithm by estimating additive white Gaussian noise (AWGN) measure. Kumar et al. deployed multi layer feed forward neural network (MLFF) for diabetes classification and validated it with Monte-Carlo cross method [20].

11.5 DEEP LEARNING APPROACH IN HEALTHCARE

Doctors and radiologists analyze the medical images for the diagnosis of various diseases. However, these interpretations are limited due to the complexity of the image and human factors like eye fatigue. Deep learning technology provides a solution with reasonable accuracy for medical imaging. Initially, in the 1980s, medical image inspection was accomplished with mathematical modeling and low-degree pixel processing. Mathematical models are used to construct an expert system which is a rule-based system. Later, for medical image scrutiny, researchers have used many handcrafted features for extraction.

The past ten years have observed a gigantic rise in medical data. Moreover, it has been generated in the mode of diagnostic images, genomic sequences, and protein structures. The diagnostic images from various sources like fundus and endoscopy images can make use for disease identification, anomaly detection, organ dissection, and reconstruction. There should be an efficient framework to save, inspect, and elucidate such data. Deep learning (DL), a subset of ML, will shed the light for these challenging problems. The advancements in machine learning and deep learning together with the use of ANN creates a paradigm shift in every sector of the healthcare industry and turns out to be the research that garners a majority of the limelight. Deep learning techniques play a key role in reshaping the medical area with the necessary improvements and innovations. It has wide applications in the spheres of clinical imaging, bioinformatics, medical information science, and communal well-being. Table 11.1 describes some domains of healthcare with deep learning techniques.

TABLE 11.1
Deep Learning in Healthcare Applications

Dermatology [21]	Used deep learning algorithms trained with convolutional neural network to classify suspicious lesions
Radiology [22]	With variants of convolutional neural networks, developed a DL architecture, machine assisted bone age labeling (MABAL)
Oncology [23]	Analyzed three types of malignant growths, namely tubercular cancer, abdomen adenocarcinoma, and mammary glands carcinoma, with proposed deep learning ensemble model
Ophthalmology [24]	Developed Caffe-AlexNet based deep neural network for computer-aided diagnosis (CAD) based diabetic retinopathy
Angiology [25]	Using deep learning techniques, the pathogenesis of rheumatoid arthritis (RA) with cardiovascular (CV) events and atherosclerosis imaging were analyzed
Pediatrics [26]	Developed a prognosis system to record auscultation of heart sounds to find out pediatric congenital heart diseases (CHDs)
Nephrology [27]	Deep learning based convolutional neural network for segmentation of digitized kidney tissue sections by calculating dice coefficients for ten tissue classes
Neurology [28]	Deep learning technique was used to determine seizure control after epilepsy surgery on examining the whole brain structural connectome
Cardiology [29]	Deep learning framework which detects automated cardiogram arrhythmia by categorizing sufferer's signal with AlexNet, a variant of convolutional neural network, into corresponding cardiac conditions

(Continued)

TABLE 11.1 (Continued)
Deep Learning in Healthcare Applications

Obstetrics-Gynecology [30]	To detect preterm birth (PTB) early, deep learning was used for characteristics extraction and distribution of electro hysterogram between gestation and labour class
Anesthesiology [31]	Recurrent neural network based deep learning framework for immediate prediction of future blood pressures after the induction of anesthesia
Otolaryngology [32]	Deep learning system was developed for the treatment of auricle disease by training 10,544 otoendoscopic images with CNN which classifies ear infections
Plastic Surgery [33]	A novel deep CNN called RhinoNet for classifying rhinoplasty images to predict the status of rhinoplasty
Sports Medicine [34]	A DL framework using 3D CNN was developed for detecting complete anterior cruciate ligament (ACL) tears
Pathology [35]	Deep learning framework with CNN for automatic topographical information extraction from a collection of thoracic and breast tumor pathology descriptions
Precision Medicine [36]	Early detection of disease findings and medical image computing can be incorporated with DL in precision and preventive medicine
Psychiatry [37]	Deep learning approach for predicting and assessing the outcome of antidepressant treatment in major depressive disorder (MDD)
Surgery [38]	Deep learning system was proposed to detect and track surgical instruments by CNN for minimally invasive surgery
Anthropology [39]	A deep neural network was implemented for the gender identification of human remains from cranium images and attained an accuracy of 95 percentage
Gastroenterology [40]	A deep neural network with deep Boltzmann machine (DBM) was used to predict accurate morbidity of gastrointestinal infection based on 129 types of pollutants contained in soil and water with Gaussian mixture model (GMM)
Histopathology [41]	A single system was developed to reveal colorectal cancer and mammary cancer by segmenting epithelial (EP) and stromal (ST) regions from histopathological images
Veterinary Medicine [42]	Deep learning framework to differentiate diverse tumors on canine MRI using GoogLeNet, a variant of CNN
Dental Medicine [43]	Deep learning system was proposed to diagnose tooth decay with GoogLeNet Inception v3 CNN network

Deep learning techniques have gained significant attention in the research world for two main reasons: first, the advancement of big data techniques has resolved the overfitting problem, and secondly, deep neural networks undergo pretraining procedures.

11.6 DEEP NEURAL NETWORK ARCHITECTURES IN THE MEDICAL FIELD

Research on ANN stagnated after the 1960s owing to the short competence of trivial architectures and restriction in computational capability. Formerly, the system of deep learning was constructed in the late 1980s. With the improvement of the computational facilities, ANN with efficient backpropagation was introduced for pattern recognition. As the backpropagation with gradient descent approach often gets trapped at local optima and it also suffers from the dilemma of overfitting because of small size of the data, adding more hidden layers to the neural network results in the creation of deep neural network (DNN) capable of solving more complex and non-linear problems. Hence, DNN has provided a new evolutionary approach to deep learning, and it can be trained with supervised as well as unsupervised methods.

The high computational demand for training and processing with hardware limitations have made DNNs impractical for many real world applications. Recent advances in hardware, parallelization through GPU acceleration, and multi-core processing enable the introduction of various DNNs, which is considered a significant breakthrough in artificial intelligence.

11.6.1 Convolutional Neural Network

A convolutional neural network (CNN) is a class of deep neural networks mainly used for the examination of images. By representative attributes, CNN learns the relationship among pixels of images using convolution and pooling layers. Suppose an image matrix of dimension $a \times b \times d$ and a filter of size $fa \times fb \times fd$ and convolution operation performs dot products between the weights. The main advantages of the convolution operation are weight sharing mechanism, local connectivity of input topology, and shift invariance. Weight distribution procedure is useful to associate with excessive spatial data such as two dimensional or three dimensional images and videos. Rectified linear unit (ReLU), the activation function is applied to introduce non-linearity in CNN and represented as $f(x) = max(0, x)$. The pooling layer uses multiple filters to perform feature extraction from images, and it also reduces a wide variety of criterion when the images are too big. For dimensional reduction, spatial pooling or downsampling is used. The fully connected layer is responsible for the final result of CNN and performs image recognition.

For fetching comparable images and medical history, a medical image retrieval system with CNN is used, allowing the medical practitioners to decide important findings of diseases. Sulieman et al. used CNN to construct features from patient portal messages consisting of multi-set words and multi-set phrases [44]. The messages were classified into different categories such as logistical, social, informational, and medical. With the advancement of endoscopic surgery, the recorded videos of performed surgery can be revisited to be used for analysis, documentation and education. For these purposes, doctors need to manually search the video shots and annotate them, which is a tedious and time consuming process.

Alexnet, a variant of CNN, is used to classify video shots that were evaluated on gynecologic surgery videos. A new system was proposed by Nadimi et al. using ZF-Net, which is an improved version of CNN, to detect and locate colorectal polyps from images of wireless colon capsule endoscopy; this proposed DNN has gained much greater accuracy [45].

11.6.2 Restricted Boltzmann Machine

A restricted Boltzmann machine (RBM) is the graphical representation of probability distribution with respect to the inputs. It is a divergent of Boltzmann machines, by a condition that the neurons should be in the form of a bipartite graph and this architecture is successful for dimensionality reduction and collaborative filtering. RBM is considered as a stochastic model with Markov random fields consisting of visible and hidden layers. For training the RBM, Boltzmann sampling is adopted and weights are calculated by maximum likelihood estimate (MLE).

A spatio-temporal feature extraction model was used for establishing medical motion sequences of the human skeleton configured with RBM [46]. Tran et al. implemented electronic medical record (EMR)–based non-negative RBM (eNRBM) for representing medical object which involves minimal human supervision [47]. For learning image features, RBM is used with an unsupervised learning approach. Nguyen et al. introduced a novel model, tensor-variate RBM (TvRBM), for EEG-based alcoholic diagnosis with fewer parameters [48]. A deep learning system based on RBM was introduced for classifying motor imagery which is an important aspect of BCI that EEG can measure.

11.6.3 Deep Belief Networks

Deep belief network (DBN) is a deep network with a stack of various RBMs introduced to discover the relationship between hidden and visible variables. In DBN, the visible layers of all RBM is linked to hidden layers of preceding ones. Sequential training of different RBM layers is performed from lower to upper layers with two main stages: pretraining and fine tuning. The former phase is an unsupervised algorithm used for feature extraction and carries out in bottom-up fashion. The latter stage contains a supervised learning algorithm performing further adjustment of network parameters in an up-down order. After extracting features from the upper layer, it is propagated back to the lower ones. The most significant advantage with DBN is that unlabeled data can be processed effectively and underfitting and overfitting problems can be circumvented. The principle behind DBN is weight and prior distribution over hidden vectors. The probability of producing visible vector can be represented in equation (11.7).

$$p(v) = \sum_{h} (p(h|w)p(v|h, w)) \tag{11.7}$$

where w indicates weight and $p(h|w)$ is prior distribution in hidden vectors. The expectation of visible and hidden units can be calculated using gibbs sampling, but this computation is time consuming to update all visible units. So a faster gradient-based algorithm was introduced to pretrain DBN as contrastive divergence (CD) algorithm by Hinton in 2012. DBN becomes competent when compared to other neural networks because it is a fine-tuned NN with multiple nonlinear hidden layers and generally pretrained.

An automated system for confirmation of breast carcinoma was developed using a pretrained unsupervised neural network with DBN which was tested on relevant data sets. The supremacy of the method is that it does not require the manifold space to be locally linear and a predefined similarity measure. DBN, which consists of a three-layered stack of RBMs, was used to classify electrocardiogram signal quality as noisy and clean signals. Wan et al. instigated a prediction algorithm based on DBN for the early detection of intestinal cancer [49]. DBN was used to help doctors discriminate autism spectrum disorders in young children or infants even before the exhibition of the behavioral symptoms and suggest better medication. An investigation of DBN was conducted for electroencephalography for various applications of medicine like seizure detection, sleep stage classification, and emotion recognition.

11.6.4 Autoencoder

Autoencoder (AE), or auto associator, is an unsupervised learning model which is mainly used for the dimensionality reduction of the data set. AEs are composed of an encoder, which converts input data into latent representation and a decoder, which performs reconstruction over this code. The conventional autoencoder is ANN, which allows minimal reconstruction error. The key distinction between MLP and AE is that the former predicts outputs based on inputs, whereas AE will reconstruct the inputs. Consider the input vector $x \in [0,1]^a$ and input-output mapping is represented in equation (11.8).

$$y = f_{\beta}(x) = \sigma(W_x + b_v) \tag{11.8}$$

where $\beta = \{W, bv\}$, W is weight vector, σ represents sigmoid activation function, and b_v is bias vector.

Since image denoising is a significant step in medical image processing, denoising autoencoders were constructed with convolutional layers for efficient denoising of medical images. Autoencoders have a wide mixture of operations on health services especially in medical image processing techniques like medical images segmentation, image reconstruction, and analysis of tomographical images to diagnose various diseases. To solve image reconstruction problem in electrical capacitance tomography (ECT), an autoencoder was proposed with an encoder and decoder unit of four layers each. Computer-aided diagnostic (CAD) classification system was developed to predict the chance of rejection of kidney transplant, which may result in complications like bleeding and infection, by distinguishing between repudiated and competent kidney transplantation. Stacked sparse autoencoder (SSAE) was designed for automatic nuclei revelation to predict mammary gland carcinoma from cellular pathology images by grading tissue specimens [50].

11.6.5 Recurrent Neural Networks

India has 18% of the world's population, but according to the Global Burden of Disease Study (GBD), India bears 32% of the global burden of respiratory diseases. Pollution is the biggest contributor to this disease burden. If the doctor thinks that there is an issue with the lungs, the location and type of certain breathing sounds can possibly help figure out the cause. Auscultation of the lungs is an important respiratory examination and helps diagnose various lung diseases. The high-pitched whistling noise that can occur while breathing in or out is known as wheezing. Doctors typically use a stethoscope to detect the breath sounds of the patient. Faint heart murmurs and rales in the lungs might lead to a false diagnosis. The recurrent neural network (RNN) is trained with analyzing the breathing sounds to ease the examination by the cardiologists. RNN has the ability to remember the events that happened in the past, and that can be used to predict future outcomes. This principle can be used in medical diagnosis to ascertain the status of the patient based on previous clinical data sets. The output of the RNN can be calculated as

$$y = \sigma(W_O h_t) \tag{11.9}$$

where W_O is a matrix contains parameters of the model, h_t a vector contains hidden states of the neural network, σ is the logistic sigmoid activation function. The hidden state of the RNN, based on current input, x_t can be represented as

$$h_t = f(h_{t-1}, x_t) \tag{11.10}$$

The major drawback to the standard RNN is that it cannot track the long term dependencies because of the vanishing gradient problem. Long short term memory (LSTM) resolves this issue and is suitable for many applications, especially in sequential data involving the medical diagnosis. Sequential data, like sounds, involve certain challenges and these were addressed with the use of sequence to sequence autoencoders with RNN. RNN-based deep learning framework was developed to detect chronic respiratory diseases by detecting abnormal respiratory sounds like wheezes and crackles. Kwon et al. successfully implemented a visual analytics tool on electronic medical records known as RetainVis based on interpretable deep learning, XAI (explainable artificial intelligence), and interactive artificial intelligence for increasing interactivity and interpretability of RNN [51].

11.6.6 Long Short Term Memory

Long short term memory (LSTM) is a variant of RNN mainly used to capture long-term dependency problems and also reduces the problem of the vanishing gradient. The architecture of LSTM consists of multiple gates and is generally referred to as vanilla LSTM. The mathematical model of LSTM can be represented in equation (11.11):

$$s_i = x_i W_{xh} + x_{i-1} W_{hh} + b \tag{11.11}$$

The output of the hidden units can be calculated as

$$h_i = \sigma(s_i) \tag{11.12}$$

where x_i indicates the input variable.

$$z_i = hW_{h0} + b \tag{11.13}$$

The expected output of LSTM can be calculated and represented in equation (11.14):

$$y = \sigma(z_i) \tag{11.14}$$

where W_{xh}, W_{hh}, and W_{h0} are weight matrices; b indicates bias vectors; and s_i and z_i represent the temporary variables.

LSTM structures' variants include unidirectional LSTM, bidirectional LSTM, stack LSTM, and fully connected LSTM. An integrated architecture of LSTM and CRF was proposed to extract the necessary information from electronic medical records (EMRs). A novel architecture with bidirectional LSTM proposed is bidirectional LSTM model with symptoms frequency position attention (BLSTM-SFPA) in healthcare as a networked clinical smart query responding system [52]. It performs experiments on the NCBI Disease data set and gained a higher F1 score. To annotate medical concepts like diseases and drugs, an integrated architecture of LSTM and conditional random fields was presented with three layers: CRF layer, word-based Bi-LSTM, and character-based Bi-LSTM layer [53]. A comparative evaluation of RNN and LSTM was made to diagnose dyslipidemia in steel workers and found out that LSTM outperforms RNN [54].

11.6.7 Generative Adversarial Nets

Goodfellow et al. put forward an advanced framework, generative adversarial nets (GANs), which was inspired by game theory, for estimating a generative model with an adversarial process corresponding to a minmax two-player game [55]. The architecture consists of dual paradigms: generator and discriminator, the former taking over the data distribution (d_{dis}), whereas the latter calculates the probability of a sample (S) occurring from the training input. The speciality of GAN is that it does not require any unrolled approximate inference networks or Markov chains during training or generation of samples. Radford et al. proposed deep convolutional GAN (DCGAN), a variant of GAN, where both the generative and discriminator models are CNNs [56]. The job of the discriminator is to distinguish between real and fake images.

Consider an input sample x, following a data distribution of P_{data}, and the probability of output being real is $R(x)$. The generator, G, gets an input sample z out of a known probability distribution $prob_z$ typically a rectangular function and maps $G(z)$ into the image volume with distribution P_I. The generator's objective is to make the distribution of image space and data distribution of sample space equal($P_I = P_{data}$). For images, input sample approximates to data distribution, the D maximizes $R(x)$, else it minimizes $R(x)$. To trick the discriminator, the generator produces images $G(z)$ such that it is trained to maximize the probability, $R(G(Z))$. As the training progresses, the generator will generate more realistic images and the discriminator, D will have the ability to discriminate real and fake images. The D receives images from the generator and creates the probability distribution as $p(S|X) = D(X)$.

Odena et al. introduced a variant of GAN which involves label conditioning called auxiliary classifier GAN(AC-GAN) [57]. For assessing image quality, AC-GAN generates image samples with 128×128 resolution which exhibits global coherence. GAN was employed effectively to learn insanity in humans from the generated images of the brain and this method attained better accuracy [58]. Bellemo et al. discussed the advantages, trends, and limitations of GANs in retinal fundus image synthesis [59].

11.7 HYBRID APPROACH OF MACHINE LEARNING AND DEEP LEARNING TECHNIQUES

The advanced development of deep learning and machine learning techniques has made a significant place in the healthcare industry for the diagnosis of very complex diseases. CNN deals with spatial data, whereas RNN works with temporal kind of data, and a combination of these networks can be used effectively for classifying various diseases. The combined architectures is mainly used for the applications like image captioning and video captioning. The combination of CNN and LSTM was used in the field of brain computer interface (BCI) for analyzing EEG signals with the help of motor imagery. In order to make the segmentation more consistent and robust, a hybrid architecture that includes both deep convolutional and recurrent neural networks was used for the detection and tracking of surgical scenes with semantic segmentation. This architecture outperforms the many current methods because it addresses certain issues like the presence of shadows, reflection, occlusion, and blurriness.

To fully exploit the long term dependencies between image and image labels Liang et al. designed an Xception-LSTM framework for blood cell image classification [60]. For efficient processing of medical data, the techniques of machine learning and deep learning can be combined for better results. Data pre-processing mechanisms like dimensionality reduction and noise removal can be exerted over the patients' data sets. Khamparia et al. utilized four various pretrained deep learning architectures for effective detection and classification of skin cancer [61]. The composite algorithms can be applied over the data and their performance can be evaluated based on various measures. A comparative analysis of results can be made for efficient and better decision making. The experimental results of hybrid models using deep learning and machine learning for disease diagnosis and clinical operations is shown in Table 11.2.

TABLE 11.2
Hybrid Models in the Medical Field

References	Hybrid Models	Disease Diagnosis	Experimental Results
[62]	CNN + DBN	Lung Cancer	Sensitivity = 94%
[63]	CNN + SVM	Oesophageal Cancer	Average precision = 92.74%
[64]	CNN + XGBoost algorithm	Skin Cancer	Mean sensitivity = 89%
[65]	Autoencoder + Deconvolution NN	Liver Metastasis	Average execution time = 3.68 seconds
[66]	Genetic Algorithm + Random Forest	Oesophageal cancer	Accuracy = 82% AUC = 0.823
[67]	Neural network + Genetic Algorithm	Coronary Artery Disease	Accuracy = 93.85% Sensitivity = 97% Specificity = 92%
[68]	Simple Recurrent Units + Gated Recurrent Units	Activity recognition of physically impaired/ elderly people	Accuracy = 99.80%
[69]	CNN + PSO + Fuzzy C-Means	Malignant melanoma	Dice score = 87.03%
[70]	CNN+Random Forest (RF) classifier	Gastrointestinal Stromal Tumor	AUC= .882 Sensitivity = 73.7% Specificity = 95.4% Accuracy = 83.2%
[71]	DNN based on automated Hyperparameter Optimization(AutoHPO) + Random Forest Regression	Cerebral Stroke	Accuracy = 71.6% Sensitivity = 67.4%
[72]	Chronological sine cosine Algorithm based DNN + Fuzzy C Means Algorithm	Acute Lymphocytic Leukemia (ALL)	Accuracy = 98.7%
[73]	AlexNet + VGG16 + VGG19 + DT + kNN + SVM	Pneumonia	Accuracy = 99.41%
[74]	ANFIS + Multiple Kernel Learning(MKL)	Heart Disease	Sensitivity = 98% Specificity = 99%
[75]	DNN + SVM	Retinal Diseases	Accuracy = 89.73%
[76]	MLP + Lagrangian Support Vector Machine (LSVM)	Parkinson's Disease	AUC = 1
[77]	CNN + GMM	Alzheimer's disease	Accuracy = 90.47% Recall = 86.66% Precision = 92.59%
[78]	VGG16 + MobileNet	Lymphoblastic Leukemia	Accuracy = 96.17% Sensitivity = 95.17% Specificity = 98.58%
[79]	CNN + RNN	Alzheimer's Disease	AUC = 0.91
[80]	AlexNet + SVM	Alzheimer's Disease	Accuracy = 96.39%
[81]	CNN + GAN	Lung Cancer	Specificity =77.8% Sensitivity = 93.9%

11.8 MATHEMATICAL MODEL OF MULTIMODAL NEURAL NETWORK FOR DISEASE PREDICTION AND LABELING

Accurate prediction of diseases by selecting a region of interest and corresponding labeling of medical images is a crucial step in disease diagnosis and clinical applications. The labeling of a large set of medical images is quite a tough task since it is time consuming and requires well-experienced doctors. To tackle these concerns, a conceptual framework was proposed for disease prediction and labeling from the medical image data set.

Our aim is to semantically label each pixel of CT images to one of the semantic classes with integrated deep neural network architecture. The framework is represented in Figure 11.3, where restricted Boltzmann machine (RBM) can be used to extract unique features of the pixels [82], and unidirectional LSTM can be used to label the image sequences [83]. The input image is transferred to the RBM and their pixel wise variations are used for disease prediction and LSTM processes that image to generate corresponding labels of the disease. Let I be the input image such that $I \in \mathbb{R}^{wxhxc}$ where $w \times h \times c$ are width, height, and channels. The CT image $I = \{I_1, I_2, \ldots, I_m\}$, which is a voxel-based label indicator, can be illustrated as a random variable vector $X = \{X_1, X_2, \ldots, X_m\}$ which is constrained on I. The (X, I) can be characterized by Boltzmann distribution [84] and represented in equation (11.15):

$$P(X = x) = \frac{1}{F(I)} e^{-En(x)} \tag{11.15}$$

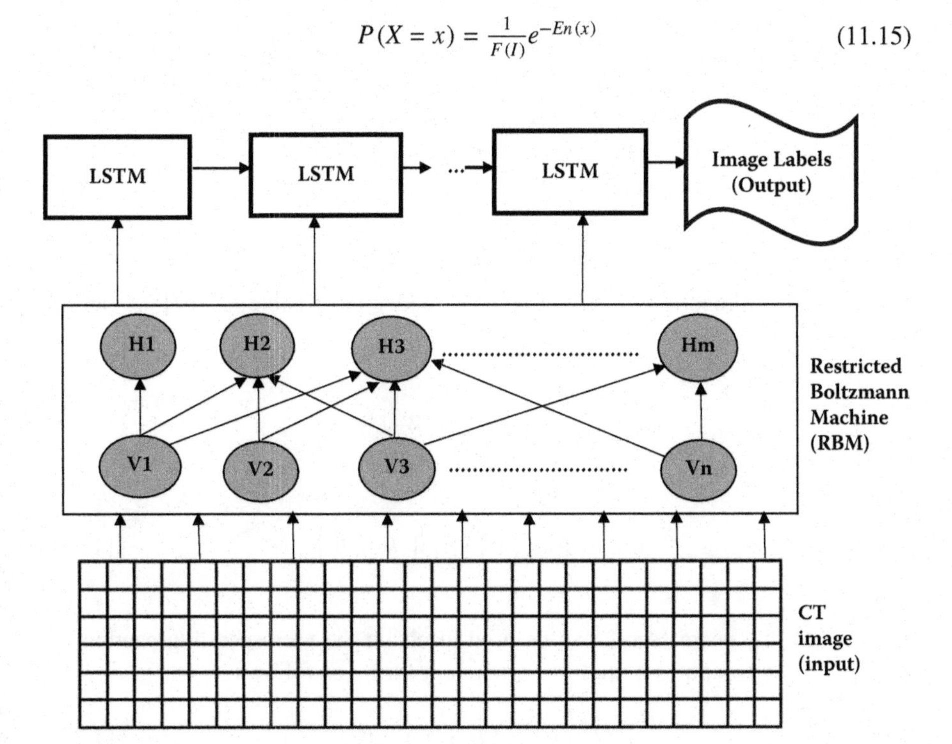

FIGURE 11.3 Multimodal NN architecture with RBM and LSTM.

where *En* indicates energy of random variable, *F(I)* is the partition function. The proposed multimodal NN can be represented with respect to energy function *En*. Restricted Boltzmann machine (RBM) is used for obtaining the combined relation among pixel values and LSTM is used for labeling.

RBM consists of *n* visible units, $V = (V_1, ..., V_n)$ and *m* hidden units, $H = (H_1, ... H_m)$ to represent observable data and captures the dependencies between observed values. The random variable *(V, H)* takes the values such that

$$(x, y) \in \{0, 1\}^{n+m} \tag{11.16}$$

Using Gibbs distribution [84], joint probability distribution for the system can be calculated as in equation (11.17):

$$P(x, y) = \frac{1}{F(I)} e^{-En(x,y)} \tag{11.17}$$

where *En* is the energy function. But pairwise dependencies between pixels of the images [82] can be denoted by Laplace Gaussian distribution where *En(x, y)* is computed as

$$En(x, y) = \sum_{i=1}^{m} \sum_{j=1}^{n} W_{ij} h_i v_j - \sum_{j=1}^{n} b_j v_j - \sum_{i=1}^{m} c_i h \tag{11.18}$$

$\forall\, j \in \{1, ..., n\}$ and $i \in \{1, ..., m\}$. W_{ij} is a real valued weight associated with V_j, and H_i, b_j, and c_i are bias values associated with *j*th visible and *i*th hidden variable. The proposed model can be modelled as a stochastic neural network [84], and the neuron's rate of firing can be computed in equation (11.19):

$$\sigma(\mathrm{x}) = \frac{1}{1 + e^{-x}} \tag{11.19}$$

The conditional probability distribution over hidden and visible layers [84] can be represented as

$$p(H_i = 1|x) = \sigma\left(\sum_{j=1}^{n} W_{ij} v_j + c_i\right) \tag{11.20}$$

$$p(V_j = 1|y) = \sigma\left(\sum_{i=1}^{m} W_{ij} h_i + b_j\right) \tag{11.21}$$

With LSTM, the beam search can be used to obtain the corresponding caption of images. LSTM computes output information at time *t* as follows

$$O_t = \sigma(W_0(h_{t-1}, x_t) + b_0 \tag{11.22}$$

In this model, the conditional probability of output sequence $(O_1, \ldots, O_m)$ for the given input sequence can be represented as $p(O_1, \ldots O_m | I_1, \ldots I_m)$.

11.9 CONCLUSION

Artificial intelligence techniques have the ability to analyze and provide appropriate medical care to patients with minimum interference from doctors, clinicians, and surgeons. Machine learning–based technologies can assist with medical emergencies and increase accuracy in disease diagnosis and clinical applications. Depending on relevant observations, a mathematical model was contributed, which involves a combination of a restricted Boltzmann machine and long short term memory, and is expected to aid in disease prognosis and labeling of medical images. Exploring these in the future through empirical studies will help doctors and clinicians improve medical diagnosis and decision making. Since the handling of immense amounts of healthcare data is difficult, deep learning has evolved as a dominant mechanism in the last few years. It will be a promising solution that will reshape the future of clinical applications. Here we presented an up-to-date review of research employing the techniques of artificial intelligence in the medical arena. We have outlined the advances of machine learning and deep learning techniques in medical management applications.

Deep learning techniques overruled the medical field due to the impact of deep neural network architectures. This chapter explores the latest deep learning architectures: convolutional neural network, restricted Boltzmann machine, deep belief network, autoencoder, recurrent neural network, long short term memory, generative adversarial network, and their recent progress in research are summarized. The hybrid frameworks for medical diagnosis, which involve machine learning and deep learning, are highlighted.

REFERENCES

[1] Haleem, Abid, Javaid, Mohd, and Khan, Ibrahim Haleem. "Current status and applications of artificial intelligence (AI) in medical field: An overview." *Current Medicine Research and Practice* (Elsevier) 9, no. 6 (2019): 231–237.

[2] Alsuliman, Tamim, Humaidan, Dania and Sliman, Layth. "Machine learning and artificial intelligence in the service of medicine: Necessity or potentiality?" *Current Research in Translational Medicine* (Elsevier) 68, no. 4 (2020): 245–251.

[3] Sharma, Nikhil, Kaushik, Ila, Bhushan, Bharat, Gautam Siddharth, and Khamparia, Aditya. "Applicability of WSN and Biometric Models in the Field of Healthcare." In Deep Learning Strategies for Security Enhancement in Wireless Sensor Networks, 304–329. IGI Global, 2020

[4] Jindal, Mansi, Gupta, Jatin, and Bhushan, Bharat. "Machine learning methods for IoT and their Future Applications." In *2019 International Conference on Computing, Communication, and Intelligent Systems (ICCCIS)*. pp. 430–434. IEEE, Greater Noida, India, 2019.

[5] Goyal, Sukriti, Sharma, Nikhil, Bhushan, Bharat, Shankar, Achyut, and Sagayam, Martin. "IoT Enabled Technology in Secured Healthcare: Applications, Challenges and Future Directions." In Cognitive Internet of Medical Things for Smart Healthcare, 25–48. Springer, Cham, 2020.

[6] Guo, Kehua, Ren, Sheng, Bhuiyan, Md Zakirul Alam, Li, Ting, Liu, Dengchao, Liang, Zhonghe, and Chen, Xiang. "MDMaaS: Medical-assisted diagnosis model as a service with artificial intelligence and trust." *IEEE Transactions on Industrial Informatics* (IEEE) 16, no. 3 (2019): 2102–2114.
[7] Chassagnon, Guillaume, Vakalopoulou, Maria, Paragios, Nikos, and Revel, Marie-Pierre. "Artificial intelligence applications for thoracic imaging." *European Journal of Radiology* (Elsevier) 123, (2020): 108774.
[8] Ma, Yang, Zhang, Ping, Tang, Yingxin, Pan, Chao, Li, Gaigai, Liu, Na, Hu, Yang, and Tang, Zhouping. "Artificial intelligence: The dawn of a new era for cutting-edge technology based diagnosis and treatment for stroke." *Brain Hemorrhages* (Elsevier) 1, no. 1 (2020): 1–5.
[9] Barricelli, Barbara Rita, Casiraghi, Elena,and Fogli, Daniela. "A survey on digital twin: Definitions, characteristics, applications, and design implications." *IEEE Access*(IEEE) 7, (2019): 167653–167671.
[10] Bouletreau, P, Makaremi, M, Ibrahim, B, Louvrier, A, and Sigaux, N. "Artificial intelligence: applications in orthognathic surgery." *Journal of Stomatology, Oral and Maxillofacial Surgery* (Elsevier) 120, no. 4 (2019): 347–354.
[11] Pattnayak, Parthasarathi, and Jena, Om Prakash. "Innovation on Machine Learning in Healthcare Services—An Introduction." *Machine Learning for Healthcare Applications* 1, (2021).
[12] Paramesha, K., H. L. Gururaj, and Om Prakash Jena. "Applications of Machine Learning in Biomedical Text Processing and Food Industry." *Machine Learning for Healthcare Applications* 1, (2021): 151–167. https://doi.org/10.1002/9781119792611.ch10
[13] Panigrahi, Niranjan, Ayus Ishan, and Jena Om Prakash. "An Expert System-Based Clinical Decision Support System for Hepatitis-B Prediction & Diagnosis." *Machine Learning for Healthcare Applications* 1, (2021): 57–75. https://doi.org/10.1002/9781119792611.ch4
[14] Orphanou, Kalia, Dagliati, Arianna, Sacchi, Lucia, Stassopoulou, Athena, Keravnou, Elpida,and Bellazzi, Riccardo. "Incorporating repeating temporal association rules in naive bayes classifiers for coronary heart disease diagnosis." *Journal of Biomedical Informatics* (Elsevier) 81, (2018): 74–82.
[15] Sinha, Arvind Kumar, Singh, Pradeep, Prakash, Anand, Pal, Dharm, Dube, Anuradha, and Kumar, Awanish. "Putative drug and vaccine target identification in leishmania donovani membrane proteins using naive bayes probabilistic classifier." *IEEE/ACM Transactions on Computational Biology and Bioinformatics* (IEEE) 14, no. 1 (2017): 204–211.
[16] Joloudari, Javad Hassannataj, Saadatfar, Hamid, Dehzangi, Abdollah and Shamshirband, Shahaboddin. "Computer-aided decision-making for predicting liver disease using PSO-based optimized SVM with feature selection." *Informatics in Medicine Unlocked* (Elsevier) 17, (2019): 100255.
[17] Vijayarajeswari, R, Parthasarathy, P, Vivekanandan, S and Basha, A Alavudeen. "Classification of mammogram for early detection of breast cancer using SVM classifier and Hough transform." *Measurement* (Elsevier) 146, (2019): 800–805.
[18] Zhang, Zhifei, Song, Yang, Cui, Haochen, Wu, Jayne, Schwartz, Fernando and Qi, Hairong. "Topological analysis and Gaussian decision tree: Effective representation and classification of biosignals of small sample size." *IEEE Transactions on Biomedical Engineering* (IEEE) 64, no. 9 (2016): 2288–2299.
[19] Zabihi, Morteza, Rad, Ali Bahrami, Katsaggelos, Aggelos K, Kiranyaz, Serkan, Narkilahti, Susanna and Gabbouj, Moncef. "Detection of atrial fibrillation in ECG hand-held devices using a random forest classifier." *2017 Computing in Cardiology (CinC)*. IEEE 44, 1–4. 2017.

[20] Kumar, Santosh, Bhusan Bharat, Singh Debabrata, and Choubey Dilip Kumar. "Classification of Diabetes using Deep Learning." In *2020 International Conference on Communication and Signal Processing (ICCSP)*, pp. 0651–0655. IEEE, 2020

[21] Brinker, Titus J., Hekler Achim, Enk Alexander H., Klode Joachim, Hauschild Axel, Berking Carola, Schilling Bastian et al. "Deep learning outperformed 136 of 157 dermatologists in a head-to-head dermoscopic melanoma image classification task." *European Journal of Cancer* (Elsevier) 113, (2019): 47–54.

[22] Mutasa, Simukayi, Chang, Peter D, Ruzal-Shapiro, Carrie and Ayyala, Rama. "MABAL: a novel deep-learning architecture for machine-assisted bone age labeling." *Journal of Digital Imaging* (Springer) 31, (2018): 513–519.

[23] Xiao, Yawen, Wu, Jun, Lin, Zongli and Zhao, Xiaodong. "A deep learning-based multi-model ensemble method for cancer prediction." *Computer Methods and Programs in Biomedicine* (Elsevier) 153, (2018): 1–9.

[24] Mansour, Romany F. "Deep-learning-based automatic computer-aided diagnosis system for diabetic retinopathy." *Biomedical Engineering Letters* (Springer) 8, no. 1 (2018): 41–57.

[25] Khanna, Narendra N., Jamthikar Ankush D., Gupta Deep, Piga Matteo, Saba Luca, Carcassi Carlo, Giannopoulos Argiris A. et al. "Rheumatoid arthritis: atherosclerosis imaging and cardiovascular risk assessment using machine and deep learning based tissue characterization." *Current Atherosclerosis Reports* (Springer) 21, no. 2 (2019): 7.

[26] Xiao, Bin, Xu, Yunqiu, Bi, Xiuli, Li, Weisheng, Ma, Zhuo, Zhang, Junhui and Ma, Xu. "Follow the sound of children's heart: a deep-learning-based computer-aided pediatric CHDs diagnosis system." *IEEE Internet of Things Journal* (IEEE) 7, no. 3 (2019): 1994–2004.

[27] Hermsen, Meyke, de Bel Thomas, Den Boer Marjolijn, Steenbergen Eric J., Kers Jesper, Florquin Sandrine, Roelofs Joris JTH et al. "Deep learning–based histopathologic assessment of kidney tissue." *Journal of the American Society of Nephrology* (Am Soc Nephrol) 30, no. 10 (2019): 1968–1979.

[28] Gleichgerrcht, Ezequiel, Munsell, Brent, Bhatia, Sonal, Vandergrift III, William A, Rorden, Chris, McDonald, Carrie, Edwards, Jonathan, Kuzniecky, Ruben and Bonilha, Leonardo. "Deep learning applied to whole-brain connectome to determine seizure control after epilepsy surgery." *Epilepsia* (Wiley Online Library) 59, no. 9 (2018): 1643–1654.

[29] Isin, Ali and Ozdalili, Selen. "Cardiac arrhythmia detection using deep learning." *Procedia Computer Science* (Elsevier) 120, (2017): 268–275.

[30] Chen, Lili and Hao, Yaru. 2017. "Feature extraction and classification of EHG between pregnancy and labour group using Hilbert-Huang transform and extreme learning machine." *Computational and Mathematical Methods in Medicine* (Hindawi).

[31] Jeong, Young-Seob, Kang, Ah Reum, Jung, Woohyun, Lee, So Jeong, Lee, Seunghyeon, Lee, Misoon, Chung, Yang Hoon, Koo, Bon Sung and Kim, Sang Hyun. "Prediction of blood pressure after induction of anesthesia using deep learning: a feasibility study." *Applied Sciences* (Multidisciplinary Digital Publishing Institute) 9, no. 23 (2019): 5135.

[32] Cha, Dongchul, Pae, Chongwon, Seong, Si-Baek, Choi, Jae Young and Park, Hae-Jeong. "Automated diagnosis of ear disease using ensemble deep learning with a big otoendoscopy image database." *EBioMedicine* (Elsevier) 45, (2019): 606–614.

[33] Borsting, Emily and DeSimone, Robert and Ascha, Mustafa and Ascha, Mona.

2020. "Applied deep learning in plastic surgery: Classifying rhinoplasty with a mobile app." *Journal of Craniofacial Surgery* (LWW) 31 (1): 102–106.

[34] Chang, Peter D, Wong, Tony T and Rasiej, Michael J. "Deep learning for detection of complete anterior cruciate ligament tear." *Journal of Digital Imaging* (Springer) 32, no. 6 (2019): 980–986.

[35] Qiu, John X, Yoon, Hong-Jun, Fearn, Paul A and Tourassi, Georgia D. "Deep learning for automated extraction of primary sites from cancer pathology reports." *IEEE Journal of Biomedical and Health Informatics* (IEEE) 22, no. 1 (2017): 244–251.

[36] Lu, Le and Harrison, Adam P. "Deep medical image computing in preventive and precision medicine." *IEEE MultiMedia* (IEEE) 25, no. 3 (2018): 109–113.

[37] Lin, Eugene, Kuo, Po-Hsiu, Liu, Yu-Li, Yu, Younger W-Y, Yang, Albert C and Tsai, Shih-Jen. "A deep learning approach for predicting antidepressant response in major depression using clinical and genetic biomarkers." *Frontiers in Psychiatry* 9, (2018): 290.

[38] Zhao, Zijian, Voros, Sandrine, Weng, Ying, Chang, Faliang and Li, Ruijian. "Tracking-by-detection of surgical instruments in minimally invasive surgery via the convolutional neural network deep learning-based method." *Computer Assisted Surgery* (Taylor & Francis) 22 (sup1) (2017): 26–35.

[39] Bewes, James, Low, Andrew, Morphett, Antony, Pate, F Donald and Henneberg, Maciej. "Artificial intelligence for sex determination of skeletal remains: application of a deep learning artificial neural network to human skulls." *Journal of Forensic and Legal Medicine* (Elsevier) 62, (2019): 40–43.

[40] Song, Qin, Zhao, Mei-Rong, Zhou, Xiao-Han, Xue, Yu and Zheng, Yu-Jun. "Predicting gastrointestinal infection morbidity based on environmental pollutants: Deep learning versus traditional models." *Ecological Indicators* (Elsevier) 81, (2017): 76–81.

[41] Xu, Jun, Luo, Xiaofei, Wang, Guanhao, Gilmore, Hannah and Madabhushi, Anant. "A deep convolutional neural network for segmenting and classifying epithelial and stromal regions in histopathological images." *Neurocomputing* (Elsevier) 191, (2016): 214–223.

[42] Banzato, Tommaso, Bernardini, Marco, Cherubini, Giunio B and Zotti, Alessandro. "A methodological approach for deep learning to distinguish between meningiomas and gliomas on canine MR-images." *BMC Veterinary Research* (BioMed Central) 14, no. 1 (2018): 1–6.

[43] Lee, Jae-Hong, Kim, Do-Hyung, Jeong, Seong-Nyum and Choi, Seong-Ho. "Detection and diagnosis of dental caries using a deep learning-based convolutional neural network algorithm." *Journal of Dentistry* (Elsevier) 77, (2018): 106–111.

[44] Sulieman, Lina, Gilmore, David, French, Christi, Cronin, Robert M, Jackson, Gretchen Purcell, Russell, Matthew and Fabbri, Daniel. "Classifying patient portal messages using Convolutional Neural Networks." *Journal of Biomedical Informatics* (Elsevier) 74, (2017): 59–70.

[45] Nadimi, Esmaeil S, Buijs, Maria M, Herp, Jurgen, Kroijer, Rasmus, Kobaek-Larsen, Morten, Nielsen, Emilie, Pedersen, Claus D, Blanes-Vidal, Victoria and Baatrup, Gunnar. "Application of deep learning for autonomous detection and localization of colorectal polyps in wireless colon capsule endoscopy." *Computers & Electrical Engineering* (Elsevier) 81, (2020): 106531.

[46] Su, Yanfeng. "Implementation and rehabilitation application of sports medical deep learning model driven by big data." *IEEE Access* (IEEE) 7, (2019): 156338–156348.

[47] Tran, Truyen, Nguyen, Tu Dinh, Phung, Dinh and Venkatesh, Svetha. "Learning vector representation of medical objects via EMR-driven nonnegative restricted

Boltzmann machines (eNRBM)." *Journal of Biomedical Informatics* (Elsevier) 54, (2015): 96–105.
[48] Nguyen, Tu, Tran, Truyen, Phung, Dinh and Venkatesh, Svetha. "Tensor-variate restricted Boltzmann machines." *Proceedings of the AAAI Conference on Artificial Intelligence* 29, no. 1 (2015).
[49] Wan, Jing-Jing, Chen, Bo-Lun, Kong, Yi-Xiu, Ma, Xing-Gang and Yu, Yong-Tao. "An early intestinal cancer prediction Algorithm Based on Deep Belief network." *Scientific Reports* (Nature Publishing Group) 9, no. 1 (2019): 1–13.
[50] Madabhushi, Anant . "Stacked sparse autoencoder (SSAE) for nuclei detection on breast cancer histopathology images." *IEEE Transactions on Medical Imaging* no. 1 (2015): 119–130.
[51] Kwon, Bum Chul, Choi, Min-Je, Kim, Joanne Taery, Choi, Edward, Kim, Young Bin, Kwon, Soonwook, Sun, Jimeng and Choo, Jaegul. "Retainvis: Visual analytics with interpretable and interactive recurrent neural networks on electronic medical records." *IEEE Transactions on Visualization and Computer Graphics* (IEEE) 25, no. 1 (2018): 299–309.
[52] Bi, Mingwen, Zhang, Qingchuan, Zuo, Min, Xu, Zelong, Jin, Qingyu. "Bi-directional LSTM Model with Symptoms-Frequency Position Attention for Question Answering System in Medical Domain." *Neural Processing Letters* (Springer) 51, no. 2 (2020): 1185–1199.
[53] Xu, Kai, Zhou, Zhanfan, Hao, Tianyong and Liu, Wenyin. "A bidirectional LSTM and conditional random fields approach to medical named entity recognition." *International Conference on Advanced Intelligent Systems and Informatics*, pp. 355–365. Springer, 2017.
[54] Cui, Shiyue, Li, Chao, Chen, Zhe, Wang, Jiaojiao and Yuan, Juxiang. "Research on risk prediction of dyslipidemia in steel workers based on recurrent neural network and lstm neural network." *IEEE Access* (IEEE) 8, (2020): 34153–34161.
[55] Goodfellow, Ian J, Pouget-Abadie, Jean, Mirza, Mehdi, Xu, Bing, Warde-Farley, David, Ozair, Sherjil, Courville, Aaron and Bengio, Yoshua. "Generative adversarial networks." *arXiv preprint arXiv:1406.2661*. 2014.
[56] Radford, Alec, Metz, Luke and Chintala, Soumith. "Unsupervised representation learning with deep convolutional generative adversarial networks." *arXiv preprint arXiv:1511.06434*. 2015.
[57] Odena, Augustus and Olah, Christopher and Shlens, Jonathon. "Conditional image synthesis with auxiliary classifier gans." *International Conference on Machine Learning*, pp. 2642–2651. PMLR, 2017.
[58] Zhao, Jianlong, Huang Jinjie, Zhi Dongmei, Yan Weizheng, Ma Xiaohong, Yang Xiao, Li Xianbin et al. "Functional network connectivity (FNC)-based generative adversarial network (GAN) and its applications in classification of mental disorders." *Journal of Neuroscience Methods* (Elsevier) 341, (2020): 108756.
[59] Bellemo, Valentina, Burlina, Philippe, Yong, Liu, Wong, Tien Yin and Ting, Daniel Shu Wei. "Generative adversarial networks (GANs) for retinal fundus image synthesis." *Asian Conference on Computer Vision*, pp. 289–302. Springer, 2018.
[60] Liang, Gaobo, Hong, Huichao, Xie, Weifang and Zheng, Lixin. "Combining convolutional neural network with recursive neural network for blood cell image classification." *IEEE Access* (IEEE) 6, (2018): 36188–36197.
[61] Khamparia, Aditya, Singh Prakash Kumar, Rani Poonam, Samanta Debabrata, Khanna Ashish, and Bhushan Bharat. "An internet of health things-driven deep learning framework for detection and classification of skin cancer using transfer learning." *Transactions on Emerging Telecommunications Technologies* e3963, (2020).
[62] Jiang, Hongyang, Ma, He, Qian, Wei, Gao, Mengdi and Li, Yan. "An automatic detection system of lung nodule based on multigroup patch-based deep learning

network." *IEEE Journal of Biomedical and Health Informatics* (IEEE) 22, no. 4 (2017): 1227–1237.

[63] Xue, Di-Xiu, Zhang, Rong, Feng, Hui and Wang, Ya-Lei. "CNN-SVM for microvascular morphological type recognition with data augmentation." *Journal of Medical and Biological Engineering* (Springer) 36, no. 6 (2016): 755–764.

[64] Hekler, Achim, Utikal Jochen S., Enk Alexander H., Hauschild Axel, Weichenthal Michael, Maron Roman C., Berking Carola et al. "Superior skin cancer classification by the combination of human and artificial intelligence." *European Journal of Cancer* (Elsevier) 120, (2019): 114–121.

[65] Chen, Hu, Zhang, Yi, Kalra, Mannudeep K, Lin, Feng, Chen, Yang, Liao, Peixi, Zhou, Jiliu and Wang, Ge. "Low-dose CT with a residual encoder-decoder convolutional neural network." *IEEE Transactions on Medical Imaging*(IEEE) 36, no. 12 (2017): 2524–2535.

[66] Paul, Desbordes, Su, Ruan, Romain, Modzelewski, Sébastien, Vauclin, Pierre, Vera and Isabelle, Gardin. "Feature selection for outcome prediction in oesophageal cancer using genetic algorithm and random forest classifier." *Computerized Medical Imaging and Graphics* (Elsevier) 60, (2017): 42–49.

[67] Arabasadi Z, Alizadehsani R, Roshanzamir M, Moosaei H, Yarifard A. A. Computer aided decision making for heart "Computer aided decision making for heart disease detection using hybrid neural network-Genetic algorithm." *Computer Methods and Programs in Biomedicine* (Elsevier) 141, (2017): 19–26.

[68] Gumaei, Abdu, Hassan, Mohammad Mehedi, Alelaiwi, Abdulhameed and Alsalman, Hussain. "A hybrid deep learning model for human activity recognition using multimodal body sensing data." *IEEE Access* (IEEE) 7, (2019): 99152–99160.

[69] Tan, Teck Yan, Zhang, Li, Lim, Chee Peng, Fielding, Ben, Yu, Yonghong and Anderson, Emma. "Evolving ensemble models for image segmentation using enhanced particle swarm optimization." *IEEE Access* (IEEE) 7, (2019): 34004–34019.

[70] Ning, Zhenyuan, Luo, Jiaxiu, Li, Yong, Han, Shuai, Feng, Qianjin, Xu, Yikai, Chen, Wufan, Chen, Tao and Zhang, Yu. "Pattern classification for gastrointestinal stromal tumors by integration of radiomics and deep convolutional features." *IEEE Journal of Biomedical and Health Informatics* (IEEE) 23, no. 3 (2018): 1181–1191.

[71] Liu, Tianyu, Fan, Wenhui and Wu, Cheng. "A hybrid machine learning approach to cerebral stroke prediction based on imbalanced medical dataset." *Artificial Intelligence in Medicine* (Elsevier) 101, (2019): 101723.

[72] Jha, Krishna Kumar and Dutta, Himadri Sekhar. "Mutual information based hybrid model and deep learning for acute lymphocytic leukemia detection in single cell blood smear images." *Computer Methods and Programs in Biomedicine* (Elsevier) 179, (2019): 104987.

[73] Toğaçar, M., B. Ergen, Z. Cömert, and F. Özyurt. "A deep feature learning model for pneumonia detection applying a combination of mRMR feature selection and machine learning models." *Irbm* (Elsevier) 41, no. 4 (2020): 212–222.

[74] Manogaran, Gunasekaran, Varatharajan, Ramachandran and Priyan, Malarvizhi Kumar "Hybrid recommendation system for heart disease diagnosis based on multiple kernel learning with adaptive neuro-fuzzy inference system." *Multimedia Tools and Applications* (Springer) 77, no. 4 (2018): 4379–4399.

[75] Yang, C-H Huck, Huang, Jia-Hong, Liu, Fangyu, Chiu, Fang-Yi, Gao, Mengya, Lyu, Weifeng and Tegner, Jesper. 2018. "A novel hybrid machine learning model for auto-classification of retinal diseases." *arXiv preprint arXiv:1806.06423.*

[76] Parisi, Luca and Ravi Chandran, Narrendar and Manaog, Marianne Lyne. "Feature-driven machine learning to improve early diagnosis of Parkinson's disease." *Expert Systems with Applications* (Elsevier) 110, (2018): 182–190.

[77] Basheera, Shaik and Ram, M Satya Sai. "Convolution neural network-based Alzheimer's disease classification using hybrid enhanced independent component analysis based segmented gray matter of T2 weighted magnetic resonance imaging with clinical valuation." *Alzheimer's & Dementia: Translational Research & Clinical Interventions* (Elsevier) 5, (2019): 974–986.

[78] Kassani, Sara Hosseinzadeh, Kassani, Peyman Hosseinzadeh, Wesolowski, Michal J, Schneider, Kevin A and Deters, Ralph. "A hybrid deep learning architecture for leukemic B-lymphoblast classification." *2019 International Conference on Information and Communication Technology Convergence (ICTC)*, pp. 271–276. IEEE, 2019.

[79] Li, Fan, Liu, Manhua and Alzheimer's Disease Neuroimaging Initiative. "A hybrid convolutional and recurrent neural network for hippocampus analysis in Alzheimer's disease." *Journal of Neuroscience Methods* (Elsevier) 323, (2019): 108–118.

[80] Shakarami, Ashkan, Tarrah, Hadis and Mahdavi-Hormat, Ali. "A CAD system for diagnosing Alzheimer's disease using 2D slices and an improved AlexNet-SVM method. " *Optik* (Elsevier) 212, (2020): 164237.

[81] Onishi, Yuya, Teramoto, Atsushi, Tsujimoto, Masakazu, Tsukamoto, Tetsuya, Saito, Kuniaki, Toyama, Hiroshi, Imaizumi, Kazuyoshi and Fujita, Hiroshi. "Multiplanar analysis for pulmonary nodule classification in CT images using deep convolutional neural network and generative adversarial networks." *International Journal of Computer Assisted Radiology and Surgery* (Springer) 15, no. 1 (2020): 173–178.

[82] Ranzato, Marc'Aurelio and Hinton, Geoffrey E. "Modeling pixel means and covariances using factorized third-order Boltzmann machines." *2010 IEEE Computer Society Conference on Computer Vision and Pattern Recognition*, pp. 2551–2558. IEEE, 2010.

[83] Oura, Soichiro, Matsukawa, Tetsu and Suzuki, Einoshin "Multimodal Deep Neural Network with Image Sequence Features for Video Captioning." *2018 International Joint Conference on Neural Networks (IJCNN)*, pp. 1–7. IEEE, 2018.

[84] Fischer, Asja and Igel, Christian. "An introduction to restricted Boltzmann machines." *Iberoamerican Congress on Pattern Recognition*. Springer. 14–36, 2012.

12 A Temporal JSON Model to Represent Big Data in IoT-Based e-Health Systems

Zouhaier Brahmia, Safa Brahmia, and Rafik Bouaziz
Department of Computer Science, University of Sfax, Sfax, Tunisia

Fabio Grandi
University of Bologna, Bologna, Italy

CONTENTS

DOI: 10.1201/9781003189053-12

12.1 INTRODUCTION

Electronic health, or e-Health, systems [1,2] are playing an increasingly crucial role in our lives, especially in pandemic periods like that of COVID-19, by facilitating health monitoring and remotely providing medical services including virtual consultations. They benefit from recent advances in medical informatics, data management, networks and telecommunications technologies, and allow patients to enjoy such services in a secure, autonomous and personalized manner.

On the other hand, the Internet of Things (IoT) technologies [3,4] are being used in many contemporary application fields like video surveillance, weather monitoring, air pollution control, smart road traffic, in addition to e-Health. In IoT-based e-Health systems [5–7], personal devices or wearable IoT sensors are transmitting data concerning the state of patients (e.g., body temperature, heart rate, oxygen saturation, glycemia) continuously, to collection points that can be computer systems of networked physicians or hospitals. These data streams are heterogeneous in nature due to the use of a variety of remote sensors, involve structured, semistructured and unstructured data and, in some cases, may also include multimedia content (e.g., videos, sounds, images). They are generated at unprecedented and ever-increasing scales, are stored and shared in different data formats and are generally processed in distributed systems. Hence, they can be considered for all intents as big data [8–12]. For big data, NoSQL (Not Only SQL) data stores [13] have been advocated as the most suitable repositories to record them, and the JSON (JavaScript Object Notation) format [14] is being considered as the best data format to represent them and facilitate their management, storage and exchange [15,16].

Moreover, e-Health IoT sensor data represent entities that are evolving over time, and several healthcare applications require keeping a full history of such data, which is necessary for monitoring the evolution of patients and diseases, diagnostic and therapeutic decision making and experimental/scientific purposes (e.g., detection of correlations between medical parameters, follow-up of efficacy and adverse reactions of drugs, study of the spreading of a disease). However, to the best of our knowledge, there is no standard/consensual *temporal* model for e-Health IoT nor NoSQL data, including JSON that lacks explicit support of time-varying data. Therefore, in order to manage NoSQL data histories and temporal e-Health IoT data, applications developers have to proceed in an ad hoc manner, also reducing the potential for e-Health data, software and system interoperability and reuse.

In this chapter, we first propose (in Section 12.3) the TJeH (Temporal JSON e-Health) data model, a temporal extension of the JSON data model, which supports the representation of temporal aspects of IoT big data [12] in e-Health systems. Furthermore, and since TJeH as an extension of JSON is a logical model, in order to make life easier for both designers and database administrators of e-Health applications, we have also defined (in Section 12.4) a graphical conceptual model for time-varying e-Health IoT data, named C-TJeH, where the "C" stands for conceptual, associated to our logical model. C-TJeH simplifies the design of temporal e-Health JSON IoT data with a conceptual model which equipped with a graphical user-friendly representation. The implementation of an editor supporting C-TJeH is planned to become the graphical user interface for the conceptual design of temporal e-Health IoT data based on the TJeH model. Before going into the details of our proposals, we present the background of our work in the section that follows.

12.2 RELATED WORK

In this section, we first present the IoT, the Internet of Medical Things (IoMT) and IoT-based e-Health systems. Then, we deal with machine learning, deep learning and their applications in healthcare systems. Next, we study big data modeling. Finally, we provide some temporal database concepts that are necessary for the understanding of our proposed models.

It is worth mentioning that, with regard to our approach, some of the machine/deep learning applications must perform temporal analytics tasks and have to manage temporal data (e.g., for continuous monitoring) and, therefore, conceptual modeling of temporal e-Health IoT data is an important component of the design of a large e-Health IoT database that could support such applications. Moreover, conceptual modeling also enables reuse and interoperability of such data.

12.2.1 IoT, IoMT and IoT-Based e-Health Systems

The IoT, also known as the Web of Things, is a global environment built upon wireless sensor networks (WSNs) where billions of objects (e.g., sensors, actuators, RFID tags, smart phones, computers, security cameras, cars, refrigerators) are connected to the Internet and are exchanging information in an autonomous and interoperable manner. In 2030, the number of IoT devices is expected to be around 50 billion [17]. Therefore, these devices will be the most important producers and consumers of data. Moreover, from a data management point of view, an increasing effort will be required for the definition and implementation of models, languages and systems for the management of IoT data and of their different aspects (e.g., uncertainty, temporality).

The application of the IoT in the healthcare field has been called the "Internet of Medical Things" (IoMT) [18] or the "Healthcare IoT". It is a secure network of medical devices (e.g., wearable sensors, implantable devices, ambient sensors, stationary devices), software applications and people that are involved in the healthcare management (e.g., patients, doctors, nurses, technicians). The core tasks of the IoMT are: (i) collecting healthcare data (e.g., weight, blood pressure, glucose level) from connected medical devices and maintaining them in databases located on some servers; (ii) storing collected data in formats that are suitable for analytical purposes and decision making; (iii) exchanging information between different IoMT stakeholders; (iv) remotely providing medical services for patients.

A typical and simplified IoT-based e-Health system, like that presented in [2], is composed of four elements: user, client, server, and device. The user can be either a patient or a healthcare professional (i.e., doctor, nurse, guardian ...). He/she could access the system, with permissions, while using devices like mobile smartphones or specific e-health devices. Moreover, the user resorts to the client to consume the e-health services (e.g., monitoring, e-consultation, data querying and saving) that are deployed on the server. The server hosts a NoSQL database for the storage of all data that are produced and exchanged in this system like users' personal data, devices' data, health sensing data and patients' health data; the choice of NoSQL is mainly for high scalability of the whole e-Health system and for providing high availability and extensibility of services. The client allows the user to interact with the server (which includes the database and the e-Health services) and to control the e-Health devices. A single e-Health device allows to configure several sensors for collecting patients health status data. Notice that, in general, sensors are made by different companies and generate data in different proprietary formats. Nevertheless, e-Health devices must be portable and interoperable.

12.2.2 Machine Learning and Deep Learning in Healthcare Systems

In [19], the authors have proposed a framework for deep learning internet of health and things (IoHT), which allows detecting and classifying skin lesions in skin images using the concept of transfer learning. Moreover, they experimentally evaluated the performances of their proposal and discussed them in a transfer learning environment.

Kumar et al. [20] have used deep learning to classify diabetes, by applying the multi-layer feed forward neural networks (MLFNN) [21] on the Pima Indian Diabetes data set. Before experiencing their MLFNN-based model, the authors have handled the missing values encountered in such a data set, since they can affect the accuracy of the classification. The experimental results, which are produced by the performance evaluation of the MLFNN model, have been compared to those obtained from the application of two machine learning classifiers: Naïve-Bayes and random forest. These results show that the introduced model provides better accuracy than the two other models.

Sharma et al. [22] study the role of wireless sensor networks and biometric-based models (like two-factor remote authentication, and user verification and authorization using fingerprint biometrics) in healthcare systems. In particular, the authors have presented a comparative table that provides advantages and disadvantages of several biometric-based models applied in healthcare. Notice that such models are efficient tools for controlling access to electronic health records, securing patient data and therefore protecting both patient data confidentiality and privacy. As for biometrics, it is the science of analyzing physical (e.g., fingerprints, eye (iris and retina), and the shape of the hand, of the finger, or of the face) or behavioral (e.g., speech recognition, and signature dynamics) characteristics of each individual and enabling the authentication of his/her identity.

Goyal et al. [23] have dealt with the use of IoT technologies in a secured healthcare context. Indeed, they started by defining the notion of Internet of Health Things (IoHT). Then, they have presented a model for future IoHT systems, with topologies, applications and services of IoHT. Notice that IoHT applications are user-oriented, whereas IoHT services are developer-oriented. Furthermore, each IoHT application is classified into either a single-condition application, concerning a single disease or illness or weakness, or a clustered-condition application, dealing with a number of circumstances together as a whole. After that, the authors have described the classes (ambient assisted living, remote healthcare monitoring, wearable gadgets, and solutions for healthcare using smartphones) and challenges (e.g., an IoHT-based system must fulfill safety, robustness, and flexibility issues) of IoHT. Next, they have studied the security requirements (resiliency, availability, defect tolerance, data freshness, self-healing, privacy, integrity, and verification) and security challenges (energy limitations, dynamic security updates, multiplicity of gadgets, scalability, memory limitations, multi-protocol network, and computational limitations) in IoHT. Finally, the authors have provided a list of technologies (ambient intelligence, augmented reality, big data, cloud computing, grid computing, wearables and networks like 6LoWPANs, WBANs, WSNs, WPANs and WLANs) that could revolutionize the services of IoHT, and some open research issues in the IoHT area (identification, cost analysis, business prototype, data security and continuous monitoring).

12.2.3 Big Data Modeling

In [24], the authors have tried to answer to the question: "can conceptual modeling come to the rescue of big data?". Indeed, they show that *"conceptual modeling can help by conceptual-model-based extraction for handling volume and velocity with automation, by inter-conceptual-model transformations for mitigating variety, and by conceptualized constraint checking for increasing veracity"*.

Chebotko et al. [25] propose a big data modeling methodology for the NoSQL database management system Apache Cassandra. This methodology is query-driven and covers the three traditional data modeling levels: conceptual, logical and physical levels. The authors also present a tool that supports such a methodology and automates the full process of data modeling.

To support the conceptual modeling of big data extract process, Martinez-Mosquera et al. [26] have extended the meta-model of the unified modeling language (UML) with five new stereotypes (structured data; semi-structured data; unstructured data; text files and binary files), in addition to the use of two other stereotypes (conversion and loader) already proposed in a previous research paper [27]. The extension has been specified at the deployment diagram of UML. To illustrate the use of their proposal, the authors have used the proposed stereotypes to conceptually model three tools that support the big data extract process: Sqoop, Flume and Data Click. Notice that a UML stereotype is a UML extensibility mechanism that allows a designer to extend the concepts/vocabulary of UML, by defining a new modeling component that is not covered by UML and that satisfies some specific requirements.

Storey and Song [28] show how conceptual modeling can contribute to the five "Vs" (volume, velocity, variety, veracity and value) of big data. In fact, with regard to the "volume", conceptual modeling can help organizing, identifying and describing important data. As for "velocity", conceptual modeling can help extracting important data. With respect to the "variety", conceptual modeling can help representing the variety, hierarchies, and networks of data and integrating data. Concerning the "veracity", conceptual modeling can help checking quality, completeness and consistency of data. In regard to the "value", conceptual modeling can help analyzing big data projects to extract value and evaluate the results.

In [29], the authors propose a modeling methodology for NoSQL databases, which is composed of three phases: the first phase, named "conceptual data modeling and aggregate design", produces a conceptual model (a UML class diagram in this case) of the application domain. Such a model defines the entities, their attributes and the relationships between these entities. Notice that related entities are grouped into aggregates. The second phase, named "aggregate partitioning and high-level NoSQL database design", partitions aggregates into smaller data elements and after that mapped them to the abstract data model NoAM (NoSQL abstract model); this latter allows defining a system-independent data model. The third phase, named "implementation", converts the NoAM model into the specific model of a given NoSQL database system (e.g., MongoDB, HBase, Amazon DynamoDB, Couchbase, Redis, Oracle NoSQL and Cassandra).

Martinez-Mosquera et al. [30] have provided a systematic literature review for big data modeling and management. In their work, the authors tried to answer three questions: "*how the number of published papers about big data modeling and management has evolved over time*?", "*whether the research is focused on semi-structured and/or unstructured data and what techniques are applied*?", and "*what trends and gaps exist according to three key concepts: the data source, the modeling and the database*?". For that purpose, they collected and studied 36 important scientific papers that have been published between 2010 and 2019. At the end of this study, the authors discovered (among others) that the entity-relationship model is the most researched model at the conceptual modeling level, the document-oriented NoSQL data model is the most researched model at the logical modeling level and MongoDB is the most NoSQL DBMS used at the physical modeling level, for implementations and technical solutions.

Recently, Pastor et al. [31] have proposed a framework that is based on a conceptual schema of the human genome, and used it to show, through a case study, how conceptual models are very helpful in the efficient understanding, communication and management (organization, storage, processing, analyze, extracting knowledge, identifying relationships between data, visualization …) of genomic data. Notice that the authors have also defined a data quality methodology for genomic data, to support this framework.

12.2.4 Temporal Database Concepts

A temporal database is a database with built-in support for defining, storing, manipulating, querying and controlling time-varying data [32–35]. Two time dimensions have been introduced for timestamping time-varying data: transaction time [36], which represents the time when data are current in the database, and valid time [37], which represents the time when data are valid in the real world. Thus, four types of temporal databases can be found: (i) transaction-time databases, which support only transaction time; (ii) valid-time databases, which support only valid time; (iii) bitemporal databases, which support both transaction time and valid time; and (iv) multitemporal databases in which coexist data of different temporal formats. Notice that, in a temporal setting, conventional (i.e., non-temporal) databases are called snapshot databases. Moreover, the timestamp of a temporal datum can be either a time interval or a time point [38].

Besides, a temporal data model [39] is a data model for representing time-varying data. Several temporal data models have been proposed in the last three decades like HRDM [40], BCDM [41], TEER [42], TEMPOS [43], XBiT [44], τXSchema [45] and TempoXDM [46].

12.3 TJEH: OUR TEMPORAL JSON MODEL FOR E-HEALTH IOT DATA

In this section, we propose our temporal JSON data model, named TJeH, which allows representing temporal aspects of e-Health IoT big data [12]. TJeH is a temporal extension of the JSON data model [14]. Such an extension consists of extending the JSON data model to support the representation of the temporal aspects of JSON components that are evolving over time and for which the DBA or the application developer/designer wants to keep the history of their evolution in the database. Notice that a JSON component is a JSON object, a JSON object member, a JSON array or a JSON array element.

The temporal dimensions that are supported by TJeH are transaction time and valid time. Therefore, a temporal JSON component may have a transaction-time, valid-time, or bitemporal format, according to the temporal dimension(s) along which its history is kept.

If a JSON component is not temporal (i.e., its value is not time-varying), it is called a snapshot JSON component.

In our temporal JSON data model, TJeH, the semantics of JSON component version timestamping is as follows:

- a transaction-time JSON component version has two timestamping object members that represent the bounds of its transaction-time interval: TTbegin (transaction time begin) and TTend (transaction time end);
- a valid-time JSON component version has two timestamping object members that represent the bounds of its valid-time interval: VTbegin (validity time begin) and VET (validity time end);
- a bitemporal JSON component version has four timestamping object members that denote the bounds of its transaction-time interval and those of its valid-time interval: VTbegin, VTend, TTbegin and TTend.

The management of timestamping object members is performed automatically and in an implicit manner by the JSON NoSQL DBMS, transparently to the user. Obviously, a snapshot JSON component has no timestamping object members.

Moreover, like XML [47,48], JSON is suitable to support temporally grouped data models [49–51], which have always been advocated as the most appropriate tools to model temporal data [38,52,53]. Thus, we have defined our TJeH model as a temporally grouped extension of JSON. In fact, it groups and represents the evolution of any mono-temporal (i.e., transaction-time or valid-time) or bitemporal

JSON component in a JSON object that in turn could contain nested sub-objects, each of which could be independently defined as transaction-time, valid-time or bitemporal (if the temporal format is not locally redefined, the temporal format of the container JSON object is inherited).

In TJeH, an individual snapshot JSON component, named "Component", is made temporal by converting it into an ordered list of temporally homogeneous "Component" versions, each of which is defined as a JSON object with four (in case of a mono-temporal component) or six (in case of a bitemporal component) JSON object members, grouped together into a container JSON array named "Component" as follows:

```
"Component": [ { "Vid":1, "value":…, "VTbegin":…, "VTend":… },
        { "Vid":2, "value":…, "VTbegin":…, "VTend":… },
        { "Vid":3, "value":…, "VTbegin":…, "VTend":… }]
```

The object member "Vid" (Version identifier) identifies a timestamped version of "Component" and has been added to make easy version access and manipulation when processing temporal and multi-version queries. The object member "value" provides the value of a version. The object members "VTbegin" and "VTend" represent the valid-time timestamps. If "Component" is of transaction-time format, two timestamp object members will be used instead: "TTbegin" and "TTend". Besides, if "Component" is of bitemporal format, four timestamp object members will be used: "VTbegin", "VTend", "TTbegin" and "TTend".

The "VTend" object member of a bitemporal or a valid-time JSON component version can have the special value "now" [38,54], which means that such a component version is currently valid when it is accessed and, thus, continues to be valid in the real world until replaced. Furthermore, the "TTend" object member of a transaction-time or a bitemporal JSON component version can have the special value "UC" [38], which means Until Changed and denotes a component version is the current one in the database until some change occurs.

In addition, although the "value" object member is usually an atomic value (i.e., a value of the string, boolean, number, integer or null JSON type), it could also be a complex/structured value (i.e., a value of the object or array JSON type), like the blood pressure that is represented/recorded by two numbers (i.e., the systolic and the diastolic blood pressures), or the position of a place/person/thing on the Earth, which is represented by three numbers (latitude, longitude and altitude coordinates).

12.3.1 Running Example

In order to illustrate our model, let us consider the example of a JSON document that stores the data of patients (i.e., their Social Security Number (SSN), name, birthdate, body temperature, blood pressure, blood glucose, cholesterol, heart rate, weight), which belongs to the NoSQL database of an IoT-based e-Health system. It is clear that the first three data describing a patient (i.e., SSN, name and birthdate) are static, whereas the last six data are evolving over time. Since all these six data are important for monitoring the health status of patients, the history of each one of them should be maintained. For the sake of simplicity, in this example we focus only on the four following time-varying data: body temperature, blood pressure, blood glucose and heart rate. Figure 12.1 shows an instance of our temporal JSON model, which stores the information of one patient (Layla Ahmad), whose health status is continuously monitored and any change to his/her body temperature, blood pressure, blood glucose or heart rate is recorded. The evolution over time of these time-varying data is maintained along the transaction time dimension, since each new value is automatically sensed and stored in the database without any intervention of the user (the patient or a healthcare professional) or the database administrator. Time-varying data and their temporal versions are presented in blue bold type.

Notice that, in the example of Figure 12.1, we assume that the unit of temperature is "degree Celsius" (°C) and that of blood glucose is "milligrams per deciliter" (mg/dL). If an application or a user requires, for instance, the temperature to be in "degree Fahrenheit" (°F), or the blood glucose in "millimoles per liter" (mmol/L), suitable conversion formulae [°F] = [°C] $*$ 9/5 + 32 and [mmol/L] = [mg/L] $*$ 1/18, respectively, can be applied.

12.4 C-TJEH: OUR GRAPHICAL CONCEPTUAL MODEL FOR TEMPORAL JSON E-HEALTH IOT DATA

In this section, we propose C-TJeH, a graphical temporal data model for conceptual modeling of time-varying eHealth IoT big data in JSON format. It provides a conceptual view of the logical data model TJeH defined as temporal extension of the conventional JSON format to represent e-Health IoT big data. Therefore, C-TJeH allows to conceptually model either conventional aspects and temporal aspects of e-Health IoT data, whereas the conventional aspects are the JSON components (i.e., objects, object members, arrays and array elements) usually appearing in a traditional JSON document, the temporal aspects are the transaction time and the valid time of such JSON components.

12.4.1 Conceptual Modeling of Conventional Aspects of e-Health IoT Data under C-TJeH

Based on the specification of the JSON format [14] and the JSON schema language [55], we have defined a minimal and complete set of six operations for the creation of conventional JSON components: object, array, Member(string), Value(type), Combinator(keyword), and subschema.

- **Object**

In place of a null-type value x, it draws an empty rectangular box (as shown in Figure 12.2) that represents an empty JSON object.

```
{ "patients":[
    { "patient":{
        "SSN":112233445566,
        "name":"Layla Ahmad",
        "birthdate":"1960-03-26",
        "bodyTemperature":[
           { "TTbegin":"2021-03-15:02:10:45",
             "TTend":"2021-03-15:08:33:27",
             "value":36.5 },
           { "TTbegin":"2021-03-15:08:33:28",
             "TTend":"UC",
             "value":37.2 } ],
        "bloodPressure":[
           { "TTbegin":"2021-03-15:02:10:45",
             "TTend":"2021-03-15:06:49:07",
             "value":{ "systolic":"133",
                       "diastolic":"82" } },
           { "TTbegin":"2021-03-15:06:49:08",
             "TTend":"UC",
             "value":{ "systolic":"119",
                       "diastolic":"79" } } ],
        "bloodGlucose":[
           { "TTbegin":"2021-03-15:02:10:45",
             "TTend":"2021-03-15:06:31:08",
             "value":90 },
           { "TTbegin":"2021-03-15:06:31:09",
             "TTend":"UC",
             "value":130 } ],
        "heartRate":[
           { "TTbegin":"2021-03-15:02:10:45",
             "TTend":"2021-03-15:03:37:19",
             "value":141 },
           { "TTbegin":"2021-03-15:03:37:20",
             "TTend":"UC",
             "value":128 } ]
      } }
  ] }
```

FIGURE 12.1 A temporal JSON document representing an instance of our TJeH model.

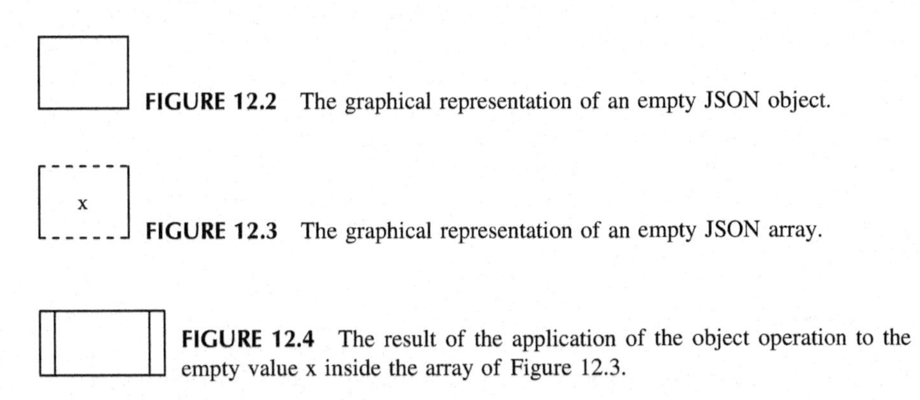

FIGURE 12.2 The graphical representation of an empty JSON object.

FIGURE 12.3 The graphical representation of an empty JSON array.

FIGURE 12.4 The result of the application of the object operation to the empty value x inside the array of Figure 12.3.

- **Array**

In place of a null-type value x, it draws: [x], where the edges of the square brackets are joined with two horizontal dashed lines (as shown in Figure 12.3), to represent an empty JSON array.

Notice that an array of objects, as shown by Figure 12.4, is obtained by applying the object operation to the empty value x inside the array.

- **Member(string)**

Inside an object box, it draws: string x, where the line goes out of the box (as shown in Figure 12.5), to represent an object member with a null-type value x.

- **Value(type)**

In place of a null-type value x, it draws: o (type), where type is string, number, integer, boolean or date, to represent either the value of an object member or an array element, which is of simple and not null type. Figure 12.6 shows two examples of applications of this operation.

Notice that although the "date" is not provided by JSON Schema [55] as a built-in data type (but as a format of the "string" type), we add it to our model since such

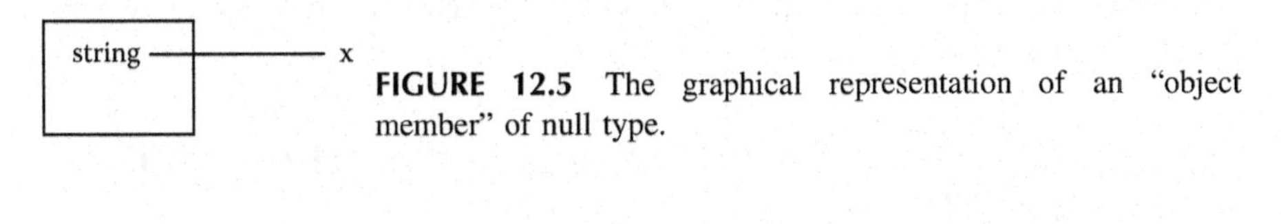

FIGURE 12.5 The graphical representation of an "object member" of null type.

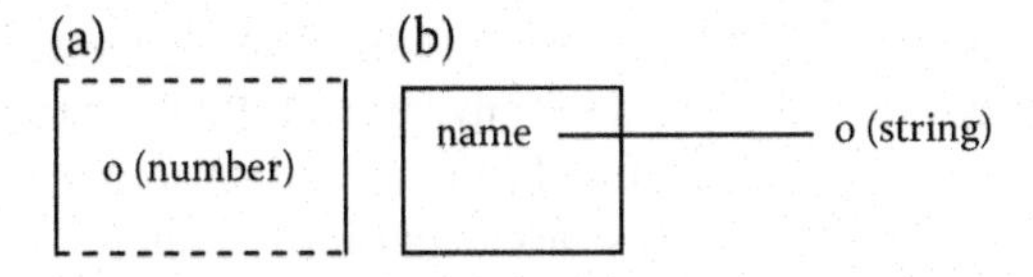

FIGURE 12.6 The result of the application of (a) Value(number) on an empty array, and (b) a Value(string) on an object member called "name".

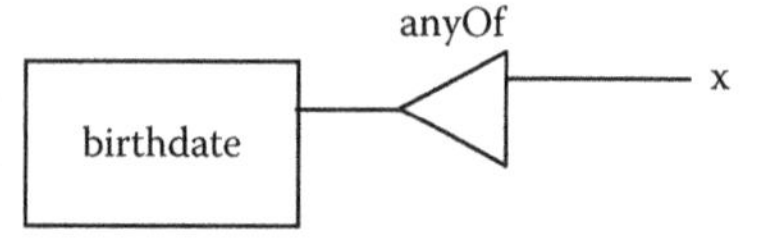

FIGURE 12.7 The effect of the application of the Combinator(anyOf) operation on the null-type value x of an object member named "birthdate".

a type is widely used (by designers) at conceptual level (and also to represent timestamps at physical level).

- **Combinator(keyword)**

In place of a null-type value x, it draws: a triangle with label keyword and a single null subschema, where keyword is "allOf", "anyOf", "oneOf" or "not", to represent a combination of schemas.

Figure 12.7 shows an example of an application of the "Combinator(anyOf)" operation on an object member.

Notice that since the "keyword" stands for a boolean combination, we propose, as alternative notation, that the NoSQL database designer can also use logical operator names (or symbols) inside the combinator triangle: AND (or $\wedge$) for "allOf", OR (or $\vee$) for "anyOf", XOR (or $\oplus$) for "oneOf" and NOT (or $\neg$) for "not".

- **Subschema**

It adds a single null subschema to an existing schema combinator. For example, if the designer wants to define a "birthdate" object member whose value could be of date type or of string type, he/she starts by applying the "Combinator(anyOf)" operation on the null-type value x of "birthdate", as shown in Figure 12.7. Then, he/she should apply Subschema on the "anyOf" combinator. After that, he/she should apply Value(date) on one of the two null-type values x and Value(string) on the other.

Moreover, we propose six deletion operations as the inverse operations of those presented above: DelObject, DelArray, DelMember, DelValue, DelCombinator and DelSubschema.

Notice also that our operations (unless they are used in a graphical environment) have JSONPath [56] arguments to denote the C-TJeH schema components to which they have to be applied.

12.4.2 Conceptual Modeling of Temporal Aspects of e-Health IoT Data under C-TJeH

As far as temporal aspects are concerned, C-TJeH supports the specification of the transaction time and valid time of the conventional JSON components. To this purpose, C-TJeH is equipped with the TemporalFormat(format) operation, to be applied to a selected component, whose argument format can be TT (for transaction time), VT (for valid time) or BT (for bitemporal).

- **TemporalFormat(TT)**
The assignment of the transaction-time format to a JSON component means that each of its versions will be labeled with a transaction-time timestamp (i.e., a transaction-time interval or a transaction-time point) automatically assigned by the database management system.
Graphically, the transaction time format is represented via a circle inside which it is written "TT", placed near the corresponding JSON component: (TT)
- **TemporalFormat(VT)**
The assignment of the valid-time format to a JSON component means that each of its versions will be labeled with a valid-time timestamp (as a temporal interval or a temporal point) provided by the user.
The graphical representation of the valid time format is a circle inside which it is written "VT": (VT) It should be placed near the corresponding JSON component.
- **TemporalFormat(BT)**
When a JSON component is assigned the bitemporal format, it means that its representation evolves along both time dimensions and its versions will be assigned both a transaction-time and a valid-time timestamp.
Graphically, the bitemporal format is represented via a circle inside which it is written "BT", put near the corresponding JSON component: (BT)

Furthermore, it should be mentioned that although the life span of a JSON component (i.e., the time when the component exists) is considered a temporal aspect in some temporal database research works, like [38,57,58], we have not taken it into account in our conceptual model, as it can be derived from the valid time aspects of such a component. In fact, the life span of a JSON component *jcomp* is equivalent to the valid time of the fact "the JSON component *jcomp* exists" and can be computed as the union of the valid timestamps of its constituent versions.

We also underline that timestamping is inherited by nested components. For example, when an object is declared with a valid time format, each one of its object members is automatically considered having a valid-time format and, unless redefined, inherits the valid timestamp values from the container object. If some of its members are also declared with a transaction-time format, such members acquire a bitemporal format.

We would also remark that a C-TJeH schema is actually a sort of meta-schema, which can be translated into a plain JSON Schema [55] document, by expliciting the versioning structures and timestamp value representations.

12.4.3 Running Example Reprise

In order to illustrate the use of our C-TJeH model, let us resume our example of Section 12.3.1 and assume that the NoSQL database designer has defined the C-TJeH model, as shown in Figure 12.8, and used it (as a conceptual schema) to create and validate the TJeH JSON document of Figure 12.1.

In this C-TJeH model, he/she has graphically declared, as transaction time, the body temperature, the blood pressure, the blood glucose and the heart rate of a patient.

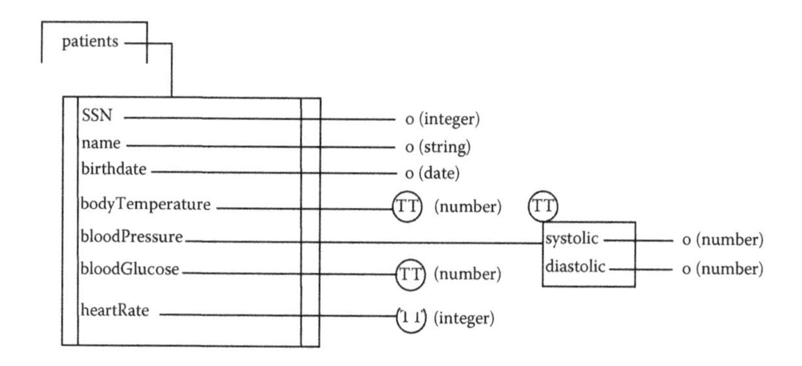

FIGURE 12.8 A C-TJeH model for patient data management in an e-Health system.

12.5 CONCLUSION

In this chapter, we have proposed TJeH, a temporal JSON model for the representation of big data in IoT-based e-Health systems. It extends JSON to support temporal aspects (transaction time and valid time) of e-Health IoT data. Furthermore, in order to facilitate the creation of TJeH databases and to simplify the work of application designers and NoSQL database administrators, we have also proposed a graphical conceptual model, named C-TJeH, associated to the TJeH logical model. Thus, C-TJeH (TJeH, respectively) is filling a gap at the conceptual (logical, respectively) level, due to the lack of temporal conceptual (logical, respectively) models for e-Health IoT JSON data in the current state of the art.

In order to show the feasibility of our two proposed models, we plan to develop a tool that allows users (i) to design a graphical conceptual model for temporal JSON-based e-Health IoT data, according to the C-TJeH model, and (ii) to create temporal JSON documents (i.e., the temporal instances), according to the TJeH model (i.e., the logical temporal schema) and conforming to C-TJeH (i.e., the conceptual temporal schema). Moreover, since both conceptual and logical data models are not static and evolve over time to reflect changes in the modeled reality or in the users' requirements, we also envisage to extend TJeH and C-TJeH to also support schema changes, while benefiting from our previous work dealing with schema versioning [59–61] in time-varying JSON-based NoSQL databases [62–64].

REFERENCES

[1] Eysenbach, Gunther. "What is e-health?." *Journal of Medical Internet Research* 3, no. 2 (2001): e20.

[2] Jin, Wenquan, and Kim Do H. "Design and Implementation of e-Health System Based on Semantic Sensor Network Using IETF YANG." *Sensors* 18, no. 2 (2018): 629.

[3] Lombardi, Marco, Pascale Francesco, and Santaniello Domenico. "Internet of Things: A General Overview between Architectures, Protocols and Applications." *Information* 12, no. 2 (2021): 87.
[4] Wang, Jianxin, Lim Ming K., Wang Chao, and Tseng Ming-Lang. "The evolution of the Internet of Things (IoT) over the past 20 years." *Computers & Industrial Engineering* 155 (2021): paper 107174.
[5] Huang, Jinbo, Wu Xianjun, Huang Wendong, Wu Xiaoli, and Wang S. "Internet of things in health management systems: A review." *International Journal of Communication Systems* 34, no. 4 (2021): e4683.
[6] Pathak, Nidhi, Misra Sudip, Mukherjee Anandarup, and Kumar Neeraj. "HeDI: Healthcare Device Interoperability for IoT-Based e-Health Platforms." *IEEE Internet of Things Journal*, IEEE, 2021. 10.1109/JIOT.2021.3052066
[7] Rayan, Rehab A., Tsagkaris Christos, and Iryna Romash B. "The Internet of Things for Healthcare: Applications, Selected Cases and Challenges." In *IoT in Healthcare and Ambient Assisted Living* (Gonçalo Marques, Akash Kumar Bhoi, Victor Hugo C. de Albuquerque, and Hareesha K.S., eds.), pp. 1–15. Singapore: Springer, 2021.
[8] Dimitrov, Dimiter V. "Medical internet of things and big data in healthcare." *Healthcare Informatics Research* 22, no. 3 (2016): 156.
[9] Ge, Mouzhi, Bangui Hind, and Buhnova Barbora. "Big data for internet of things: a survey." *Future Generation Computer Systems* 87 (2018): 601–614.
[10] Aceto, Giuseppe, Persico Valerio, and Pescapé Antonio. "Industry 4.0 and health: Internet of things, big data, and cloud computing for healthcare 4.0." *Journal of Industrial Information Integration* 18 (2020): paper 100129.
[11] Rghioui, Amine, Lloret Jaime, and Oumnad Abedlmajid. "big data Classification and Internet of Things in Healthcare." *International Journal of E-Health and Medical Communications* 11, no. 2 (2020): 20–37.
[12] Bansal, Maggi, Chana Inderveer, and Clarke Siobhán. "A Survey on IoT big data: Current Status, 13 V's Challenges, and Future Directions." *ACM Computing Surveys (CSUR)* 53, no. 6 (2020): Article 131.
[13] Davoudian, Ali, Chen Liu, and Liu Mengchi. "A survey on NoSQL stores." *ACM Computing Surveys (CSUR)* 51, no. 2 (2018): Article 40.
[14] IETF. The JavaScript Object Notation (JSON) Data Interchange Format. *Internet Standards Track document* (2017), December 2017. https://tools.ietf.org/html/rfc8259 (accessed: 2021-04-13).
[15] Rao, T. Ramalingeswara, Mitra Pabitra, Bhatt Ravindara, and Goswami A. "The big data system, components, tools, and technologies: a survey." *Knowledge and Information Systems* 60, no. 3 (2019): 1165–1245.
[16] Davoudian, Ali, and Liu Mengchi. "big data Systems: A Software Engineering Perspective." *ACM Computing Surveys (CSUR)* 53, no. 5 (2020): Article 110.
[17] Statista Research Department. Number of IoT connected devices worldwide 2019-2030 (2021), January 22, 2021. https://www.statista.com/statistics/802690/worldwide-connected-devices-by-access-technology/ (accessed: 2021-04-13).
[18] Al-Turjman, Fadi, Nawaz Muhammad Hassan, and Ulusar Umit Deniz. "Intelligence in the Internet of Medical Things era: A systematic review of current and future trends." *Computer Communications* 150 (2020): 644–660.
[19] Khamparia, Aditya, Singh Prakash Kumar, Rani Poonam, Samanta Debabrata, Khanna Ashish, and Bhushan Bharat. "An Internet of Health Things-driven Deep Learning Framework for Detection and Classification of Skin Cancer using Transfer Learning." *Transactions on Emerging Telecommunications Technologies* (2020). 10.1002/ett.3963
[20] Kumar, Santosh, Bhusan Bharat, Singh Debabrata, and Choubey Dilip kumar. "Classification of Diabetes using Deep Learning." In *Proceedings of the 2020*

International Conference on Communication and Signal Processing (ICCSP 2020), pp. 0651–0655, IEEE, 2020.

[21] Svozil, Daniel, Kvasnicka Vladimír, and Pospichal Jiří. "Introduction to multi-layer feed-forward neural networks." *Chemometrics and Intelligent Laboratory Systems* 39, no. 1 (1997): 43–62.

[22] Sharma, Nikhil, Kaushik Ila, Bhushan Bharat, Gautam Siddharth, and Khamparia Aditya. "Applicability of WSN and Biometric Models in the Field of Healthcare." In *Deep Learning Strategies for Security Enhancement in Wireless Sensor Networks* (Sagayam K. Martin, Bhushan Bharat, Andrushia A. Diana, and de Albuquerque Victor Hugo C., eds.), pp. 304–329, Hershey, PA: IGI Global, 2020.

[23] Goyal, Sukriti, Sharma Nikhil, Bhushan Bharat, Shankar Achyut, and Sagayam Martin. "IoT Enabled Technology in Secured Healthcare: Applications, Challenges and Future Directions." In *Cognitive Internet of Medical Things for Smart Healthcare* (Aboul Ella Hassanien, Aditya Khamparia, Deepak Gupta, K. Shankar, and Adam Slowik, eds.). Studies in Systems, Decision and Control, vol. 311, pp. 25–48. Cham: Springer, 2021.

[24] Embley, David W., and Liddle Stephen W. "big data—Conceptual Modeling to the Rescue." In *Proceedings of the 32nd International Conference on Conceptual Modeling (ER 2013), LNCS* vol. 8217, pp. 1–8, Springer, (2013). 10.1007/978-3-642-41924-9_1

[25] Chebotko, Artem, Kashlev Andrey, and Lu Shiyong. "A big data modeling methodology for Apache Cassandra." In *Proceedings of the 2015 IEEE International Congress on big data (BigData Congress 2015)*, pp. 238–245, IEEE, (2015).

[26] Martinez-Mosquera, Diana, Luján-Mora Sergio, and Recalde Henry. "Conceptual modeling of big data extract processes with UML." In *Proceedings of the 2017 International Conference on Information Systems and Computer Science (INCISCOS 2017)*, pp. 207–211, IEEE, (2017).

[27] Trujillo, Juan, and Luján-Mora Sergio. "A UML Based Approach for Modeling ETL Processes in Data Warehouses." In *Proceedings of the 22nd International Conference on Conceptual Modeling (ER'2003), LNCS* vol. 2813, pp. 307–320, Springer, (2003).

[28] Storey, Veda C., and Song Il-Yeol. "Big data technologies and Management: What conceptual modeling can do." *Data & Knowledge Engineering* 108 (2017): 50–67. 10.1016/j.datak.2017.01.001

[29] Atzeni, Paolo, Bugiotti Francesca, Cabibbo Luca, and Torlone Riccardo. "Data modeling in the NoSQL world." *Computer Standards & Interfaces* 67 (2020): 103149. 10.1016/j.csi.2016.10.003

[30] Martinez-Mosquera, Diana, Navarrete Rosa, and Lujan-Mora Sergio. "Modeling and Management big data in Databases—A Systematic Literature Review." *Sustainability* 12, no. 2 (2020): 634. 10.3390/su12020634

[31] Pastor, Óscar, León Ana Palacio, Reyes José Fabián Román, Simón García Alberto, Rodenas Casamayor Juan Carlos. "Using conceptual modeling to improve genome data management." *Briefings in Bioinformatics* 22, no. 1 (2021): 45–54. 10.1093/bib/bbaa100

[32] Grandi, Fabio. "Temporal Databases." In *Encyclopedia of Information Science and Technology* (3rd edition), (Mehdi Khosrow-Pour, ed.), pp. 1914–1922, Hershey, PA: IGI Global, (2015).

[33] Böhlen, Michael H., Dignös Anton, Gamper Johann, and Jensen Christian S. "Temporal Data Management - An Overview." In *Business Intelligence and big data: Proceedings of eBISS 2017, LNBIP* vol. 324, (Zimányi Esteban, ed.), pp. 51–83. Cham: Springer, (2018).

[34] Jensen, Christian S., and Snodgrass Richard T. "Temporal Database." In *Encyclopedia of Database Systems* (2nd edition), (Liu Ling, and Özsu M. Tamer, eds.). New York: Springer, (2018a). 10.1007/978-1-4614-8265-9_395

[35] Lu, Wei, Zhao Zhanhao, Wang Xiaoyu, Li Haixiang, Zhang Zhenmiao, Shui Zhiyu, Ye Sheng, Pan Anqun, and Du Xiaoyong. "A Lightweight and Efficient Temporal Database Management System in TDSQL." *PVLDB* 12, no. 12 (2019): 2035–2046.

[36] Jensen, Christian S., and Snodgrass Richard T. "Transaction Time." In *Encyclopedia of Database Systems* (2nd edition), (Ling Liu, and M. Tamer Özsu, eds.). New York: Springer, (2018b). 10.1007/978-1-4614-8265-9_1064

[37] Jensen, Christian S., and Snodgrass Richard T. "Valid Time." In *Encyclopedia of Database Systems* (2nd edition), (Ling Liu, and M. Tamer Özsu, eds.) New York: Springer, (2018c). 10.1007/978-1-4614-8265-9_1066

[38] Jensen, Christian S., Dyreson Curtis E., Böhlen Michael, Clifford James, Elmasri Ramez, Gadia Shashi K., Grandi Fabio, Hayes Pat, Jajodia Sushil, Käfer Wolfgang, Kline Nick, Lorentzos Nikos, Mitsopoulos Yannis, Montanari Angelo, Nonen Daniel, Peressi Elisa, Pernici Barbara, Roddick John F., Sarda Nandlal L., Scalas Maria Rita, Segev Arie, Snodgrass Richard T., Soo Mike D., Tansel Abdullah, Tiberio Paolo, and Wiederhold Gio. "The consensus glossary of temporal database concepts – February 1998 version." In *Temporal Databases – Research and Practice, LNCS* vol. 1399, (Etzion Opher, Jajodia Sushil, and Sripada Suryanarayana, eds.), pp. 367–405, Berlin: Springer, (1998).

[39] Jensen, Christian S., and Snodgrass Richard T. "Temporal Data Models." In *Encyclopedia of Database Systems* (2nd edition), (Ling Liu, and M. Tamer Özsu, eds.). New York: Springer, (2018d). 10.1007/978-1-4614-8265-9_394

[40] Clifford, James, and Croker Albert. "The historical relational data model (HRDM) revisited." In *Temporal Databases: Theory, Design and Implementation*, (Tansel Abdullah Uz, Clifford James, Gadia Shashi, Jajodia Sushil, Segev Arie, and Snodgrass Richard, eds.), pp. 6–27, Redwood City: Benjamin/Cummings Publishing Company, (1993).

[41] Jensen, Christian S., Soo Michael D., and Snodgrass Richard T. "Unifying temporal data models via a conceptual model." *Information Systems* 19, no. 7 (1994): 513–547.

[42] Gregersen, Heidi, and Jensen Christian S. "Temporal Entity-Relationship models-a survey." *IEEE Transactions on Knowledge and Data Engineering* 11, no. 3 (1999b): 464–497.

[43] Dumas, Marlon, Fauvet Marie-Christine, and Scholl Pierre-Claude. "TEMPOS: a platform for developing temporal applications on top of object DBMS." *IEEE Transactions on Knowledge and Data Engineering* 16, no. 3 (2004): 354–374.

[44] Wang, Fusheng, and Zaniolo Carlo. "XBiT: An XML-based bitemporal data model." In *Proceedings of the 23rd International Conference on Conceptual Modeling (ER 2004)*, pp. 810–824, Berlin, Heidelberg: Springer, (2004).

[45] Currim, Faiz, Currim Sabah, Dyreson Curtis, and Snodgrass Richard T. "A tale of two schemas: Creating a temporal XML schema from a snapshot schema with τXSchema." In *Proceedings of the 9th International Conference on Extending Database Technology (EDBT 2004)*, pp. 348–365, Berlin, Heidelberg: Springer, (2004).

[46] Brahmia, Zouhaier, Hamrouni Hind, and Bouaziz Rafik. "TempoX: A disciplined approach for data management in multi-temporal and multi-schema-version XML databases." *Journal of King Saud University – Computer and Information Sciences* (2019). in press. 10.1016/j.jksuci.2019.08.009

[47] Wang, Fusheng, and Zaniolo Carlo. "Temporal queries and version management in XML-based document archives." *Data and Knowledge Engineering* 65, no. 2 (2008): 304–324.

[48] Dyreson, Curtis E., and Grandi Fabio. "Temporal XML." In *Encyclopedia of Database Systems* (2nd edition), (Ling Liu, and M. Tamer Özsu, eds.). New York: Springer, (2018). 10.1007/978-1-4614-8265-9_411

[49] Brahmia, Safa, Brahmia Zouhaier, Grandi Fabio, and Bouaziz Rafik. "τJSchema: A Framework for Managing Temporal JSON-Based NoSQL Databases." In *Proceedings of the 27th International Conference on Database and Expert Systems Applications (DEXA'2016), Part 2, LNCS vol. 9828*, (Sven Hartmann, and Hui Ma, eds.), pp. 167–181, Cham: Springer, (2016).

[50] Brahmia, Safa, Brahmia Zouhaier, Grandi Fabio, and Bouaziz Rafik. "A disciplined approach to temporal evolution and versioning support in JSON data stores." In *Emerging Technologies and Applications in Data Processing and Management* (Zongmin Ma, and Li Yan, eds.), pp. 114–133, Hershey: IGI Global, (2019).

[51] Goyal, Aayush, and Dyreson Curtis. "Temporal JSON." In *Proceedings of the 5th IEEE International Conference on Collaboration and Internet Computing (CIC 2019)*, pp. 135–144, (2019).

[52] Clifford, James, Croker Albert, and Tuzhilin Alexander. "On Completeness of Historical Relational Query Languages." *ACM Transactions on Database Systems (TODS)* 19, no. 1 (1994): 64–116.

[53] Clifford, James, Croker Albert, Grandi Fabio, and Tuzhilin Alexander. "On Temporal Grouping." In *Proceedings of the 1995 International Workshop on Temporal Databases*, pp. 194–213, (1995).

[54] Clifford, James, Dyreson Curtis E., Isakowitz Tomás, Jensen Christian S., and Snodgrass Richard T. "On the Semantics of "Now" in Databases." *ACM Transactions on Database Systems (TODS)* 22, no. 2 (1997): 171–214.

[55] IETF. JSON Schema: A Media Type for Describing JSON Documents. Internet-Draft, (2018). 19 March 2018. https://json-schema.org/latest/json-schema-core.html (accessed: 2021-04-13).

[56] Gössner, Stefan. JSONPath – Xpath for JSON. (2007). 21 February 2007. http://goessner.net/articles/JsonPath/ (accessed: 2021-04-13).

[57] Gregersen, Heidi, and Jensen Christian S. "On the ontological expressiveness of temporal extensions to the entity-relationship model." In *Proceedings of the 18th International Conference on Conceptual Modeling Workshops (ER 1999 Workshops)*, pp. 110–121, (1999a).

[58] Gregersen, Heidi. "TimeERplus: a temporal EER model supporting schema changes." In *Proceedings of the 22nd British National Conference on Databases (BNCOD 2005), LNCS* vol. 3567, pp. 41–59, (2005).

[59] Brahmia, Zouhaier, Grandi Fabio, Oliboni Barbara, and Bouaziz Rafik. "Schema Versioning." In *Encyclopedia of Information Science and Technology* (3rd edition), (Mehdi Khosrow-Pour, ed.), pp. 7651–7661, Hershey, PA: IGI Global, (2015).

[60] Brahmia, Zouhaier, Grandi Fabio, Oliboni Barbara, and Bouaziz Rafik. "Schema Versioning in Conventional and Emerging Databases." In *Encyclopedia of Information Science and Technology* (4th edition), (Mehdi Khosrow-Pour, ed.), pp. 2054–2063, Hershey, PA: IGI Global, (2018).

[61] Roddick, John F. "Schema Versioning." In *Encyclopedia of Database Systems* (2nd edition), (Ling Liu, and M. Tamer Özsu, eds.), New York: Springer, (2018). 10.1007/978-1-4614-8265-9_323

[62] Brahmia, Safa, Brahmia Zouhaier, Grandi Fabio, and Bouaziz Rafik. "Temporal JSON Schema Versioning in the τJSchema Framework." *Journal of Digital Information Management* 15, no. 4 (2017): 179–202.

[63] Brahmia, Zouhaier, Brahmia Safa, Grandi Fabio, and Bouaziz Rafik. "Versioning Schemas of JSON-based Conventional and Temporal big data through High-level Operations in the τJSchema Framework." *International Journal of Cloud Computing* 10 (2021). 10.1504/IJCC.2021.10030585

[64] Brahmia, Safa, Brahmia Zouhaier, Grandi Fabio, and Bouaziz Rafik. "Versioning Temporal Characteristics of JSON-based big data via the τJSchema Framework." *International Journal of Cloud Computing* 10 (2021). 10.1504/IJCC.2021.10030586

13 Use of UAVs in the Prevention, Control and Management of Pandemics

Giuliana Bilotta
Iuav University, Venice, Italy

V. Barrile, E. Bernardo, and A. Fotia
Università Mediterranea di Reggio Calabria, Reggio Calabria, Italy

CONTENTS

DOI: 10.1201/9781003189053-13

13.1 INTRODUCTION

This research proposes an automated system for the management of a fleet of RPAS for the procurement/delivery of goods with high value in use such as PPE and goods for medical use managed through an Open GIS we programmed [1,2].

The project is also part of the general theme of monitoring flows and crowding of people in connection to the use of public transport, with particular reference to LPT, based on the comparison with the multitemporal data acquired on the time. Consequently, is necessary to track anonymously passenger along the origin-destination route, through an integrated system that reuses the available infrastructures in the best possible way.

Through an image processing system acquired by the security cameras present on public transport vehicles and by the cameras at the stops and drone cameras, through the use of Machine Learning, we get in the Open GIS we cited the state of the crowding.

In the future, the research will also be aimed at experimenting some actions of interest in relation to pandemic emergency problems, such as detection and acquisition of meteo-climatic data or automatic drone flight techniques for sanitation operations.

As a background for the use of drones in emergencies, the bibliography lists numerous applications of drones in emergencies [3], such as in CrisisMappers interventions [4][1] (often using the Ushahidi platform [5][2]) and, in the last ten years, of volunteers organized and coordinated by WeRobotics. In these interventions, first used were these technologies in emergencies with the support of crowdsourcing [6].

Drones were used in the search for survivors of Malaysia Airlines Flight 370 in 2014, in the April 2015 Nepal earthquake relief efforts [7]. In 2018, the Insect Pest Control Laboratory (IPCL) of the Joint FAO/IAEA Division of Nuclear Techniques in Food and Agriculture (NAFA) conducted using drones a trial to combat Zika [8] and other deadly mosquito-borne diseases such as dengue and malaria. In November 2019, on behalf of the World Food Program (WFP), WeRobotics [9][3] organized several trainings and simulations of humanitarian drone interventions on behalf of the WFP (and others) in the Dominican Republic, Peru, Myanmar, Malawi and Mozambique. From 2017, they were used as a fleet of cargo drones to transport medicine in Peru and vaccine in Papua New Guinea, Nepal, Democratic Republic of Congo, Cameroon, Uganda, Dominican Republic, Fiji Islands.

The cameras of the drones, together with those present on the LPT vehicles and at the stops, and the MAC signal of the mobile phone devices, can also be used for verification and surveillance actions, specifically to monitor people's movements [10] and gatherings. These actions give rise to delicate debates on privacy and individual rights. On the other hand, the monitoring of local public transport and the anonymous tracking of passengers along the origin-destination route does not seem to encounter any ethical obstacles.

Regarding the background of crowding and route monitoring, similar analyses related to infomobility have been pioneered by Carlo Ratti and his Senseable City

Lab at MIT (Massachusetts Institute of Technology) in Boston [11]. Among these, the Real Time Rome project of 2006, presented at the Venice Biennale of that year, analyzed in real time the dynamics of the city in relation to the movement of people on foot and on public transport. Interesting and innovative is the part played by communication technologies. In the case of the analysis of connectivity used only as a source of signal.in the case of Rome, the founding idea consisted of the tracking of the movement of signals (MAC address, MAC = Media Access Control) of mobile phone devices that, with their own speed, make it possible to distinguish pedestrian traffic from that of cars and public transport.

Our motivation is to solve the problem of distribution of medical material and monitoring of people gathering.

To do this, we organized a system that includes an automated fleet of drones for material distribution and image acquisition and for crowd monitoring in the LPT, with the use of different algorithms and machine learning all integrated in a GIS.

The major contributions of this chapter are:

- the use of a fleet of drones in an automated way for distribution of medical goods (with the genetic algorithms for multi-objective analysis to determine the flight plan of drones),
- the integration of multiple algorithms with particular reference to machine learning algorithms implemented for monitoring and therefore control of crowding (for the O/D matrix) and a GIS for visualization.

Therefore, the main novelty of this contribution is in the coordinated use of all these elements that through predictive systems provide results visualizable in a GIS that can be updated over time.

13.1.1 Chapter Organization

The organization of the subsequent parts of this chapter is as follows. Section 13.2 of this paper describes in a synthetic way the use of drones in the pandemic emergency. Section 13.3 introduces the proposed system, defining firstly what are the parameters and characteristics to optimize (through genetic algorithms) the multi-objective function useful for the definition of a flight plan to be used to create an automated drone fleet capable to distribute medical material and acquire images at bus stops. A series of interacting machine learning algorithms were then identified for the definition of the origin/destination matrix that can be updated in almost real time (on an hourly basis) for the management of the crowds and for the possible sending of additional vehicles for the management of local public transport. Everything is visualized in a GIS that can be updated over time.

Once defined algorithms and methods are to be used, Section 13.4 addresses our experimentation in a test area, and shows the results obtained. In Section 13.5, the results are discussed and commented. Section 13.6 provides the conclusion and finishes with possible future works.

13.2 THE USE OF DRONES IN THE PANDEMIC EMERGENCY: PANDEMIC DRONES

The use of drones in containment actions [12] during health emergencies appears advantageous both for their technical efficiency and for the peculiarity of minimizing human exposure.

Recent community research reports a number of experiences during the COVID-19 pandemic using SAPRs, as Table 13.1 shows.

TABLE 13.1
Comparison and Effectiveness of Pandemic Counter Actions Using Drones

Use Case	Containment Action	Results (and Locations)
Medical Drone Deliveries	Transport of medicines during the epidemic	Good and effective results (Antwork, China; Swiss Post, Matternet, Switzerland; Wing and UPS, USA, etc.)
Spraying Streets with Water and Disinfectant	Aerial disinfection operations	Poor results (Wuhan, many others village and cities in China, Seoul, many others village and cities in Korea, etc.)
Delivery and Logistics Involving Essential Goods	Food delivery	Good and effective results (Wing, Google, USA; Flytrex, AHA, Reykjavík, Iceland)
Body Temperature Scanning	Use of drones equipped with thermal sensors	Not completely reliable (Daytona Beach, FL, USA; Seattle, WA, USA; Draganfly, Canada; Global Cyberspace Governance, Shangai, China)
Situational Awareness, Lockdown/Curfew Enforcement	Use of drones equipped with night vision cameras	Effective (Wuhan, many others village and cities in China)
Situational Awareness, Lockdown/Curfew Enforcement	Use of drones equipped with zoom lenses	Effective (Wuhan, many others village and cities in China)
Broadcasting Useful Information Situational Awareness, Lockdown/ Curfew Enforcement	Use of drones equipped with speakers	Effective (Wuhan, many others village and cities in China; Seoul, South Korea, etc.)
Gathering Weather Data for Meteorologists	Using drones equipped with sensors for temperature, humidity and wind in the atmosphere	Effective, from 2013 (Oklahoma University, Norman, OK, USA; University of California, San Diego, CA, USA; NASA, FL, USA, etc.)

In addition, new research efforts aimed at enhancing the value of SAPRs as "pandemic drones" in prevention, control and emergency response activities are underway at several advanced public/private institutions.

There are many uses in which drones prove helpful, and some of these began before the pandemic. Among the containment actions listed previously, recent studies, for example, have shown that disinfection of outdoor environments leads to poor results [13]. Even remote temperature scanning may not be completely reliable.

13.3 MATERIALS AND METHODS

For the reasons described previously, in this research we focused on the development of an innovative and automated system for the deployment of drones in the distribution of medical supplies (which has proven to be effective in various cases: Antwork, China [14]; Swiss Post, Matternet, Switzerland; Wing and UPS, USA, etc.) and in the monitoring and control of movements and crowding of LPT users in order to reduce the risk of contagion, using a series of algorithms with particular reference to those of machine learning, managing the whole system through a common and updatable open GIS [15], realizing a complete system that allows in automatic way to visualize the results related to the transport of medical material and to the monitoring directly on GIS according to the flow chart in Figure 13.1.

Subsequently, according to the flow chart in Figure 13.1, the methodology as a whole, its implementation, the functioning of the algorithms explaining how they interact with each other, and an application of the method shown in a test area is explained.

13.3.1 Delivering Medical Goods

In order to solve the problems connected to the transport of medical devices, in this experiment we have created an automated system that allows it to monitor and manage through a suitable GIS any requests and transport of medical supplies.

We have created a GIS Open multi-platform (computer, tablet and smartphone) updatable and searchable, which allows it to report any requests for supplies of medical goods and allows it to manage a fleet of automated drones that, starting from the warehouses of medical supplies and delivers medical devices and drugs at the points of delivery (where users can go to pick up the devices in an orderly manner and without creating crowds). The recharging stations of the drone fleet proposed in this experiment, located in pre-established points, make it possible to reach destinations that would otherwise be impossible with the sole autonomy of the drone battery, and also allows it to transmit images taken along the way and send any new flight plans.

In this work, we used a fleet of automated drones connected to the cloud that are automatically recharged through special charging stations located in predetermined points. The data acquisition system provides for the installation of some platforms along the path to be monitored to allow the drone battery to be recharged and the

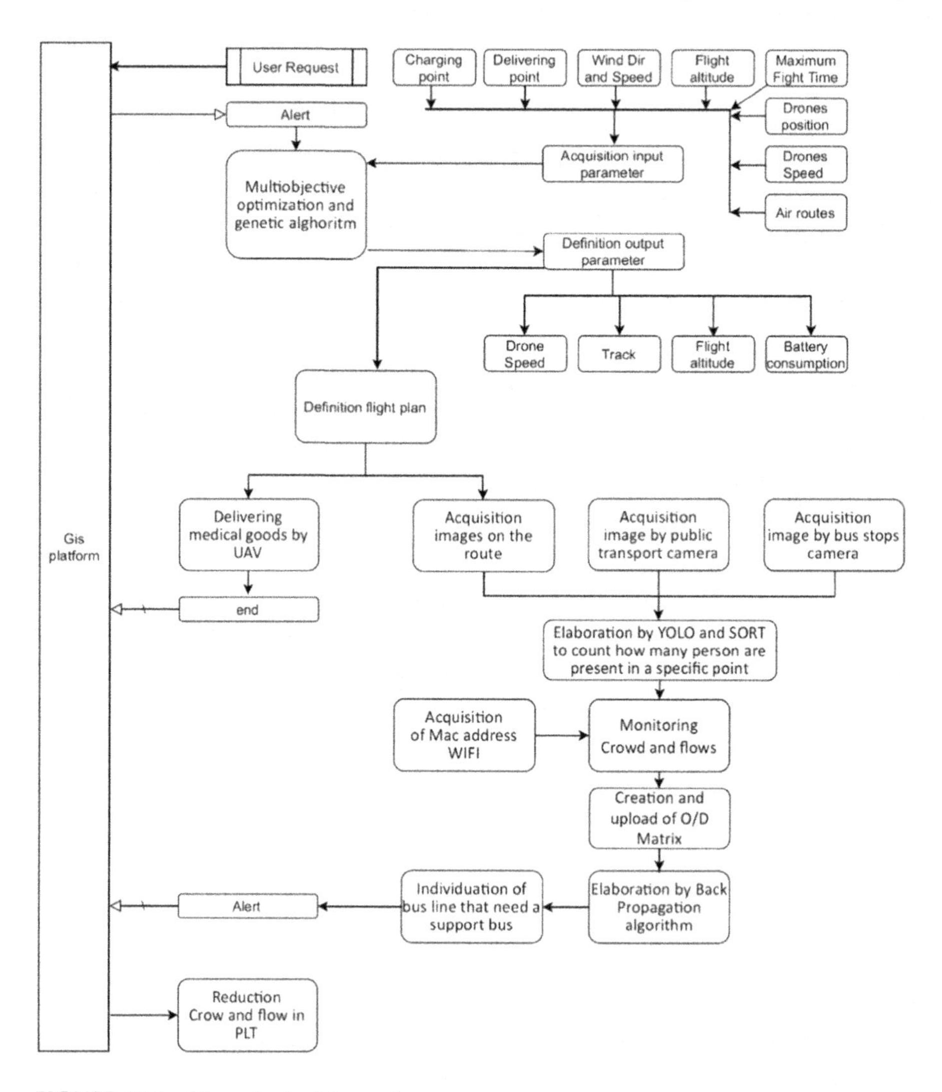

FIGURE 13.1 Flow chart of the system.

data necessary for subsequent processing to be transferred [16]. We have built an innovative monitoring system including drones, intelligent multi-landing and charging pads, automatically governed that communicate at short range with nearby drones and indicate the status of the station according to the following scheme:

1. When a drone in flight detects that the battery is running low, it looks for the nearest charging station, the latter communicates to the drone if there is a free pitch and a charged battery available.
2. Having obtained the OK to land, the drone, knowing the GPS coordinates of the station, approaches and, moving vertically, lands on the assigned stand [17].

3. Once landed, a subsystem recharges the onboard battery or swaps it, replacing the discharged battery with a charged one. During the replacement, the drone is still powered through a special connector in order not to lose communications and to allow the automatic procedure with the exchange of information [18]. After recharging, take-off takes place. The wireless charging station is made up of an "intelligent" induction plate which, when the drone lands, determines the type of batteries supplied to the aircraft, and thus establishes the correct charging parameters. This is made possible thanks to a small device on board the drone consisting of a microcircuit with a data transmission system, weighing a few tens of grams and dimensions contained in the order of a few centimeters, such that it can be installed not only on large professional drones but also on smaller commercial ones [19]. These stations are totally waterproof and weatherproof and also serve as a temporary shelter for the appliances.

Thanks to the IFTTT algorithm that guarantees once a certain battery charge threshold is reached, the choice of the nearest charging base [20] through a comparison between the distance of the point (drone coordinates) and the coordinates of the charging points present in the area, updating the flight plan. The same happens for the start of the flight following the user's request (Figure 13.2).

Considering the system of monitoring and transport of materials by UAV we have realized is completely automated and that the regulations in force in the study area allow only VLOS (visual line of sight) operations, the fleet of drones is equipped with safety parachutes, operated by an accelerometer. The parachute comes into operation when the system detects a free-fall, rollover or failure condition: it works with drones that have sensors to monitor flight interruptions: the sensor sends a command to an actuator that ejects a parachute (protected from the propellers that could otherwise damage it).

In health emergency conditions, the supply/distribution of medicines, basic necessities and PPE using SAPRs, safely and with minimal time and cost, represents a multi-objective optimization problem that requires careful strategic logistics planning [21].

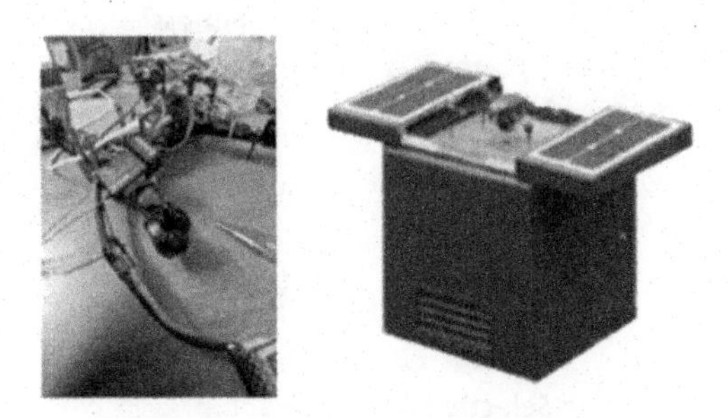

FIGURE 13.2 Automated drone system components and drone input/output wireless charging base.

For this reason, our research had as initial goal to define a drone-based system that optimizes the benefit-resource ratio, considering a set of factors and constraints (including urban context/compliance with current regulations) using a set of parameters, listed below. We also set out to explore other application potentials, related to in-flight monitoring and safety of SAPRs, in conjunction with other existing tracking and monitoring systems. To define the multi-objective function, we proceeded to use stochastic optimization algorithms capable of performing multi-objective optimizations in a simple and fast way (genetic algorithms), with particular reference to the bubble sorting algorithm [22] for sorting. The lower accuracy, acceptable in this case, is compensated by the higher robustness, not needing to calculate the gradient, but simply evaluating the value of the objective function.

The multi-objective genetic algorithm is composed of four distinct phases that are repeated at each generation (Figure 13.3): for each individual is calculated the value of the objective function (fitness) that allows to order the population following the criterion of dominance of the Pareto front. Thanks to the obtained ordering we can select the best individuals and generate a new population by means of recombination.

Genetic algorithms start from an initial population of solutions and iteratively evolve it. This population is generated randomly and at each iteration, the solutions are evaluated by a fitness function and based on this evaluation and some of them are selected, favoring the solutions with higher fitness. The selected solutions are recombined among them to generate new solutions that tend to transmit the good characteristics of the parent solutions in the following generations. The main scheme of a genetic algorithm is indicated in Figure 13.3.

In Figure 13.4, a diagram with all the phases aimed to define parameters useful for the use of the multi-objective function for the definition of the flight plan.

In particular, in Table 13.2, input and output parameters have been identified (referred to each single drone) on the basis of which the best configuration can be chosen by the multi-objective function. To indicate the parameters, we have used terms from aeronautics.

Obtaining an optimal delivery path from vehicles of different types is a classic vehicle routing problem (VRP), of which there are several variants that can be

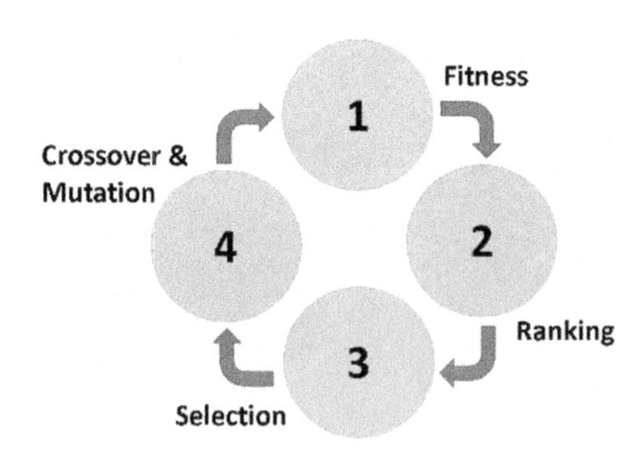

FIGURE 13.3 Main steps of the genetic algorithm for solving the multi-objective problem.

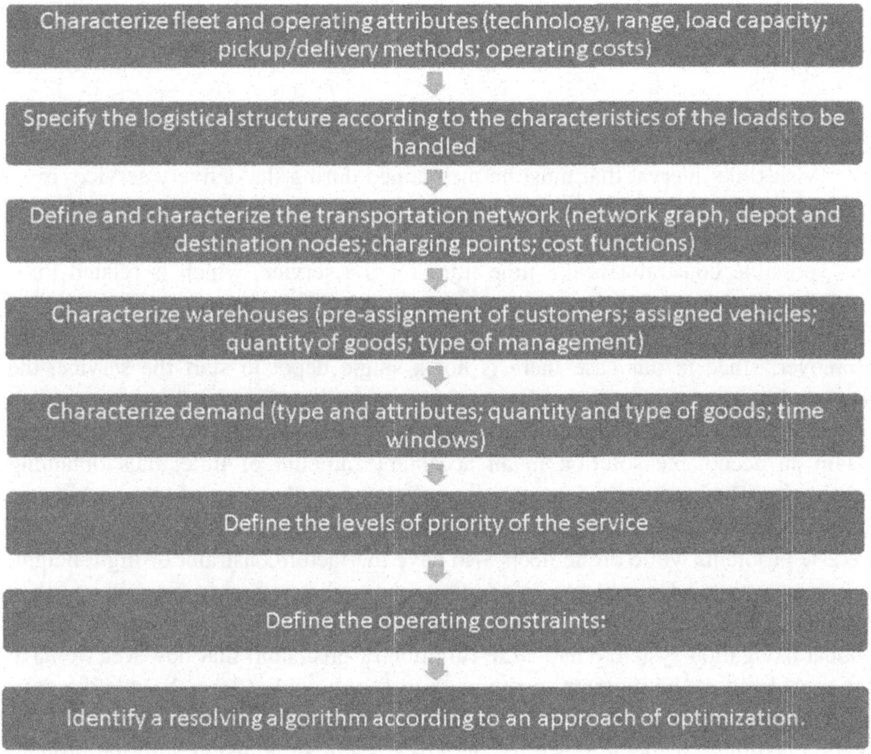

Characterize fleet and operating attributes (technology, range, load capacity; pickup/delivery methods; operating costs)

↓

Specify the logistical structure according to the characteristics of the loads to be handled

↓

Define and characterize the transportation network (network graph, depot and destination nodes; charging points; cost functions)

↓

Characterize warehouses (pre-assignment of customers; assigned vehicles; quantity of goods; type of management)

↓

Characterize demand (type and attributes; quantity and type of goods; time windows)

↓

Define the levels of priority of the service

↓

Define the operating constraints:

↓

Identify a resolving algorithm according to an approach of optimization.

FIGURE 13.4 Project phases considered for the flight plan.

TABLE 13.2
Input and Output Parameters for the Optimization

INPUT Parameters	ID	OUTPUT Parameters	ID
Maximum flight time	Tmax (in min)		
Maximum mission time	MTmax (in days)		
Radius from area center	R (in m)		
Speed	S (in km/h)		
Intersections of air routes	IAR (variable point coordinates)	Track	TR
Drone position	PSN (variable point coordinates)		
Time until intersection of air routes	TIAR (if no, ok; else change speed)	Speed	S
Track	TR		
Destination coordinates	DEST	Requested altitude	RA
Wind speed	WSPD		
Wind direction	WDI	Battery consumption	FR
Flight altitude	A	Fuel remaining	
No-fly zones	NFZ (area coordinates)		

grouped with respect to their constraints. Such constraints may relate, for example, to:

- the available number of depots,
- the size of the demand parameter, or one may impose a constraint of the visit time interval that must be maintained during the delivery service. In case the capacity constraints imposed on the vehicle fleet are exceeded, it becomes necessary to assign a new vehicle with a new route. Another possible constraint is the time limit for the service, which is related to flight time and fuel consumption (in our case of the battery).

Moreover, since in our case there is not a single depot to start the service, the scenario becomes more complex but can be faced both with exact algorithms, which however need a long computation time, and with metaheuristic approaches that can obtain an acceptable solution in an acceptable amount of time, thus obtaining "populations" of quite efficient solutions. Related to the purpose of reaching an optimal path, analogous is the traveling salesman problem (TSP). VRPs and TSPs are 2-D problems while drone fleets also have the factor/constraint of flight height, thus constituting 3-D problems. In addition, our application takes place in an urban environment; therefore, with additional problems of reduced accuracy of GNSS (global navigation systems) and DOP (dilution of precision) that however we have not considered at the moment, postponing to future applications the relative optimization, as well as at the moment we have not considered additional factors such as the maximum available power of the UAV, paths in collision with the ground, paths that require more battery power than initially available and paths that cannot be smoothed using circular arcs.

The search for the best path is often associated with the search for the shortest path. This is the case for solving the traveling salesman problem (TSP), which involves finding the shortest route that visits all given cities once. In the case of UAV route planning, the optimal route is more complex and includes many different features. To account for these features, a cost function is used and the route planning algorithm becomes a search for a route that will minimize the cost function. The cost of a route decreases with the degree to which the desired features are satisfied. A route that satisfies all features to a high degree would result in a low cost.

We define our cost function (13.1), according to constraints and parameters of Table 13.2, as follows:

$$F_{cost} = C_{Tmax} + C_{MTmax} + C_R + C_S + C_{IAR} + C_{PSN} + C_{TIAR} + C_{TR} + C_{DEST} + C_{WSPD} + C_{WDI} + C_A + C_{NFZ} \tag{13.1}$$

where C_{Tmax}, C_{MTmax} and C_R penalize routes that are temporally longer; C_S, C_{WSPD} and C_{WDI} penalize flying at higher UAV speeds, higher wind speeds and flying in the opposite direction of the wind; C_{IAR} and C_{TIAR} penalize routes with collision risk, C_{TR} and C_{DEST} penalize longer and more complex routes, C_A penalizes routes with higher average altitude and C_{NFZ} penalizes routes that cross areas that should not be flown over.

In particular, C_R, C_A and C_{NFZ} are optimization criteria and are used to improve trajectory quality.

During the optimization phase of our algorithm, a solution will be sought that minimizes the cost function and, thus, finds a trajectory that best satisfies factors and constraints represented in the cost function. The genetic algorithm will minimize the cost function by finding the four parameters (TR, S, RA and FR) that will define the best trajectory.

In case it creates a broken trajectory and therefore has a function of cost for every element, it would be necessary to have a function of total cost and sum of the single functions of cost.

GA is a non-deterministic optimization method based on Darwin's genetic theory of evolution. It simulates the evolution of a population of solutions to optimize a problem. Similar to living organisms that adapt to their environment over generations, solutions in the GA adapt to a fitness function by an iterative process using biology-like operators such as chromosome crossovers, mutations and gene reversals. GA is used here to simulate the evolution of a population of trajectories by fitting them to the cost function defined in the previous lines. The initial trajectories are then randomly generated without considering their feasibility. The suitability of each solution is then evaluated and "parent" solutions are selected. The "child" solutions are created from the selected parents using the crossover step. Mutations such as adding a new waypoint, deleting or modifying an existing node are then applied to the "child" solutions. Finally, the "parent" generation is replaced by the "child" generation and the evolutionary cycle continues until the termination criterion is met such as, for example, a fixed execution time or the maximum number of generations to be simulated. At this point, the bubble sort genetic algorithm is implemented to sort solutions.

In Figure 13.5, a diagram of the multi-objective optimization problem, with factors and constraints from which, through the genetic algorithm, we arrive at the optimized solutions.

The parameters are calculated at the beginning of each run of the code and have the task of making dimensionless calculations in order to adapt to the input files. To facilitate the reading, they are then reconverted in dimensional quantities. We can see the best sequences we were able to find in relation to factors and constraints, i.e. the best solutions in terms of speed, height, battery consumption and flight time, to optimize the flight plan. The optimal solution, once obtained on the basis of the calculation of the multi-objective function, is selected and then the flight plan of the drone is set.

13.3.2 Monitoring Crowd and Flows

In relation to the crowding monitoring phase, the same GIS is already implemented for the distribution of medical material also makes it possible to carry out up-to-date monitoring of the movements of people using the LPT and to identify the sections of the route that may require reinforcement cars to reduce

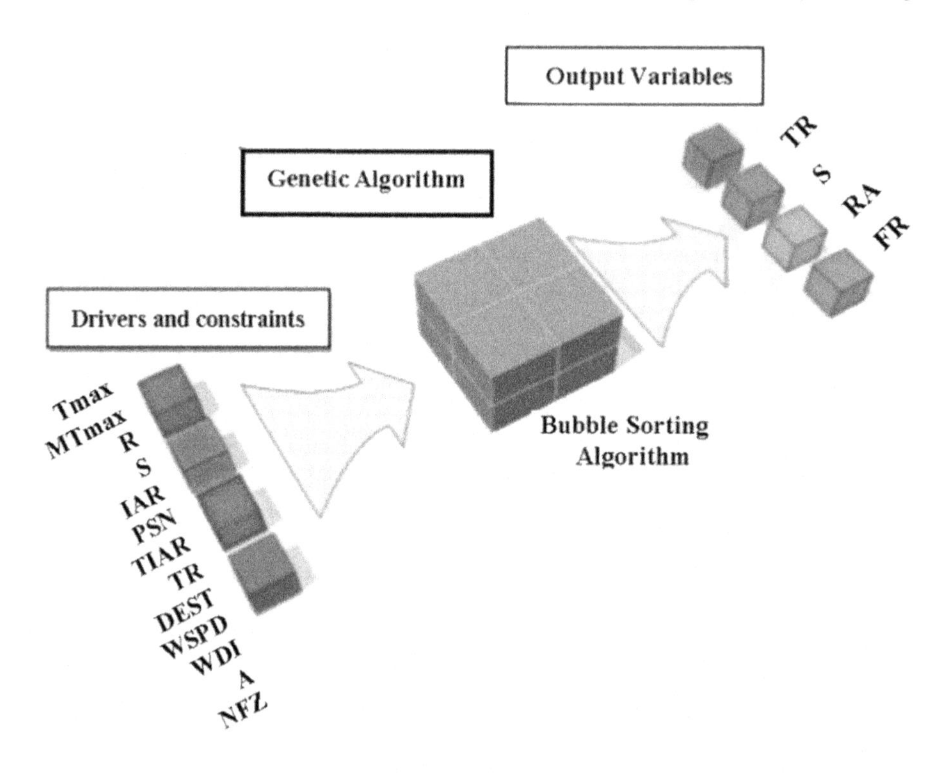

FIGURE 13.5 Multi-objective function, with factors and constraints and output variables.

crowding inside vehicles and at stops [23–25]. The objective was to obtain forecasts of flow information on an hourly basis and on a continuous cycle on trends, based on the comparison between data acquired in real time and historical data. The target is the ability to follow people along the entire route from origin to destination using mainly machine learning techniques in order to build the O/D matrix with real data (monitoring) and not estimated (traditional techniques). This result was obtained by correlating the images collected by the cameras of public transport, those installed at bus stops and those mounted on drones (processed with the YOLO algorithm for people detection and the SORT sorting algorithm for tracking, and then through machine learning applications) integrated with the tracking of the MAC address that, to respect privacy, is immediately "obfuscated" through the application of a cryptographic hash function [26]. Specifically, in order to determine the path of the single user we have built the matrix of origin-destination with the tracking obtained by processing the various images and applying the algorithms of machine learning (YOLO and SORT) and with the MAC address (a unique identifier of the personal telecommunications device that each of us now carries with him), integrating and verifying the results obtained with the classic method of construction of the matrix O/D and the use of particular models through interviews. The O/D matrix (the purpose of which is to have traffic flows in the study area inbound, outbound and internal) was therefore constructed by inserting the flows thus detected on an hourly basis.

This was necessary in order to know the actual destinations of users who use the LPT, and who stop at bus stops to wait for the bus to reach their destination. In fact, it is necessary to obtain a statistical distribution of departure-arrival points (note the departure, i.e. the bus stop). To this end, the flow present in each cell of the O/D matrix was subsequently subdivided into the number of users using a certain line of the LPT, also using the MAC address. We have therefore created an innovative tool in the management of the exercise applicable both in the current historical moment and in the ordinary management of the LPT. At present, in fact, it is not possible to obtain complete origin-destination matrices in an automatic way, since the data coming, for example, from the validation of electronic tickets (where available) provide information on the uphill stop but not on the downhill stop. The objective of the project is therefore a significant increase in knowledge in this area.

13.3.3 Machine Learning Algorithms and Codes Used for the Proposed Automated System

The whole system has been easily programmed in Python and foresees the management of the following five main blocks:

1. PC platform for data transmission to the drone, through Python programming in CoLab (user request, flight plan);
2. On-board software (ArduPilot), to acquire the signal transmitted by the PC that indicates to the drone where to fly and for the transmission from the drone to the PC with analog video transmitters with the aim of transmitting the video in real time; for this purpose, micro-controllers are used that use SPI and I2C protocols for hardware and software communication to exchange data with external peripherals in synchronous mode;
3. Antenna platform: MAC address signals from routers are tracked through an HTM code that identifies and localizes them.
4. PC platform for processing: in order to design the automatic flight plan following the user request, which determines rules fixed with IFTTT, GA organized in Python) is used. in relation to data processing, a receiver has been connected to the PC via USB OTG cable in order to pick up the video signal that will be the input for subsequent processing. It has been organized a SQL DB managed through sqlite 3 library containing the information related to the elements to be recognized (people); the application uses two main libraries of which the OpenCV manages the functionality related to pattern recognition within the image (YOLO and SORT) and the functions of writing and reading of the folder, while the other library PyQt5 manages the graphic part and then allows an integration between the user and the system;
5. Platform for transmission to the GIS and user interface: it runs a procedure called data transfer GIS (DTGIS) for the subsequent export of the data acquired within the GIS, where the "historical" update is managed in the existing database, in order to verify the effectiveness of the development.

In more detail, the DTGIS was developed to automatically transfer to the GIS the data acquired by the drone fleet in three software modules, each with specific functions:

1. The plug-in module that extends the number of objects that can be represented, recognizable and classifiable;
2. The kernel that interact with the users, coordinates the different modules, pre-processing and post- processing the input/output data of the modules themselves;
3. The GIS I/O (input/output) module that manages the interface with the GIS software.

In particular, in the GIS I/O module are given the inputs in the files (space database where the different attributes have been assigned to the objects), returning output polylines and polygons in shp-dbf format.

More in detail, a number of algorithms and methodologies have been used to implement the proposed system. Specifically:

- A multi-objective function, using genetic algorithms, previously described, was used for determining the flight plan choices of the drones.
- For the phase of transport and delivery of medical material, algorithms we have developed for charging and recognition of charging stations, of the IFTTT type, have been used.
- To determine the flows the machine learning algorithms YOLO and SORT were used, while for the origin/destination matrix, the MAC address was also acquired.
- In addition, real-time hourly and continuous cycle information on trends, based on a comparison with recent and historical data, was obtained with the application of machine learning algorithms (including the back-propagation algorithm for the historical series).

13.3.3.1 IFTTT (If This Then That)

It is a code that allows real-time creation of condition chains called applets, triggered by other services (e.g. Gmail, Facebook, Instagram, etc.) and can send a message when, for example, the user uses a hashtag in a tweet, or can send a copy of a Facebook photo to an archive when the user is tagged in it. IFTTT can automate processes related to home automation or web applications such as receiving personalized weather forecasts or alerts in case of events such as floods or other [33]. In our case, we have used this service to send alerts to request medical material and to realize the automatic flight of drones when the alert is received.

The programming logic of **applets** is in fact of the type:

- **if** a determined **event** happens (**trigger**)
- **then** execute a determined **action**

In Figure 13.6, is a simple piece of code as an example of IFTTT programming is the temporal choice of the system activity.

```
[ ] var currentHour = Meta.currentUserTime.hour()
    if (currentHour >= 8 || currentHour < 16 ) { }
    else {
    Fly.FlyFleet.skip
```

FIGURE 13.6 Part of code of IFTTT programming for the temporal choice of the system activity.

13.3.3.2 YOLO

You Only Look Once (YOLO) is a convolutional neural network [27] that can predict multiple positions and box categories simultaneously and can realize end-to-end target detection and recognition [28–30]. Its greatest advantage is its speed, which makes it suitable for applications, for example, in the field of monitoring of flight targets, but it is also widely used in case of fires, obstacles, in medicine, in sports and finally, and this is what interests us most, in the detection of vehicles and pedestrians. YOLO, for its speed of execution (it processes images in real time at 45 frames per second) is ideal in the case of real-time detection of human figures at the stops of local public transport and inside buses [25,31]. The detection is not a real recognition such as to lead to the identification of the person (which would pose problems of privacy) but, together with the SORT algorithm (a sorting algorithm, or sorting, which allows us to count the bounding boxes created by YOLO), makes it possible to track a person inscribed in the bounding box along its movement [25].

In particular, in our application, the O/D matrix is built and updated hourly through the YOLO and SORT algorithms and through MAC address counting, using the Python platform for object classification and the GIS Python console for updating the O/D matrix through MAC address counting and/or bounding boxes.

Specifically:

- Acquired the images from the cameras present either on the bus or at the stops, the same are processed through the YOLO algorithm in order only to obtain an object classification.
- The image to be examined is subdivided in a grid, and it will be examined through a convolutional neural network with the help of "convolutional" sliding windows considering every single cell as a window.

The visual interface for the individuation of the searched element consists of the restitution of a vector of the type: [pc bx by bw bh c1 c2 c3] where:

pc is the probability that the image contains one of the recognized objects, bx is the x-coordinate of the center of the object, by is y-coordinate of the center of the object, bw is width of the box containing the recognized object and bh is the height of the box containing the recognized object.

c1 is the probability that the object belongs to class 1, c2 is the probability that the object belongs to the class 2 and c3 is the probability that the object belongs to class 3.

Once this vector is returned, the visual interface would be able to draw a box containing the object (bounding box).

Each bounding box (of each cell) is predicted by the model with five values:

$$\text{x, y, w, h and the “Pr(Object)} * IOU_{\text{pred}}^{\text{truth}}\text{”,}$$

where:

(x, y) are the coordinates of the center of the bounding box with respect to the edges of the grid cell, W is the width of the bounding box, h is the height of the bounding box, Pr(Object) is the confidence score, and $IOU_{\text{pred}}^{\text{truth}}$ Intersection Over Union is a metric used in the systems of object detection in order to determine the deviation between the bounding box previewed from the model and those real ones.

Every cell of the grid, independently from the number B of bounding box generated, predicts C classes with the relative conditioned probability `(Pr(Class |Object))`

To this point, the model, for every bounding box, multiplies the conditioned probabilities of the classes (of the cell) with the confidence score of the bounding box, obtaining therefore a specific confidence score of every class for every bounding box:

$$\text{Pr(ClassilObject)} * \text{Pr(Object)} * IOU_{\text{pred}}^{\text{truth}} = \text{Pr(Classi)} * IOU_{\text{pred}}^{\text{truth}}$$

The value thus obtained encodes both the probability that an object of a given class will appear in the bounding box under consideration (Figure 13.7), and the precision with which the predicted bounding box delimits the spatial contours of the object.

The bounding boxes of the single object thus created are related in the different acquisition devices through the SORT algorithm.

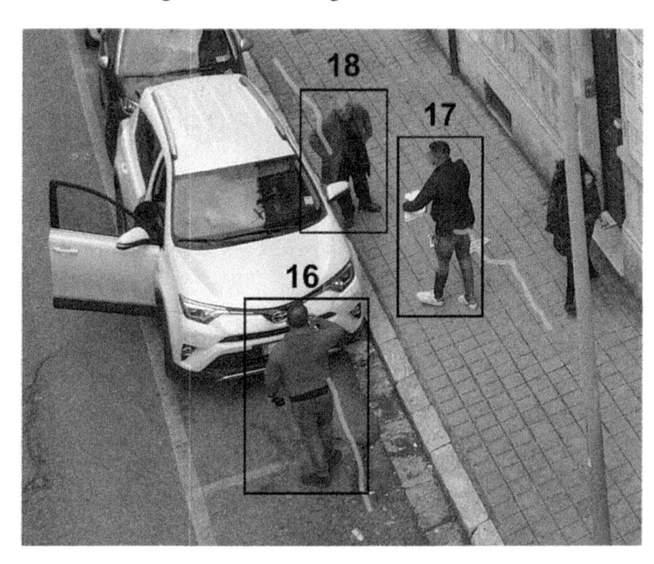

FIGURE 13.7 Bounding boxes created by YOLO algorithm and tracking by SORT.

```
import numpy as np
import time
import cv2
from darkflow.net.build import TFNet
import matplotlib.pyplot as plt
```

FIGURE 13.8 Part of YOLO code for real-time acquisition and creation of the darkflow model instance.

```
options = {
 'model': 'cfg/yolo.cfg',
 'load': 'bin/yolov2.weights',
 'threshold': 0.3

}
tfnet = TFNet(options)
```

FIGURE 13.9 Part of YOLO code for real-time acquisition and creation of the darkflow model instance defined using options.

In Figures 13.8 and 13.9 are parts of the YOLO code for real-time acquisition and creation of the darkflow model instance defined using options.

13.3.3.3 SORT

SORT is a simple, real-time algorithm for 2-D online tracking of multiple objects in video sequences, designed for online tracking applications where only past and current frames are available and the method produces object identities on the fly [32].

This data, compared to the MAC, address "wake" of cell phones, allows for verification of displacements and consequently flow calculations. These flow data, once inserted in the O/D matrix and processed, can be predicted in the short term from the time series.

Figure 13.10 shows a piece of code of the SORT algorithm.

13.3.3.4 Backpropagation

In machine learning, particularly in deep learning, backpropagation is a widely used algorithm in training neural networks for supervised learning. Neural networks are characterized by the presence of loops that have a large impact on the learning and prediction capabilities of the network:

1. The initialization of "weights" in a random manner;
2. The propagation of the initial data with relative multiplication by the "weights", and then passing the results through the activation function;
3. The comparison of the obtained results with the supervised ones;
4. The error assessment to understand the goodness of the "weights" adopted;
5. The actual backpropagation phase of adjustment of the "weights" if necessary.

```
from sort import *

#create instance of SORT
mot_tracker = Sort()

# get detections
...

# update SORT
track_bbs_ids = mot_tracker.update(detections)

# track_bbs_ids is a np array where each row contains a valid bounding box and track_id (last column)
...
```

FIGURE 13.10 Part of the code of the SORT algorithm.

The algorithm of backpropagation can be interrupted when the error becomes sufficiently small, at our discretion. To train a neural net means to modify in recursive way parameters, that is the "weights" that are initially attributed in random way and then adjusted every time we have a new epoch. The backpropagation is very useful to analyze trends and then with time series-based predictive functions; in this sense, it is used in our experimental application.

13.3.3.5 MAC Address

The MAC address isn't an algorithm but the physical address of the device. Every mobile device, if it has Wi-Fi enabled, near a Wi-Fi router leaves a trace of its MAC address in the router's log. This trace can be followed in its own path. This is necessary because users who use the LPT, and who are waiting at bus stops to reach their destination, could take any bus; for this reason, we need to obtain a statistical distribution of departure-arrival points.

Figure 13.11 shows a piece of code in HTML to count and locate the single MAC address at the arrival bus stop.

13.3.3.6 Genetic Algorithm

Those called genetic algorithms, already explained previously, are stochastic optimization algorithms that allow to evaluate different starting solutions as if they were different individuals, recombining them (analogous to biological reproduction). By introducing elements of disorder analogous to genetic mutations, new solutions (new individuals) are produced and evaluated by choosing the best ones

```
function showPosition(position) {
    var latlon = position.coords.latitude + "," + position.coords.longitude;
    var img_url = "http://maps.googleapis.com/maps/api/staticmap?center="
    +latlon+"&zoom=14&size=400x300&sensor=false";
    document.getElementById("mapholder").innerHTML = "<img src='"+img_url+"'>";
```

FIGURE 13.11 Part of code in HTML to count and locate the single MAC address at the arrival bus stop.

```
void BubbleSort(Vector a, int n)
{
    for(int j=n-1; j > 0; j--)
        for(int k=0; k < j; k++)
            if (a[k+1] < a[k])
                Swap(a,k,k+1);
}
def bubbleSort(arr):
  n = len(arr)
  # Traverse through all array elements
  for i in range(n-1):
  # range(n) also work but outer loop will repeat one time more than needed.    # Last i elements are already in place
    for j in range(0, n-i-1):
      # traverse the array from 0 to n-i-1      # Swap if the element found is greater      # than the next element
      if arr[j] > arr[j+1] :
        arr[j], arr[j+1] = arr[j+1], arr[j]
# Driver code to test above
arr = Fc
bubbleSort(arr)
print ("Sorted array is:")
for i in range(len(arr)):
  print ("%d" %arr[i]),
```

FIGURE 13.12 Part of the bubble sort code for sorting in Python.

(environmental selection). Each of these stages of recombination and selection is called generation like that of living beings [34]. Finally, it converges toward solutions "of optimal". They are then able to perform multi-objective optimizations quickly, not requiring calculation of the gradient but simply evaluating the value of the objective function with less accuracy (in our case not necessary) but with greater robustness than other algorithms used in optimization problems.

In particular, in our experimentation, the bubble sorting algorithm is used, a simple GA algorithm for sorting a list of data. Each pair of adjacent elements is compared and reversed in position if they are in a wrong order. The algorithm continues to perform these steps again throughout the list until no more swaps are performed, a situation that shows that the list is sorted. Some parts of its code for sorting in Python are shown in Figure 13.12.

13.4 CASE STUDY

The experimentation of the system we proposed has been carried out in the neighborhood between Viale Genoese Zerbi, Viale della Libertà and Viale Amendola, in the city of Reggio Calabria (RC), Italy (in Figure 13.13). The study area is defined only at the neighborhood level, not being possible at this stage the extension to the entire city, and having only research character.

It should be clarified that trials were conducted on an experimental basis only, to validate the soundness of the proposed research procedure, and that only partial and not exhaustive data were used. In fact, the data used are few or, in some cases, simulated and were used only to validate the proposed method.

The operational phases of the experimentation that, through the use of GIS, the fleet of drones and the system of cameras at the stops and on the buses together with the use of various machine learning algorithms, allows both the delivery of medical supplies and the monitoring and control of gatherings among the users of the LPT, are described below.

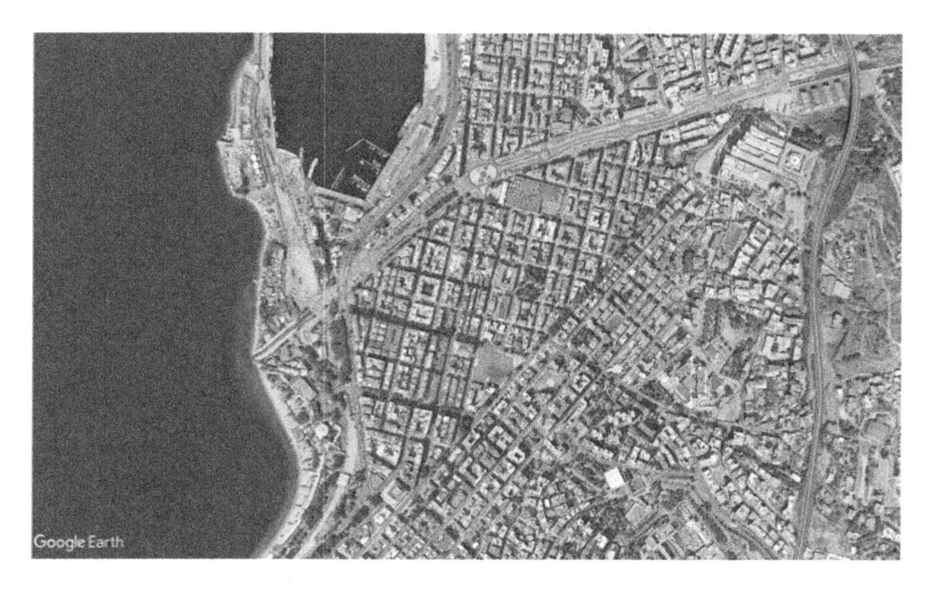

FIGURE 13.13 Study area, a neighborhood of Reggio Calabria (RC), Italy.

13.4.1 Medical Goods Delivery

In relation to the problem inherent in the transport of medical equipment, by referring to the flow chart in Figure 13.1 and the algorithms explained, the operational phases are:

- The user reports through the open GIS the medical supplies he needs, an alert is generated;
- Through IFTTT the alert is sent to the operations center;
- The flight plan is automatic: the multi-objective problem is solved (with genetic algorithms) choosing the best one according to depots, collection points, recharge columns and bus stops; the collection point is chosen with distance comparison, the minimum distance is chosen with buffer operations from the request coordinates;
- Once the flight plan is chosen and the drone is equipped, the latter leaves with the medical material;
- During the journey the drone acquires images of bus stops;
- For longer journeys, the drone recharges through the recharging columns described in 13.3.1 and transmits the images acquired along the way;
- The drone delivers medical supplies to collection points, where it transmits images;
- An alert is sent notifying the user of the successful delivery (with IFTTT);
- Once recharged, the drone returns to the original depot or to other depots (depending on any new flight plans acquired via the recharging column).

Figure 13.14

We used a system based on a fleet of four drones.

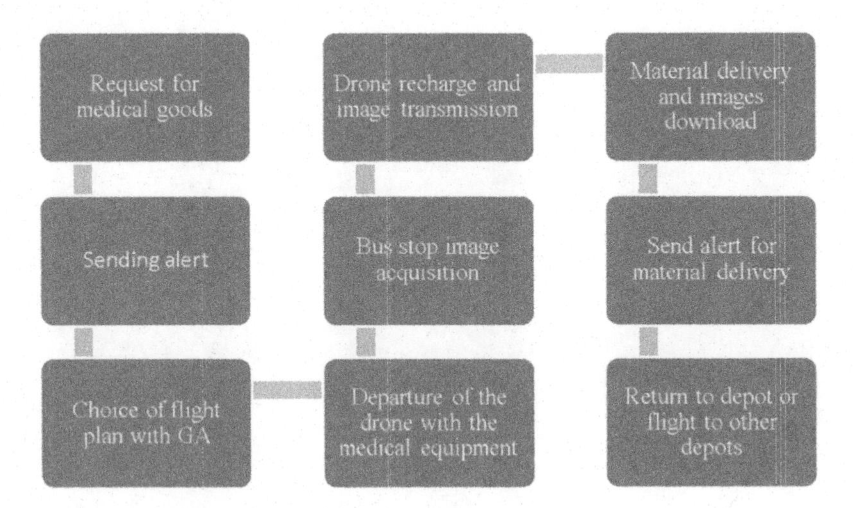

FIGURE 13.14 Operational phases of transport and delivery of medical supplies.

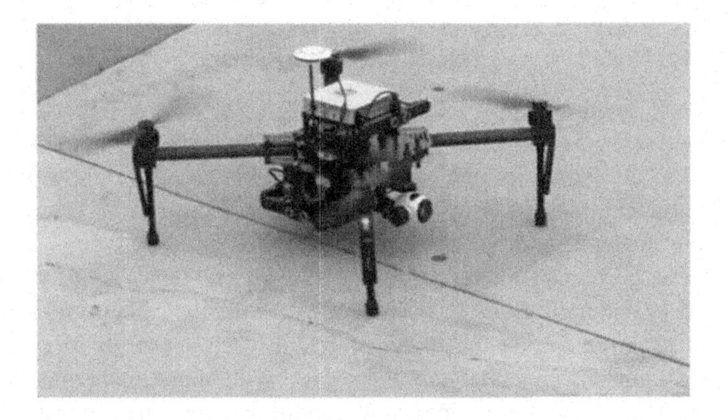

FIGURE 13.15 Drone used for the experimental system.

The drones used (DJI Matrice 100, in Figure 13.15, fully programmable and customizable), are equipped with omnidirectional vision sensors, obstacle detection system, intelligent features such as point of interest, allowing to easily create complex shooting and are equipped with a fully stabilized three-axis gimbal camera, with a 1/2-inch CMOS sensor to record 4K videos and take 20-Mpixel photos.

More in detail, we identified:

- n. 2 deposits of departure and recharge of the drones (marked in the GIS of Figure 13.16 with a man icon pushing warehouse cart) simulating the supply and distribution of material of comparable size and consistency to those respectively of:
  1. Masks
  2. Gowns
  3. Hydroxychloroquine, sanitizing gels and sprays, etc.

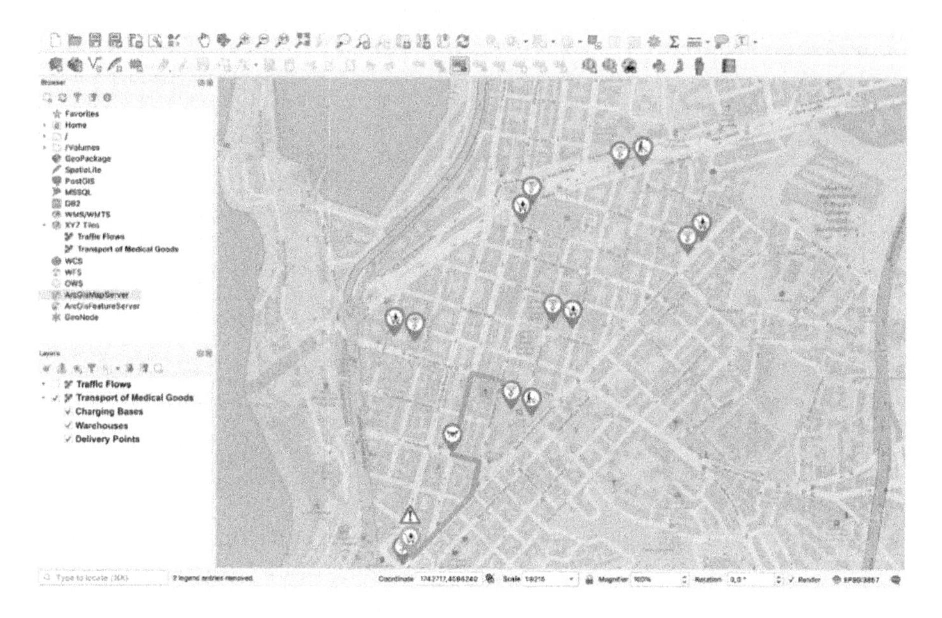

FIGURE 13.16 Flight plan with alert and delivery by drone.

- n. 5 delivery points (marked in the GIS of Figure 13.16 by a shopping cart with an arrow) located within the neighborhood to allow the end user to receive the goods in total safety and without risk of crowds. The indicator changes color when selected for delivery.
- n. 7 recharge bases (marked in the GIS of Figure 13.16 with by a thunderbolt) to recharge drone batteries, receive new flight plans and transmit images acquired during the route, placed in such a way as to guarantee the maximum distance that can be covered with single recharges, also in relation to possible environmental conditions and the weight of the transported goods.

The system built and tested works as follows:

- The external user, using the multi-platform webGIS created (computer, tablet and smartphone) alerts the requests (marked in the GIS of Figure 13.16 by a triangle) for delivery of sanitary material to the control center installed in this experiment at the geomatics laboratory.
- The center, having received the alert, displays in the GIS the request; automatically (using IFTTT applets) the drone is ready to leave according to the pre-set flight plan resulting from the multi-objective analysis with genetic algorithm (marked in the GIS of Figure 13.16 with a blue route, with the drone icon sliding on the path), which is best suited to deliver the medical supplies, taking into account the distance from the depots, collection points and recharging stations. It starts from the depot in an automated way for the delivery of the sanitary material that will be deposited

in the predetermined delivery points and captures images of bus stops along the way. The preset route requires the drone to recharge along the way through a recharge column (described in 13.3.1). A flashing alert (marked in the GIS of Figure 13.16 by a flashing triangle) is sent, notifying the user of the successful delivery. The charging station near the collection point allows the drone to recharge, transmit images, return to the depot, or acquire new flight plans to possibly head to other depots. The acquired and transmitted images are finally stored inside a DataCube.

In Figure 13.16 is the flight plan, with depots, recharge bases, delivery points and, at the bottom of the figure, location of the alert with request of material goods.

As seen, in the image is the location of the 2 depot points (man icon pushing warehouse cart), 7 charging points (thunderbolt icon) and 5 drop-off points (shopping cart icon) located in the neighborhood chosen for the case study. Each depot and drop-off point includes a charging point. Specifically, the image shows the flight plan and the path of a drone that, following the request for medical material from a user, takes off with the medical material from the recharge point and the deposit located in Piazza del Popolo, and heads towards the collection point located in front of the Archaeological Museum of Reggio Calabria (at the beginning of Viale Giovanni Amendola), where it will finally deliver the medical material, following the path obtained by solving the multi-objective problem with genetic algorithm. Depending on the state of the battery, the drone will return to the deposit, or it will recharge in the recharge column placed near the collection point. The alert shows the collection point chosen according to the position of the user who made the request for medical material.

13.4.2 Monitoring and Control of Movements and Crowding

Regarding the monitoring and control of crowding, our experimentation consisted of the experimental placement of Wi-Fi and cameras at bus stops and on the affected LPT bus lines; capturing and storing the images of the installed cameras; applying machine learning algorithms (YOLO, SORT) on the images and then detecting people at the stops detected by the bounding boxes (with YOLO) and tracking the individual paths of the users detected by the YOLO bounding boxes (with SORT). In addition, we tracked user paths anonymously with MAC addresses captured by routers at stops and on buses. Then we constructed the origin-destination matrix, also verified with interviews. We visualized the obtained results (traffic flows and crowding) in the GIS.

Said phases are indicated in Figure 13.17.

In our case study, we used the images acquired by the cameras of public transportation (simulated by us experimentally, with smartphones on poles), by the cameras installed in bus stops (also installed experimentally) and by the cameras mounted on drones (the lines and stops investigated are those that affect the neighborhood under study).

These images were processed in real time with the YOLO algorithm (which allows the detection of objects and people based on their appearance characteristics,

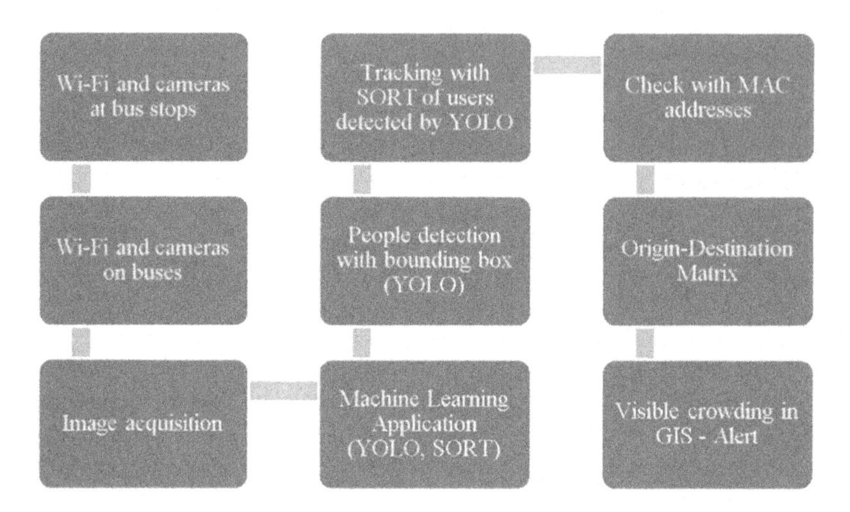

FIGURE 13.17 Operational phases of monitoring and control of movements and crowding.

i.e. geometric shape, contour, color or edge and their movement characteristics in subsequent frames) and then the SORT sorting algorithm for tracking.

The images have been integrated with the tracking of the MAC address which, in order to respect privacy, is immediately "obfuscated" through the application of a cryptographic hash function.

Regarding the data transmission to the software platform and the MAC address tracking (paragraph 13.3.2), limited to our neighborhood we have placed Wi-Fi sensors at bus stops, and provided with cameras both bus stops and buses.

The installation of Wi-Fi sensors has allowed us to verify the presence of the degree of crowding at the bus stop in a completely anonymous way and not related to the company that manages the telephone users. In addition, this experimental campaign allowed for statistically significant feedback on the number of people getting on and off the bus at the stop.

In order to determine the path of the single user we built the origin-destination matrix (Figure 13.18) with the tracking obtained by processing the images and applying the machine learning algorithms YOLO and SORT, and with the MAC address detected in the Wi-Fi log at the passage of mobile phone users. The verification monitoring was carried out through a sample analysis of the passengers present with the classic method of construction of the O/D matrix to verify the numerical veracity of the data sent by the sensors, through interviews and the use of suitable models.

Specifically, Figure 13.18 shows the origin/destination matrix obtained as described, that reports internal, interchange, crossing and intra-zonal displacements.

It is noted that the same origin/destination matrix is hourly updated via a txt as is shown in the GIS (Figure 13.19). More specifically, Figure 13.19 shows the origin/destination matrix at a peak hour (1:00 pm) in March.

Figure 13.20 shows instead the origin/destination matrix at the same peak hour in August.

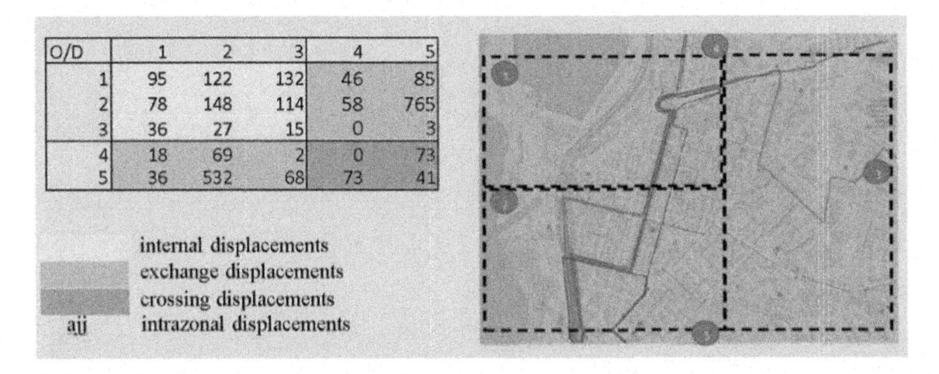

O/D	1	2	3	4	5
1	95	122	132	46	85
2	78	148	114	58	765
3	36	27	15	0	3
4	18	69	2	0	73
5	36	532	68	73	41

FIGURE 13.18 Origin-destination matrix.

	ID	Time	Flow 1	Flow 2	Flow 3	Flow 4	Flow 5	Flow
1								
2	1-2-3-5	13:00	50	97	5	0	44	196
3	1-2-3-5	13:00	33	98	7	0	41	178
4	2-3-5	13:00	0	93	6	0	50	149
5	2-3-5	13:00	0	104	8	0	49	161
6	1-2-3-5	13:00	40	90	6	0	48	184
7	1-2-3-5	13:00	55	97	5	0	47	204
8	2-3-5	13:00	0	91	6	0	44	141
9	2-3-5	13:00	0	95	9	0	49	153
10	1-2-3-5	13:00	42	98	7	0	48	195
11	1-2-3-5	13:00	45	87	8	0	43	183
12	1-2-3-5	13:00	43	92	5	0	48	188
13	1-2-3-5	13:00	54	83	8	31	53	199
14	1-2-4-5	13:00	52	9	0	40	51	142
15	1-2-4-5	13:00	24	12	0	47	44	120
16	1-2-4-5	13:00	24	7	0	44	44	171
17	1-2-4-5	13:00	20	10	0	162	47	171

FIGURE 13.19 Origin/destination matrix in the GIS.

As can be observed, the crowding is greatest on the lines leading to the beach and downtown: we have highlighted the most crowded line (circled in the figure).

From the matrix of origin-destination it is possible to individualize the area where the flows of displacement are greater and consequently to identify the lines (indicated with a greater thickness of the line) that cross that area.

As can be seen in Figure 13.21, the thicker lines, individually identified with MAC addresses, detect the bus routes with the greatest crowding based on the findings of the origin-destination matrix in the area under consideration.

It is also possible to visualize crowding at stops in the GIS. For example, in Figure 13.22, the crowds at the stops are indicated with circles of increasing size.

	ID	Time	Flow 1	Flow 2	Flow 3	Flow 4	Flow 5	Flow
1								
2	1-2-3-5	13:00	50	97	5	0	44	196
3	1-2-3-5	13:00	32	98	7	0	41	178
4	2-3-5	13:00	0	85	6	0	50	149
5	2-3-5	13:00	0	106	8	0	49	161
6	1-2-3-5	13:00	40	90	6	0	48	184
7	1-2-3-5	13:00	55	97	5	0	47	204
8	2-3-5	13:00	0	91	6	0	44	141
9	2-3-5	13:00	0	95	9	0	49	153
10	1-2-3-5	15:00	42	98	7	0	48	195
11	1-2-3-5	13:00	45	87	8	0	41	183
12	1-2-3-5	13:00	45	92	5	0	48	186
13	1-2-3-5	13:00	54	63	9	31	53	199
14	1-2-4-5	13:00	52	9	0	40	51	143
15	1-2-4-5	13:00	24	12	0	47	44	120
16	1-2-4-5	13:00	73	7	0	44	44	121
17	1-2-4-5	13:00	20	10	0	162	47	121

FIGURE 13.20 Origin/destination matrix, crowding alert for high value.

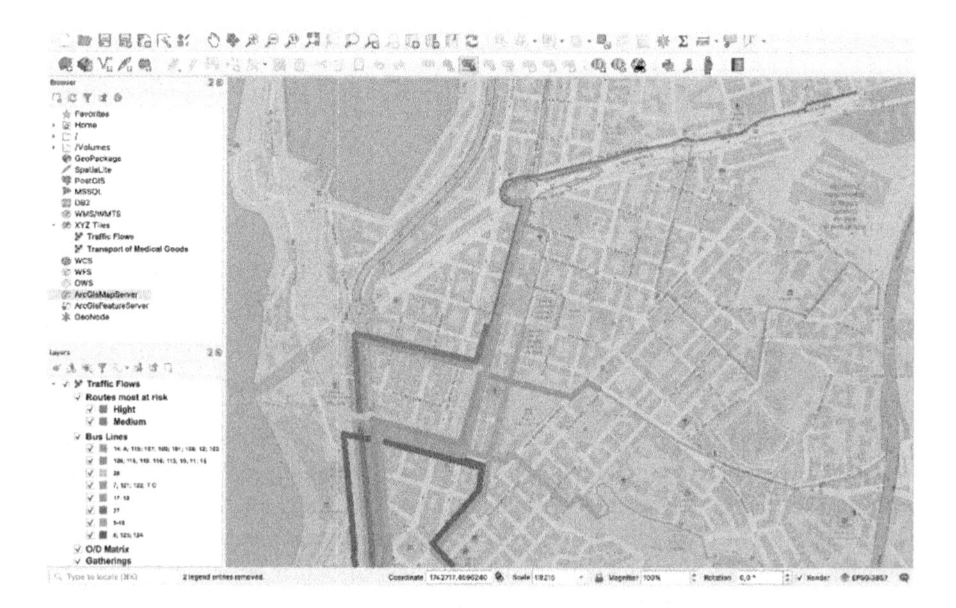

FIGURE 13.21 GIS showing the busiest LPT lines obtained from the origin-destination matrix.

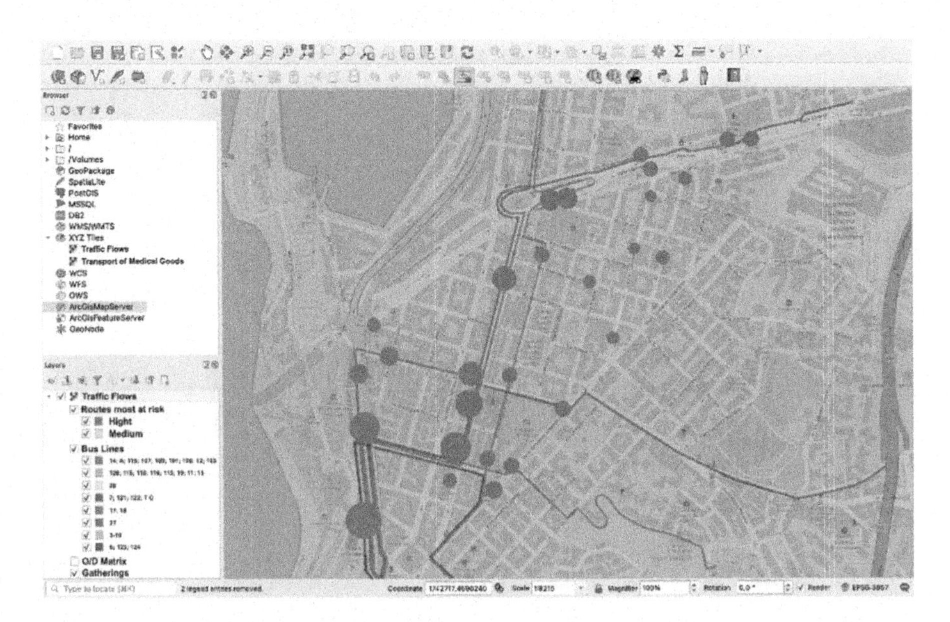

FIGURE 13.22 GIS, LPT lines with gatherings.

From Figures 13.21 and 13.22, it can be seen that the largest crowds are at the stops of the lines heading towards the center (which are represented thicker in Figure 13.21 while larger circles are seen in Figure 13.22), so the user can prefer less crowded stops or choose another time for his movements on the LPT vehicles.

Through the techniques of machine learning based on neural networks and algorithms of backpropagation are at the same time analyzed historical series to identify trends and send an alert to the LPT service. In fact, if the forecast exceeds the crowding threshold, the system signals the need for integration with another vehicle so as to distribute the LPT users correctly and at a distance and reduce crowding (Figure 13.23).

For example, in Figure 13.23, we see the thickest line visible that represents the stretch that on the basis of the predictive analysis carried out will be reinforced to meet the need that was already evident in Figure 13.21. In this way, it will be possible to intervene directly in a particular period such as this of the pandemic in which buses must travel at partial load by sending auxiliary bus, without the need to intervene in the re-planning of the entire urban transport system.

In conclusion, the GIS created, as well as doing what has been described in the previous paragraph (delivery of medical equipment), also makes it possible to monitor the movements of people using the LPT and to identify the sections of the route that require reinforcement bus to reduce congestion inside the vehicles and at stops.

In the future, in order to have reliable values and to provide certain results on the territory, it will be necessary to have more complete data, not partial time series, certain parameter values, possibly adding other parameters. Moreover, it will be necessary to have homogeneously distributed data. In fact, the data used today are

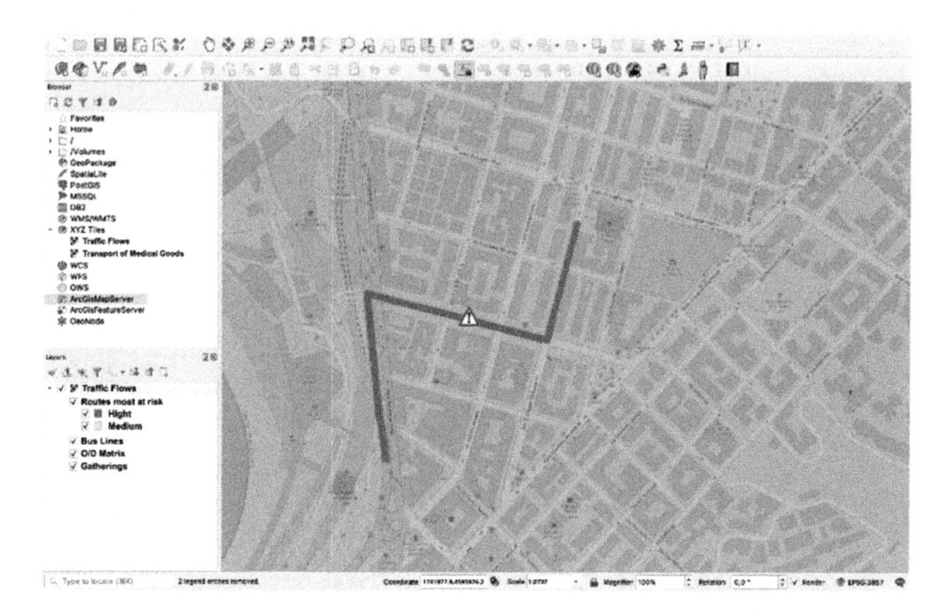

FIGURE 13.23 GIS, LPT: with machine learning, the lines that will be most crowded are identified and an alert is sent.

not sufficient to get definite answers on the territory but have only been used to test the proposed methodology.

13.5 DISCUSSION

In particular, with regard to monitoring and control, in this research we obtained:

- the monitoring of crowding (density), turnout (instant of arrival) and permanence (duration of presence) of passengers at bus line stops;
- monitoring of passenger boarding and alighting at individual stops;
- monitoring of traffic flow;
- the generation of alarms in the presence of crowding levels deemed critical.

As the research deepens, on the basis of what we experimented so far it will be possible to integrate with:

- the provision of real-time information to public transport users in relation to areas to be avoided as they are currently affected by levels of crowding judged to be critical;
- the forecast analysis of the number of passengers getting on and off the means of transport in order to be able to organize the trips (drivers and vehicles) necessary to deal with requests and to avoid the gathering of people at stops;
- the possibility of exposing the data processed via API to applications and platforms of the operator or third parties.

To date, in fact, we have created a system with great potential for research purposes. Currently, thanks to the possibilities of machine learning, it can be used for the transport of medical devices and for the monitoring and control of users who use the LPT, but in the future it can also be extended to the sanitization of critical indoor and outdoor environments, monitoring of pollutants, weather and traffic conditions.

This research may also provide a basis for suggesting new guidelines for changing current regulations regarding drones to make them an effective solution in emergency conditions.

13.6 CONCLUSIONS

The recent spread of COVID-19 has demonstrated the need to use automated solutions that require minimal personnel, both to increase cost/time efficiency and to limit physical contact (and thus limit the risk of contagion).

The normal applications of drones during the pandemic to date have been single-vehicle, one-to-one relationships. This project aims to overcome that limitation by proposing a significant advancement in industry research related to the management of a complex routing problem.

The biggest limitation is represented by the current regulations that we hope will be adapted to the needs of emergency situations.

As far as the monitoring and control of crowding is concerned, on the basis of the experimental work we have carried out, using more powerful hardware and software in the future we could improve the algorithms and extend the study area.

In the future, some of the algorithms used today can be subsequently implemented, improved, updated with other more performing and possibly more fitting.

After all, many steps forward have been made in the field of machine learning applied to medicine and health services [35–37].

It should be noted once again that in this contribution is presented mainly a method, not so much the results, unfortunately based on partial data and therefore certainly susceptible to improvement.

A dashboard platform for local public transport could also be implemented separately in the future. When fully operational, the bus driver could set up a complete monitoring of both what is happening on the bus in terms of crowding, and what may be happening at the next stop in terms of people waiting at the line. It is then also possible to report the numbers of seats available on the bus before the bus arrives at the stop. Platform and dashboard would then be used even after the health emergency for the management of the public transport line and its optimization, providing data not available today. In this way, it will be possible to study the best performance indicators to provide to users to optimize their travel choices. Platform and dashboard would be self-consistent web services, but nevertheless equipped with APIs to allow the use of the information collected and processed by third-party software. In this way, the individual operator will be able to customize the solution on their own legacy systems, optimizing its operational and applicative effectiveness in relation to their specific needs.

NOTES

1 The International Network of Crisis Mappers (Crisis Mappers Net) is an international community of experts, practitioners, policymakers, technologists, researchers, journalists, scholars, hackers and skilled volunteers engaged at the intersection of humanitarian crises, new technology, crowd-sourcing and crisis mapping.
2 Ushahidi, Inc. is a nonprofit company that develops free open source software for the collection, visualization and interactive geolocation of information. Ushahidi means "testimony" or "witness" in Swahili.
3 Patrick Meier (co-founder of the nonprofit WeRobotics) has operated numerous drone operations which he has reported on his blog https://irevolutions.org until March 2020) collaborating with Open Street Map, Google Crisis Response, OCHA (UN Office for the Coordination of Humanitarian Affairs), UNOSAT (UN Operational Satellite Applications Programme, which provides satellite imagery in support of humanitarian aid), WFP (UN World Food Programme) World Bank, Red Cross, played a key role in the foundation of Flying Labs, operational in 25 countries (Asia, Africa and Latin America).

REFERENCES

[1] Barrile, Vincenzo, Candela Gabriele, Fotia Antonino, and Bernardo Ernesto. "UAV Survey of Bridges and Viaduct: Workflow and Application." *Lecture Notes in Computer Science* 11622 (2019): 269–284. 10.1007/978-3-030-24305-0_21.

[2] Stauffer, Chris, and Grimson W. Eric L. "Learning patterns of activity using real-time tracking." IEEE *Transactions on Pattern Analysis and Machine Intelligence* 22, no. 8 (2000): 747–757. 10.1109/34.868677.

[3] Barrile, Vincenzo, Bernardo Ernesto, and Fotia Antonino. "GPS/GIS system for updating capable faults in the Calabrian territory through the use of soft computing techniques." *European Association of Geoscientists & Engineers. Conference Proceedings, International Conference of Young Professionals «GeoTerrace-2020»* 1 (2020): 1–5. 10.3997/2214-4609.20205710.

[4] CrisisMappers. (2009). Last access on March 25, 2021 http://crisismapping.ning.com

[5] Ushahidi. "At Ushahidi, we Imagine a World where Everyone is Empowered to Participate in Creating a Better World." (2009). Last access on March 23, 2021. https://www.ushahidi.com/

[6] Meier, Patrick. *Digital Humanitarians. How Big Data Is Changing the Face of Humanitarian Response*. Routledge, New York, (2015). 10.1201/b18023.

[7] Ofli, Ferda, Meier Patrick, Imran Muhammad, Castillo Carlos, Tuia Devis, Rey Nicolas, Briant Julien, Millet Pauline, Reinhard Friedrich, Parkan Matthew and Joost Stéphane. "Combining Human Computing and Machine Learning to Make Sense of Big (Aerial) Data for Disaster Response." *Big Data* 4, no. 1 (2016): 47–59.

[8] Meier, Patrick. "How Mosquitos are Hitching a Ride on Drones to Reduce Zika." (January 11, 2018). Last access on March 24, 2021 https://irevolutions.org/2018/01/11/drones-to-control-zika/

[9] WeRobotics. "It's Not About The Robots. It's about who gets to use them. It's about power. We shift power back to local experts in Africa, Asia, Latin America and beyond." (2016). Last access on March 23, 2021. https://werobotics.org/

[10] Prati, Andrea, Mikic Ivana, Trivedi Mohan M., and Cucchiara Rita. "Detecting moving shadows: algorithms and evaluation." *IEEE Transactions on Pattern Analysis and Machine Intelligence* 25, no. 7 (2003): 918–923. 10.1109/TPAMI.2003.1206520.

[11] Ratti, Carlo, Frenchman Dennis, Pulselli Riccardo M., and Williams Sarah. “Mobile Landscapes: Using Location Data from Cell Phones for Urban Analysis.” *Environment and Planning B: Planning and Design* 33, no. 5 (2006): 727–748. 10.1068/b32047.

[12] Bernardo, Ernesto, Barrile Vincenzo, Fotia Antonino and Bilotta Giuliana. “Landslide susceptibility mapping with fuzzy methodology”. *European Association of Geoscientists & Engineers Conference Proceedings, International Conference of Young Professionals «GeoTerrace-2020»* 1 (2020): 1–5. 10.3997/2214-4609.20205712.

[13] The Lancet Journal on Infectious Diseases of March 5, 2020.

[14] Terra Drone/Started transporting pharmaceutical drones in Zhejiang Province, China, (February 14, 2020). Last access on March, 25, 2021 https://dpcajapan.org/latest-technology/technology/%E3%83%86%E3%83%A9%E3%83%89%E3%83%AD%E3%83%BC%E3%83%B3%EF%BC%8F%E4%B8%AD%E5%9B%BD%E3%83%BB%E6%B5%99%E6%B1%9F%E7%9C%81%E3%81%A7%E5%8C%BB%E8%96%AC%E5%93%81%E9%A1%9E%E3%81%AE%E3%83%89%E3%83%AD%E3%83%BC/

[15] Barrile, Vincenzo, Candela Gabriele, and Fotia Antonino. “Point cloud segmentation using image processing techniques for structural analysis.” *ISPRS Annals of the Photogrammetry, Remote Sensing and Spatial Information Sciences* 42, no. 2/W11 (2019): 187–193. 10.5194/isprs-Archives-XLII-2-W11-187-2019.

[16] Barrile, Vincenzo, Bilotta Giuliana, D’Amore Enzo, Meduri Giuseppe M. and Trovato Sandro. “Structural modeling of a historic castle using close range photogrammetry.” *International Journal of Mathematics and Computers in Simulation* 10 (2016): 370–380.

[17] Barrile, Vincenzo, and Bilotta Giuliana. “Self-localization by Laser Scanner and GPS in automated surveys.” *Lecture Notes in Electrical Engineering*, 307 (2014): 293–313. 10.1007/978-3-319-03967-1.

[18] Fotia, Antonino, and Pucinotti Raffaele. “Applying 3D and Photogrammetric Scanning Systems to the Case of Cultural Heritage”. In *New Metropolitan Perspectives. NMP 2020. Smart Innovation, Systems and Technologies* (Bevilacqua C., Calabrò F., Della Spina L., eds.), 178, pp. 1532–1540, Cham: Springer, (2021). 10.1007/978-3-030-48279-4_143.

[19] Bernardo, Ernesto, Musolino Marialisa and Maesano Mariangela. “San Pietro di Deca: From Knowledge to Restoration. Studies and Geomatics Investigations for Conservation, Redevelopment and Promotion.” In *New Metropolitan Perspectives. NMP 2020. Smart Innovation, Systems and Technologies*, (Bevilacqua C., Calabrò F., Della Spina L., eds.) 178, Cham: Springer, (2021). 10.1007/978-3-030-48279-4_147.

[20] Bernardo, Ernesto, and Bilotta Giuliana. “Monumental Arc 3D Model Reconstruction Through BIM Technology”. In *New Metropolitan Perspectives. NMP 2020. Smart Innovation, Systems and Technologies*, (Bevilacqua C., Calabrò F., Della Spina L., eds.). 178. Cham: Springer, (2021). 10.1007/978-3-030-48279-4_148.

[21] Bernardo, Ernesto, Barrile Vincenzo and Fotia Antonino. “Innovative UAV methods for intelligent landslide monitoring.” *European Association of Geoscientists & Engineers Conference Proceedings, International Conference of Young Professionals «GeoTerrace-2020»* 1 (2020): 1–5. 10.3997/2214-4609.20205713.

[22] Astrachan, Owen L. “Bubble sort: An archaeological algorithmic analysis.” *SIGCSE Bulletin(Association for Computing Machinery, Special Interest Group on Computer Science Education)*, (2003): 1–5.

[23] Nadimi, Sadegh, and Bhanu Bir. “Physical models for moving shadow and object detection in video.” in *IEEE Transactions on Pattern Analysis and Machine Intelligence* 26, no. 8 (2004): 1079–1087. 10.1109/TPAMI.2004.51.

[24] Gupta, Pratishtha, Rathore Manisha, and Kumari Saroj. "A Survey Of Techniques And Applications For Real Time Image Processing." *International Journal of Global Research in Computer Science* 4, no. 8 (2013): 30–39.

[25] Gadde, Raghudeep, Jampani Varun, and Gehler Peter V. "Semantic Video CNNs through Representation Warping." *ICCV 2017* (2017). abs/1708.03088.

[26] Lei, Ming, Qi ZiJie, Hong Xiaoyan, and Vrbsky Susan. "Protecting Location Privacy with Dynamic Mac Address Exchanging in Wireless Networks." *2007. IEEE Intelligence and Security Informatics*. New Brunswick, NJ, USA. (2017): pp. 377–377, 10.1109/ISI.2007.379513.

[27] Lan, Wenbo, Dang Jianwu, Wang Yangping, and Wang Song. "Pedestrian Detection Based on YOLO Network Model." *2018 IEEE International Conference on Mechatronics and Automation (ICMA)*, Changchun, China, (2018): pp. 1547–1551. 10.1109/ICMA.2018.8484698.

[28] Cucchiara, Rita, Costantino Grana, Massimo Piccardi, and Andrea Prati. "Detecting moving objects, ghosts, and shadows in video streams." *IEEE Transactions on Pattern Analysis and Machine Intelligence* 25, no. 10 (2003): 1337–1342. 10.1109/TPAMI.2003.1233909.

[29] Dalal, Navneet, and Triggs Bill. "Histograms of oriented gradients for human detection." In *Computer Vision and Pattern Recognition* (2005), CVPR 2005. IEEE Computer Society Conference on 1:886-893. 10.1109/CVPR.2005.177.

[30] Ćorović, Aleksa, Ilić Velibor I., Đurić Sinica, Marijan Mališa, and Pavković Bogdan. "The Real-Time Detection of Traffic Participants Using YOLO Algorithm." *2018 26th Telecommunications Forum (TELFOR)*. (2018): 1–4. 10.1109/TELFOR.2018.8611986.

[31] Heikkila, Marko, and Pietikainen Matti. "A texture-based method for modeling the background and detecting moving objects." *IEEETransactions on Pattern Analysis and Machine Intelligence* 28, no. 4 (2006): 657–662. 10.1109/TPAMI.2006.68.

[32] Marszałek, Zbigniew. "Parallelization of Modified Merge Sort Algorithm." *Symmetry* 9, no. 9 (2017): 176. 10.3390/sym9090176.

[33] Kauling, Dylan, and Mahmoud Qusay H. "Sensorian Hub: An IFTTT-based platform for collecting and processing sensor data." *14th IEEE Annual Consumer Communications & Networking Conference (CCNC)*, Las Vegas, NV, (2017): pp. 504–509. 10.1109/CCNC.2017.7983159.

[34] Postorino, Maria Nadia, Barrile Vincenzo, and Cotroneo Francesco. "Surface movement ground control by means of a GPS–GIS system." *Journal of Air Transport Management* 12, no. 6 (2006): 375–381. 10.1016/j.jairtraman.2006.09.003.

[35] Pattnayak, Parthasarathi, and Jena, Om Prakash. "Innovation on Machine Learning in Healthcare Services–An Introduction." In: *Machine Learning for Healthcare Applications*, (2021): pp. 1–15. 10.1002/9781119792611.ch1.

[36] Paramesha, K., Gururaj, H.L. and Jena, Om Prakash. "Applications of Machine Learning in Biomedical Text Processing and Food Industry.". In: *Machine Learning for Healthcare Applications*, (2021): pp. 151–167. 10.1002/9781119792611.ch10.

[37] Panigrahi, Niranjan, Ayus, Ishan, and Jena, Om Prakash. "An Expert System-Based Clinical Decision Support System for Hepatitis-B Prediction & Diagnosis." In: *Machine Learning for Healthcare Applications* (2021): 57–75. 10.1002/9781119792611.ch4.

14 Implicit Ontology Changes Driven by Evolution of e-Health IoT Sensor Data in the τOWL Semantic Framework

Zouhaier Brahmia, Abir Zekri, and Rafik Bouaziz
University of Sfax, Sfax, Tunisia

Fabio Grandi
University of Bologna, Bologna, Italy

CONTENTS

14.1 INTRODUCTION

In the semantic web [1], applications are using ontologies to deal with semantic aspects. An ontology [2] allows conceptualizing a domain into a machine-understandable format that could be used for automated knowledge management in intelligent systems, like expert systems, decision support systems or recommender systems. Moreover, ontologies are not static, since they accordingly change each time

DOI: 10.1201/9781003189053-14

the underlying domain changes [3]. Advanced ontology-based systems (e.g., e-health, e-commerce and e-government systems, online social networks) must keep track of the full history of ontology changes, at both "instance" and "structure" levels, in order to be able to satisfy some temporal requirements like processing time-slice queries [4], recovering past ontology versions [5], and tracking ontology changes [6].

Nowadays, the use of Internet of Things (IoT) systems in many areas, like smart cities, environmental protection, intelligent transport, industry 4.0, and e-Health, is growing up rapidly [7]. IoT sensors are generating data measuring different desired quantities (e.g., in an IoT-based weather station: air temperature, humidity and pressure, wind speed and direction, rainfall level). Furthermore, IoT sensor data [8] are also time-varying at both "value" and "structure" levels. In particular, changes in their "structure" may be a consequence of the replacement of sensors and/or upgrades of the supported data format (e.g., new HW and SW versions, alternate sensor models, different producers).

Besides, electronic health (e-Health) [9,10] systems are being widely used and are playing an increasingly crucial role in our lives, especially in pandemic periods like that of COVID-19, by facilitating health monitoring and remotely providing medical services including consultations without direct contact. They benefit from recent advances in medical informatics, data management, networks and telecommunications technologies, and allow patients to enjoy such services in a secure, autonomous and personalized manner. In particular, currently several e-Health systems are using both IoT technologies for remote monitoring of the evolution of patients states, and ontologies, for semantic interoperability with other systems based on the conceptualization of the domain of each system (as in, e.g., [11], [12] and [13]). The deployment of shared ontologies allows different systems to reliably exchange information and to enable the integration of their functionalities in a transparent way. In recent years, several ontologies have been proposed for IoT-based e-Health systems [14,15]. Such ontologies are in general ontologies for the e-Health domain, which are augmented with concepts and relationships from ontologies developed in the IoT field [16,17].

In an ontology-based IoT e-Health system, data instances generated by IoT sensors (e.g., body temperature, blood pressure, blood glucose, oxygen saturation, cholesterol and heart rate measures) have to comply with the adopted ontology. Each new instance "$I(d)_t$" of a datum "d" (e.g., an air temperature), generated at an instant t, is updating the last instance "$I(d)_{t'}$" of the same datum "d", generated at the instant $t' < t$. Additionally, the two instances "$I(d)_t$" and "$I(d)_{t'}$" are considered as two successive versions of the datum "d"; the last instance of "d" is called the current version of this datum.

However, some new instance versions could be structurally inconsistent with respect to the current ontology. In this situation, we talk about *non-conservative* instance updates and we say that the new data instances are replacing the previous ones in a non-conservative manner; on the contrary, instance updates are considered as *conservative* when the new instances are conformant to the current ontology. In order to be accomplished, non-conservative instance updates require that some changes be applied to the current ontology in order to generate a new ontology version which could consistently accommodate also the new data instances.

In this chapter, we first propose (in Section 14.3) an approach that supports ontology changes which are triggered by non-conservative instance updates, giving rise to an ontology schema versioning driven by the arrival of unusual instances, unexpected at the initial ontology design time. Then, we apply (in Section 14.4) this approach to our established semantic framework τOWL (Temporal OWL 2), already proposed for managing the definition of temporal OWL 2 ontologies and their evolution, in a context where both schemas and instances of ontologies are temporally versioned. Moreover, as a proof-of-concept of the proposed approach, we released a new version of our τOWL-Manager tool that also supports the management of non-conservative ontology instance updates (as described in Section 14.5). Finally, we provide (in Section 14.6) conclusions and some remarks about our future work. Before going into the details of the approach, we survey research works that are related to our work, in the section that follows.

14.2 RELATED WORK

In this section, first we briefly describe our τOWL framework. Then, we study ontology-based IoT e-Health systems. Finally, we deal with machine learning and deep learning in healthcare systems.

14.2.1 The τOWL Framework

τOWL [18,19] is an infrastructure that allows a knowledge base administrator (KBA) to build a temporal OWL 2 [20] ontology structure compatible with a time-varying OWL 2 ontology instance, using a conventional OWL 2 ontology structure and a set of annotations dealing with logical and physical temporal aspects of some constituents of this structure.

First, the KBA creates the conventional ontology structure, which is an OWL 2 document containing ontology axioms that describe the concepts of a domain and the relationships between these concepts, without any temporal aspect. Associated with each conventional ontology schema, a set of compatible conventional OWL 2 ontology data instances can be stored. Modifications to the conventional ontology structure are automatically propagated to the underlying conventional ontology instance in order to maintain compatibility.

Then, the conventional ontology structure is annotated by the KBA with some logical and physical annotations [21], which allow him/her to explicitly define requirements concerning how to represent and how to manage temporal aspects related to its components, as described below.

Logical annotations are used by the KBA to specify whether conventional ontology schema component variations are tracked over valid time and/or transaction time, whether its lifetime is modeled as a time interval (state) or a single time point (event), whether the component is forbidden to appear at certain times, and whether its content is allowed to change.

Physical annotations are used by the KBA to specify which representation options are chosen for timestamps, such as which is their temporal type (valid-time, transaction-time, or bitemporal), which particular representation format is adopted (e.g., slice-based or item-based representation) and where they are placed.

Next, when the KBA commands the system to commit the above described temporal ontology construction work, including the creation of a conventional ontology schema and the specification of its temporal annotations, the system generates the temporal ontology schema that associates a set of temporal annotations to the conventional schema of the ontology.

Hence, the system creates a temporal ontology document that links each conventional ontology instance document, which is conformant to a conventional ontology schema, to its temporal ontology schema, that is to its set of temporal annotations (a temporal ontology document stores the temporal evolution of a conventional ontology instance document by storing all the versions of this document, each version with a different timestamp).

Eventually, the system uses the temporal ontology document to automatically generate the squashed ontology document that stores the temporal ontology instances. Such instances are produced by applying the temporal logical and physical annotations (belonging to the temporal ontology schema) to the conventional ontology instances (recorded in the conventional ontology document versions).

14.2.2 Ontology-Based IoT e-Health Systems

The IoT, also known as the Web of Things, is a global environment where billions of objects (e.g., sensors, actuators, RFID tags, smart phones, computers, security cameras) are connected to the Internet and are exchanging information in an autonomous and interoperable manner. It is built upon an infrastructure of wireless sensor networks (WSNs).

Ontologies (and semantic web technologies, in general) are increasingly used by IoT applications, as they allow the filling of a significant gap concerning the semantics of exchanged data [22]. In fact, in the IoT we have a great number of diverse “things”, with their different networks and rapidly evolving deployment platforms (which give rise to simultaneous and frequent changes to their description data). Furthermore, the IoT things are producing enormous volumes of data with multiple heterogeneous formats, lacking a formal specification and/or a machine-readable description, whose semantics could be exploited by application programs in useful activities like query answering, knowledge discovery, and cybersecurity.

In general, an ontology is composed of the description of a consistent set of classes (or concepts) and relationships between such classes and of their instances; the description specifies that each class/relationship could have some properties. Furthermore, axioms could be used to constrain instances of classes and/or instances of relationships. An ontology is used as a high-level formalization of an application domain, whose structural part plays a role similar to a database schema. The data that are handled by such an application represent the instance of the ontology being exploited indeed.

Moreira et al. [23] have explained the need for interoperability in IoT systems, and shown how ontologies allow to accomplish such interoperability. They have also motivated, proposed, and validated a new ontology, named SAREF4Health, as an extension of SAREF (smart applications reference ontology) [16] to support IoT-based healthcare systems, and in particular healthcare use cases related to real-time electrocardiography (ECG) data. Notice that SAREF is an extensible IoT reference ontology already standardized by the European Telecommunications Standards Institute (ETSI).

In [24], the authors show how ontologies could be used as a tool for enabling the deployment of health IoT systems, by allowing comparison and contrast of medical information.

Rubí and Gondim [25] propose an interoperable IoMT platform for e-Health systems, to deal with the fact that each IoMT manufacturer builds its own architecture, devices, protocols, and data formats, and consequently software systems must be revised to interoperate within an IoMT platform. This proposal is based on jointly using an openEHR-based ontology and the semantic sensor network ontology [26,27] for IoT platforms, and extending the machine-to-machine ETSI standard that follows semantic web technologies (e.g., SPARQL) to reach IoMT and EHR (electronic health records) interoperability. Notice that openEHR [28,29] is a technology proposed by the openEHR organization for modeling EHR in a formal way.

Titi et al. [30] provide a healthcare IoT system to continuously monitor the chronically ill elderly. Such a system is based on an ontology that guarantees semantic interoperability between heterogeneous devices (e.g., sensors, cameras) and humans (e.g., patients, physicians) using the system via different hardware and/or applications. More precisely, the authors have built their ontology by integrating some existing ontologies on health (SNOMED CT, and ICD-10), IoT (SSN ontology, and SOSA), time (OWL-Time), and persons (FOAF), and by defining a set of SWRL reasoning rules. To obtain such an ontology, they have applied an ontology engineering methodology already proposed in [31]. The authors have also evaluated the efficiency of their proposal.

In [32], the authors propose a method for semantic integration of health data and home environment data, collected from heterogeneous services and devices. To this purpose, they define an integration ontology based on the web ontology language (OWL), which specifies a unifying model for health data gathered from HL7 FHIR (fast healthcare interoperability resources) standard implemented services, normal Web services, and Web of Things (WoT) services, and for linked data and home environment data acquired by means of WoT services that are described by formal ontologies.

Villanueva-Miranda et al. [33] study the state-of-the-art approaches that have been proposed to solve semantic interoperability problems between heterogeneous and isolated IoMT platforms. The authors show how semantic web technologies have been used to build such approaches. In general, two types of approaches have been defined by researchers to deal with IoMT interoperability problems: one-to-one ontology alignment and deployment of a central ontology.

In [10], the authors have dealt with the design, implementation, and evaluation of an e-Health system based on the semantic sensor network (SSN) ontology. This system is composed of e-Health users (patients and healthcare professionals), e-Health devices, an e-Health client, and an e-Health server. In order to support semantic interoperability within this system, a semantic model has been defined using the data modeling language YANG [34]. YANG had previously been used for the configuration of devices (e.g., network devices, IoT devices, and mobile devices) and for the modeling of sensors information. The semantic model plays the role of a communication protocol between the devices and the server. Any message received from a device by the server is automatically parsed according to that model and taking into account the specific format (e.g., JSON) of the message. Moreover, the e-Health system automatically generates messages, with specific formats, which describe sensing data.

Ullah et al. [35] start by studying the state of the art of applications of IoT in the medical sector. After that, they propose a new IoT-based semantic model, called k-Healthcare, for e-Health and m-Health. It is based on smartphone sensors and wearable sensors, which enable to collection of data on patient health, in order to process and send them to a central storage space in the cloud. Such stored data could then be accessed by corresponding patients or by authorized healthcare professionals. Furthermore, k-Healthcare is composed of four layers (the sensor layer, the network layer, the Internet layer, and the services layer) that collaborate with each other to allow storage, processing, and retrieval of health data of patients.

14.2.3 Machine Learning and Deep Learning in Healthcare Systems

Analyzing IoT sensor data is becoming a new source of data for e-Health systems [36], since it allows discovering new knowledge, predicting early detection of disease, and improving decision making (in particular, in important/dangerous situations).

In [37], the authors have proposed a framework for deep learning from Internet of Health and Things (IoHT) data, which allows detecting and classifying skin lesions in skin images using the concept of transfer learning. Moreover, they experimentally evaluated the performances of their proposal and discussed them in a transfer learning environment.

Kumar et al. [38] have used deep learning to classify diabetes, by applying the multi-layer feed forward neural networks (MLFNN) [39] on the Pima Indian Diabetes data set. Before experiencing their MLFNN-based model, the authors have handled the missing values encountered in such a data set, since they can affect the accuracy of the classification. The experimental results, which are produced by the performance evaluation of the MLFNN model, have been compared to those obtained from the application of two machine learning classifiers: Naïve-Bayes and random forest. These results show that the proposed model provides better accuracy than the two other models.

Sharma et al. [40] study the role of wireless sensor networks and biometric-based models (like two-factor remote authentication, and user verification and authorization using fingerprint biometrics) in healthcare systems. In particular, the authors have presented a comparative table that provides advantages and disadvantages of several biometric-based models applied in healthcare. Notice that such models are efficient tools for controlling access to electronic health records, securing patient data, and therefore protecting both patient data confidentiality and privacy.

Biometrics is the science of analyzing physical characteristics (e.g., fingerprints, eye iris and retina patterns, shape of the hand, finger, or face) or behavioral characteristics (e.g., speech recognition, signature dynamics) of each individual and enabling the authentication of his/her identity.

Goyal et al. [41] have dealt with the use of IoT technologies in a secured healthcare context. They started by defining the notion of Internet of Health Things (IoHT) and came up with the definition of a model for future IoHT systems, with proposed topologies, applications, and services for IoHT. Notice that IoHT applications are user-oriented whereas IoHT services are developer-oriented. Furthermore, each IoHT application is classified into either a single-condition application, concerning a single disease or illness or weakness, or a clustered-condition application, dealing together with a number of circumstances considered as a whole. After that, the authors have described several IoHT application classes (ambient assisted living, remote healthcare monitoring, wearable gadgets, and solutions for healthcare using smartphones) and analyzed challenges for IoHT (e.g., an IoHT-based system must fulfill safety, robustness, and flexibility issues). Next, they have studied the IoHT security requirements (i.e., resiliency, availability, defect tolerance, data freshness, self-healing, privacy, integrity, and verification) and IoHT technology challenges (i.e., energy limitations, dynamic security updates, multiplicity of gadgets, scalability, memory limitations, multi-protocol network, and computational limitations). Finally, the authors have provided a list of technologies (i.e., ambient intelligence, augmented reality, big data, cloud computing, grid computing, wearables, and networks like 6LoWPANs, WBANs, WSNs, WPANs, and WLANs) that could revolutionize the services of IoHT, and discussed some open research issues in the IoHT area (i.e., identification, cost analysis, business prototype, data security, and continuous monitoring).

14.3 IMPLICIT ONTOLOGY STRUCTURE CHANGES TRIGGERED BY NON-CONSERVATIVE UPDATES TO ONTOLOGY DATA INSTANCES

Our approach for the management of implicit ontology schema changes that are triggered by non-conservative ontology instance updates is presented in this section.

First of all, our approach is intended to be applicable to ontologies with a DBox [42,43], which mainly behave like a database following the closed world assumption (CWA) [44,45] and for which we can talk about an *ontology schema*.

Notice that the CWA means that "what is not known to be true must be false"; it is used in an environment in which data are assumed to be complete, like classical databases (which are in general supposed storing all relevant data representing true facts). On the contrary, the open world assumption (OWA) [46] means that "what is not known to be true or false is unknown"; it is adopted in a setting in which data are assumed to be incomplete, like knowledge bases and semantic web repositories. Notice also that several contemporary applications support both assumptions for the same ontology, as shown in [47], [48], and [49], in order to allow incomplete data sets to be integrated with complete data sets.

Notice that, although basically sticking to the CWA, our proposal is a way to add some kind of "openness" to the CWA by means of the implicit ontology versioning triggered by non-conservative instance updates. In practice, this happens in the same way that, in the database field, the adoption of a semistructured data model, like XML [50] or JSON [51], strongly mitigates the inability to represent incomplete data of the relational model (where the only allowed incompleteness feature is represented by the controversial use of null values) by allowing the representation of flexible and extensible data structures. New ontology data instances non conforming to the old ontology schema can be merged with the old ontology data instances by creating a new ontology schema (from the old ontology schema), both compliant with the old and the new data instances, by means of implicit schema changes automatically performed by the system (the KBA must only approve their execution) within the same transaction that adds the new data instances. The adoption of the schema versioning technique [52,53] implies that the old ontology schema version with the old associated instance is also retained and can be retrieved on demand (e.g., to be still used by legacy applications or for audit purposes).

In particular, the non-conservative (instance) update operations that we consider in this work are the following:

- rename operations (involving class names or property names, of data instances);
- insertion of data instances of a class that does not belong to the current ontology schema;
- insert, update, or delete operations that involve data instances of a class belonging to the current version of the ontology schema, but violating some constraints in this schema, like the following ones:
  - insert operations that add values for data properties which are not defined for a class in the current version of the ontology structure, or which are incompatible with the data types of such properties or violate integrity constraints specified in the current version of the ontology schema;
  - update operations that replace the value of a data property with a new one that is incompatible with the type of such property as specified in the current version of the ontology schema;
  - delete operations that act on values of mandatory data properties, or on a class instance for which a mandatory relationship exists in the current version of the ontology schema.
- delete, insert, or update operations involving instances of an object property in the current ontology schema, causing a violation of some schema constraints.

For example, assuming a functional and mandatory relationship R is defined between the two classes C1 (domain) and C2 (range), non-conservative operations on instances of R could be as follows:

- delete an instance (x1, y1) from R without deleting x1 from C1; the result of such an operation would violate the fact that R is mandatory and, in order to force it, a schema change operation that changes R from mandatory to optional must be generated and executed;
- add a new instance (x1, y1) to R, or replace x2 with x1 in the instance (x2, y1) of R, while an instance (x1, y2) already exists for R; the result of such an operation would violate the functional nature of R and could not be executed without changing R from functional to generic.

In order to exemplify the functioning of our proposal, suppose that the KBA must add to the current version of the ontology instance document Inst_Vers1, a new instance of a class C having a value V for a property P, whereas the class C has no property P, in the current ontology schema version S_Vers1 to which I_Vers1 conforms. Hence, to add the new instance of C to I_Vers1, an ontology schema change is needed to add to S_Vers1 an axiom stating that class C has the property P. Such a change produces both a new ontology schema version S_Vers2 and a new ontology instance version I_Vers2 in which the new instance of C can be stored. It is worth mentioning that the old instances of C, stored in I_Vers1, will also be conforming to S_Vers2 in case P has been added as an optional property and will not in case P has been added as mandatory. Such an option will be prompted to the KBA and the choice left to him/her. In the latter case, such instances for which a value for the P property cannot be supplied are deleted from I_Vers2 in order to guarantee the consistency of the new ontology version. On the contrary, if a value for P is supplied by the KBA, such instances are updated and left in I_Vers2.

Vice versa, if the class C has a mandatory property Q in S_Vers1 and the KBA has to add to I_Vers1 an instance of C for which a value for the property Q is not defined, an ontology schema change is needed to remove the property Q from C or to transform the property Q of C from mandatory to optional, through the deletion or substitution of the corresponding axiom in S_Vers1, respectively. Such a change produces either a new version S_Vers2 of the ontology schema and a new version I_Vers2 of the ontology instance document, where the new instance of C must be stored. Also in this case, the choice between the two options is left to the KBA and, with the aim of preserving the consistency of the new version of the ontology, it determines the destiny in I_Vers2 of the existing instances of C stored in I_Vers1. If the former option is chosen such instances will not be maintained in I_Vers2 unless, according to a further KBA specification, the values of their property Q are deleted. If the latter option is chosen, the existing instances of C in I_Vers1 will be also kept in I_Vers2 together with the new instance of C.

As far as implicit ontology schema changes are concerned (e.g., "add a property P to the class C as optional" in the first case above with the choice of former option, or "modify the property Q of the class C from mandatory to optional" in the second case above with the choice of the latter option), we can consider two different modalities for their generation depending on the way instance updates are effected: interactive mode and batch mode.

- **Interactive mode:** the instance updates are interactively effected by the KBA on the current ontology version via a graphical interface or update language; the implicit schema change generation is triggered by the schema constraint violation caused by the KBA actions which are detected on the fly; this is the modality explored in this work and whose support has been added to the τOWL-Manager.
- **Batch mode:** the new data instances are supplied by the KBA as a separate ontology instance document that must be integrated into the current ontology version; a sequence of implicit schema changes is generated by the execution of a validity checking task that verifies whether the new data instances to be integrated conform or not to the current ontology schema before adding them to the new ontology version; this modality will be explored in our future work.

In both cases, the production of the new ontology schema version, which ensures the new ontology instance to be consistent with its schema, can be automated via the execution of the generated implicit ontology schema changes (which may imply propagation, guided by the KBA, of such schema changes to the existing data instances not affected by the updates).

14.4 EXTENDING TOWL TO SUPPORT NON-CONSERVATIVE UPDATES OF ONTOLOGY INSTANCES

In τOWL, updating an ontology instance consists in updating an already existing conventional ontology instance document, or more precisely the current version of the conventional ontology instance document, as such a document is versioned only along transaction time in our framework. Updating here means adding new content to the current version of the conventional ontology instance document, modifying some contents of this document, or removing some contents from it.

When the KBA has completed his/her work session of updating a conventional ontology instance document, through a graphical and interactive language (i.e., via the user interface of our τOWL-Manager prototype), and commands the system to commit his/her work, the sub-module "Ontology Instance Document Update Processor" (of the module "Ontology Instance Document Change Manager" in the τOWL-Manager tool) is called in order to execute the algorithm listed in Figure 14.1.

This algorithm uses the following acronyms:

- COD: Conventional Ontology Instance document;
- CurVers_COD: Current Version of COD;
- NewVers_COD: New Version of COD;
- COS: Conventional Ontology Schema;
- CurVers_COS: Current Version of COS;
- NewVers_COS: New Version of COS;
- TOD: Temporal Ontology Document;
- SOD: Squashed Ontology Document;

```
Algorithm Update_Conventional_Ontology_Instance_Document
Inputs: CurVers_COD, CurVers_COS, UO, SC
        ## UO is a set of ontology instance updates produced by the
        Interaction Manager ##
        ## SC is a set of ontology schema changes produced by the
        Interaction Manager ##
Outputs: NewVers_COD, and possibly NewVers_COS
Begin
   1. Generate Copy_CurVers_COD, a copy of CurVers_COD;
   2. Apply UO to Copy_CurVers_COD to obtain NewVers_COD;
   3. Compare NewVers_COD to CurVers_COD;
   4. If (NewVers_COD == CurVers_COD) Then
   5.   Delete NewVers_COD;
   6.   Inform the KBA that actually no changes have been made to
        CurVers_COD;
   7. Else
   8.   Update the TOD corresponding to CurVers_COD;
   9.   Generate the CurVers_SOD corresponding to the CurVers_COS;
   10.  If (SC is not empty) Then ## NewVers_COD is not valid with
                                       respect to CurVers_COS ##
   11.    Apply SC to CurVers_COS to obtain NewVers_COS
   12.    Under the interactive KBA guidance, propagate schema changes in
          SC to unaffected instances in NewVers_COD;
   13.    Update the corresponding TOS;
   14.    Generate the NewVers_SOD corresponding to the NewVers_COS;
   15.  End If
   16. End If
End
```

FIGURE 14.1 The algorithm for updating a conventional ontology instance document.

- CurVers_SOD: Current Version of SOD;
- NewVers_SOD: New Version of SOD;
- TOS: Temporal Ontology Schema.

In general, our approach facilitates the instance checking task and the implicit schema change generation, and performs them in an efficient way, since the system relies either on the current version of the ontology schema definition and on the list of all instance update operations (that have been executed on the current version of the ontology instance document), to detect the KBA's actions (i) that move inside such an ontology schema definition (i.e., conservative updates) or (ii) that cross its borders (i.e., non-conservative ones) and consequently require implicit ontology schema changes. To be more precise, we explain in the following how the management of ontology instance updates is done through the user interface of our τOWL-Manager prototype system, which is based on two main components: the Interaction Manager and the ontology instance document update processor.

In order to add a new instance of a class, the KBA starts by selecting the target class from the class hierarchy to the left of the interface and clicking on the contextual menu "Create instances" or by writing the class name in a suitable text field. In case the written name actually does not correspond to an existing class, the Interaction Manager assumes the KBA wants to create a new class (recognizing it as a non-conservative update) and, after asking for confirmation, asks the KBA where the new class should be put in the hierarchy by means of the specification of its superclass; once the superclass of the new class is supplied, the Interaction Manager generates the corresponding schema changes to be added to SC (SC had been initialized to the empty set):

```
SC:= SC + {"AddClass NewClass;"};
SC:= SC + {"AddSubClass NewClass TO SuperClass;"};
```

After that, the Interaction Manager shows the Data Property Assertions displaying the properties of the selected class, or the properties that are inherited from the superclass in case of a new subclass, that the KBA can use to fill in the slots in order to specify values for the existing properties.

Notice here that when adding a new instance of an existing class, the KBA could also perform the following tasks:

- adding new properties, by clicking on the link "Add Data Property Instance(s)" and specifying a property name and possibly a set of values for the new property; then, a non-conservative update is detected and the corresponding schema change is generated:

  ```
  SC:= SC + {"AddDataProperty NewProperty TO Class;"};
  ```

  Confirmation is then asked to the KBA whether the new property has to be defined as optional and/or the number of inserted values has to be taken as a cardinality constraint; in the former case the following schema change has to be added

  ```
  SC:= SC + {"SetMinCardinality OF NewProperty TO 0;"};
  ```

  whereas in the latter case the following schema change has to be added

  ```
  SC:= SC + {"SetMaxCardinality OF NewProperty TO NewValCount;"};
  ```

- changing the data type of existing properties (e.g., from

`xsd:decimalto`
`xsd:string), since the inserted property values may be non-compatible with the type currently defined for that property; hence, a new data type (to which the existing values can possibly be converted without loss of information) is derived from the inserted values and, after asking confirmation to the KBA, the following schema change is generated:`

```
SC:= SC + {"ChangeDataType OF Property TO newDataType;"};
```

• renaming existing properties, by editing properties names, which come either from the selected class or from the specified superclass; also in this case, the Interaction Manager detects a non-conservative update and generates the corresponding schema change:

```
SC:= SC + {"RenameDataProperty PropertyName TO NewName;"};
```

• changing the minimum cardinality of existing properties (e.g., changing the property from mandatory to optional[1]), by deleting one or more values from those currently defined for the property such that the remaining values violate the current minimum cardinality constraint (this includes deleting the single value of an existing mandatory property); hence, the Interaction Manager detects a non-conservative update and builds the corresponding schema change:

```
SC:= SC + {"SetMinCardinality OF PropertyName TO NewValCount;"};
```

• changing the maximum cardinality of existing properties (e.g., to change the property from functional to generic[2]), by adding one or more values to those currently defined for the property such that the resulting values violate the current maximum cardinality constraint (this includes adding a second value for an existing functional property); hence, the Interaction Manager detects a non-conservative update and builds the corresponding schema change:

```
SC:= SC + {"SetMaxCardinality OF PropertyName TO NewValCount;"};
```

• removing some existing properties, by clicking on the link "Remove Data Property Instance(s)"; consequently, in case the data property was currently defined as mandatory, a non-conservative update is detected and the corresponding schema changes are generated after asking confirmation to the KBA whether the property has to be removed from the class definition or it has simply to be made optional: in the former case the generated schema change is

```
SC:= SC + {"RemoveDataProperty PropertyName FROM Class;"};
```

whereas in the latter case the generated schema change is

```
SC:= SC + {"SetMinCardinality OF PropertyName TO 0;"};
```

• specifying some instances of the relationships of this class, by clicking on the button labeled with the symbol "+" located to the right on top of the table reserved to Object

Property Assertions, while some range values correspond to classes that do not exist in the current version of the conventional ontology schema (using the graphical editor, the domain of a relationship instance cannot be changed since it corresponds to the chosen class on which the KBA is working). In such a case, the Interaction Manager infers that the KBA wants to change the range of some relationship and the KBA is interactively asked where to put the new classes in the class hierarchy; according to the KBA's answers, the Interaction Manager generates, for each changed range, the following required schema changes:

```
SC:= SC + {"AddClass NewClass;"};
SC:= SC + {"AddSubClass NewClass TO SuperClass;"};
SC:= SC + {"ChangeRange OF RelationshipName TO NewClass;"};
```

Automatic modifications of cardinality constraints involving object properties, triggered by non-conservative insertions, deletions, or updates of relationship instances, are managed in a way similar to cardinality constraints of data properties as listed previously.

In order to update existing class instances (with their properties and relationships), the KBA must open the "Ontology Instance Document" menu and select the "Evolve Ontology Instances" submenu. The Interaction Manager will then let him/her choose a conventional ontology schema (e.g., PersonFOAF in our case), or more precisely and implicitly the current version of this schema; according to the choice of the KBA, the current conventional ontology instance document version, corresponding to the selected conventional ontology schema, is displayed. The KBA could then perform updates (in a broad sense) on property instances and/or on relationship instances of each class instance, which can come out either conservative or not. For any option (i.e., update, delete, or insert) the KBA may choose that goes against a constraint specified in the current conventional ontology schema version, the Interaction Manager assumes he/she wants to do a non-conservative update that consequently requires an ontology schema change. Hence, the Interaction Manager uses the specifications and values provided by the KBA to compile the required list of all necessary implicit schema changes. Notice here that the schema changes generated during the interaction are not different from the ones described above for class instance insertions.

When the KBA completes the task of updating the ontology instance and asks τOWL-Manager to commit his/her work, the Interaction Manager receives his/her order and calls the sub-module "Ontology Instance Document Update Processor" (whose algorithm is listed in Figure 14.1) passing to it four arguments: the current conventional ontology schema version (CurVers_COS), the current conventional ontology instance document version (CurVers_COD) which is being "updated", the final list of all instance update operations (UO) that have been performed by the KBA, and the complete list of all generated schema change operations (SC); the former list constitute a LOG of the operations executed by the KBA in the whole instance update session and the latter has been automatically generated during the interaction of the KBA with τOWL-Manager as explained previously. Once called, the sub-module "Ontology Instance Document Update Processor" executes the steps in the algorithm of Figure 14.1. In fact, it (i) generates a copy of

CurVers_COD, (ii) applies the list of instance update operations (UO) to this copy, and (iii) compares the updated copy to CurVers_COD; in case there is no difference between them, it (iv) removes the updated copy, and (v) informs the KBA that no changes have been made. However, in case the updated copy NewVers_COD is different from CurVers_COD, it (vi) updates the temporal ontology document corresponding to CurVers_COD so that the new ontology instance document version NewVers_COD is taken into account, (vii) verifies the validity of NewVers_COD with respect to CurVers_COS, by checking if SC is empty or not. If SC is not empty, the sub-module "Ontology Instance Document Update Processor", (viii) applies SC to CurVers_COS producing the new ontology schema version NewVers_COS. If necessary, it also (ix) propagates (under the interactive guidance of the KBA) the schema changes in SC to the data instances present in CurVers_COD which have not been affected by the updates in UO. Then, it (x) updates the corresponding temporal ontology schema in order to include NewVers_COS, and (xi) generates the new version of the squashed document corresponding to CurVers_COS.

Notice that we have chosen to present the schema change operations generated by the Interaction Manager (SC) as high-level operations [54], which meet frequent ontology schema evolution requirements and consist of intuitive ontology schema changes expressed in a compact and user-friendly way. However, each one of these operations can easily be converted into a valid sequence of low-level ontology schema change operations we defined in our previous works [18,19].

14.5 PROOF-OF-CONCEPT EXTENSION OF THE TOWL-MANAGER TOOL

As a proof-of-concept, our approach has been implemented as an extension of our τOWL-Manager tool [18], which is a prototype implementation of our original τOWL framework. Such an extension consists of the following aspects:

- Revision of the module "Ontology Instance Document Change Manager" to let it also support non-conservative updates and, thus, allow the creation of new conventional ontology instance document versions that are not conforming to the current ontology schema version; in the previous version of the tool, such instance versions were automatically rejected.
- Definition of a new module, named "Implicit Ontology Schema Change Manager", which automatically (and transparently to the KBA) generates a new version of the conventional ontology schema and updates the corresponding temporal ontology schema, each time is called by the module "Ontology Instance Document Change Manager".

To illustrate the use of the new version of τOWL-Manager, we present an interaction session example that show how this tool manages non-conservative updates to ontology instance documents. We work on an ontology PersonFOAF, whose schema is initially a copy of the well-known FOAF definition[3]. In this example (see Figures 14.2 to 14.6), the non-conservative update consists in adding a new

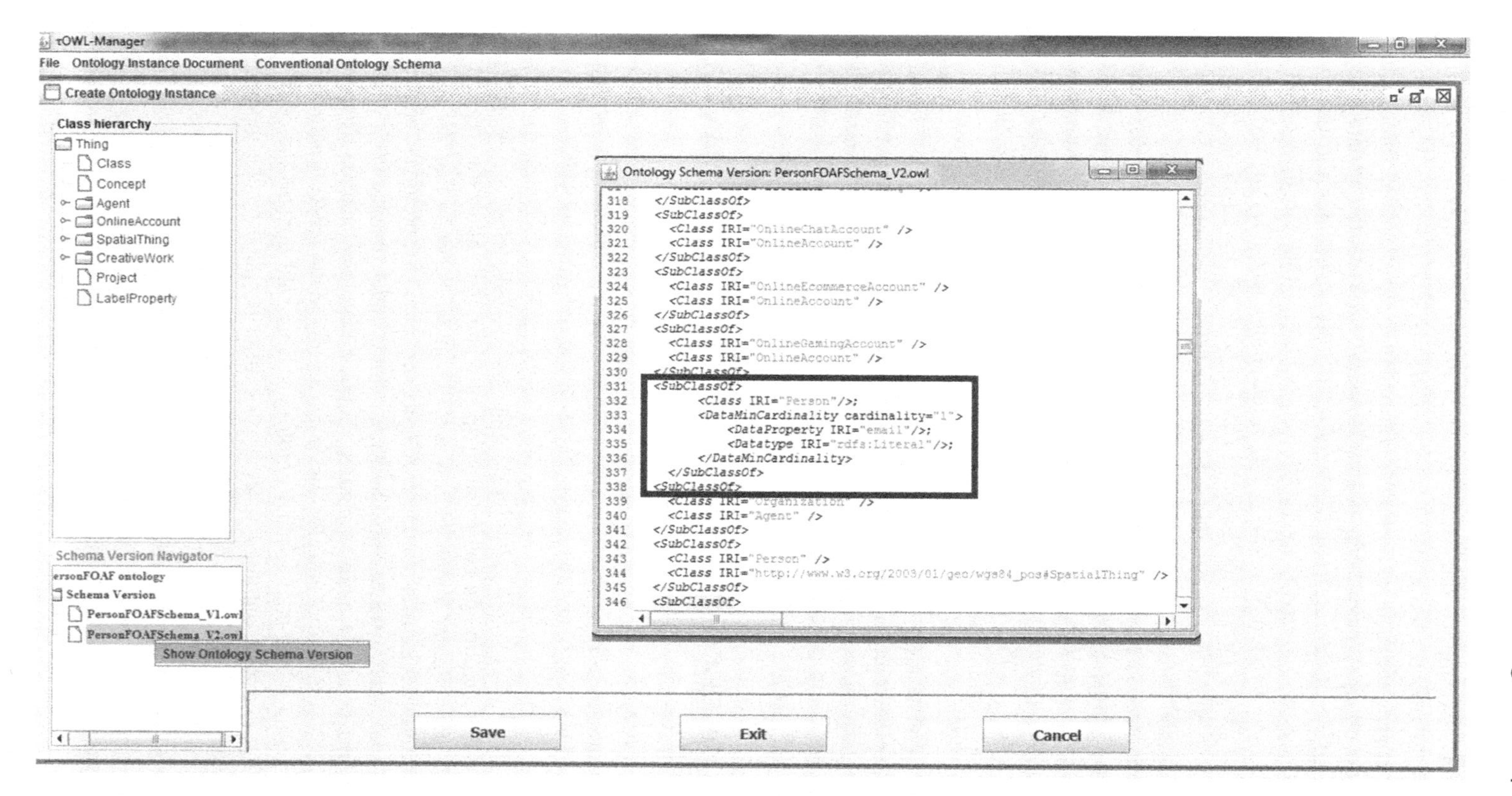

FIGURE 14.2 Step 1 of the non-conservative instance update process session of the example. The system displays the OWL 2 code of the second schema version of the PersonFOAF ontology, as an answer to a request coming from the KBA. It is clear that "email" is a mandatory data property of the Person class, as its minimum cardinality is equal to 1.

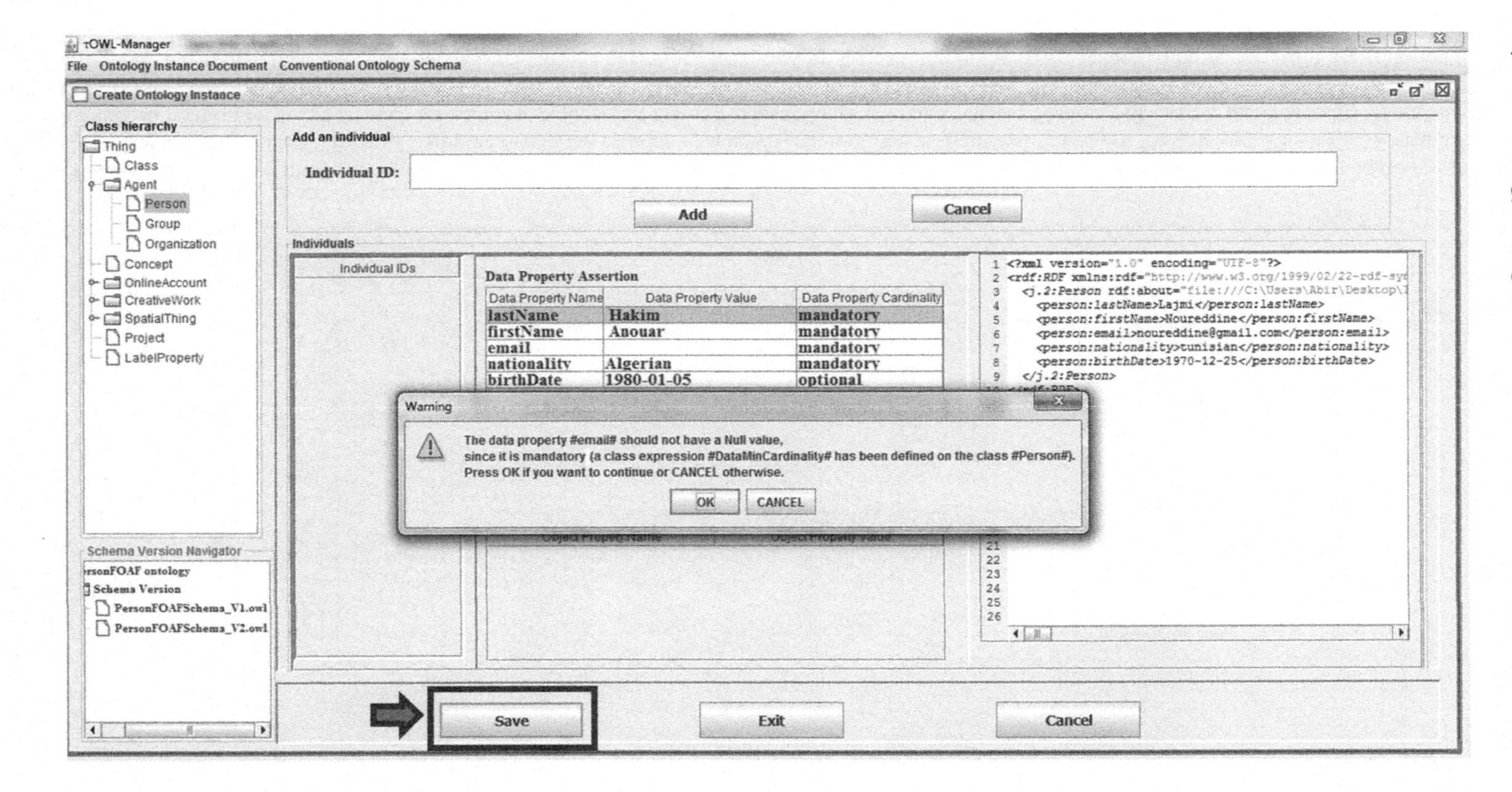

FIGURE 14.3 Step 2 of the non-conservative instance update process session of the example. The KBA enters the data of a new instance of the class Person (with the following data properties: lastName = "Hakim", firstName = "Anouar", nationality = "Algerian", and birthdate = "1980-01-05") without a value for the mandatory data property "email", and asks the system to save this new instance.

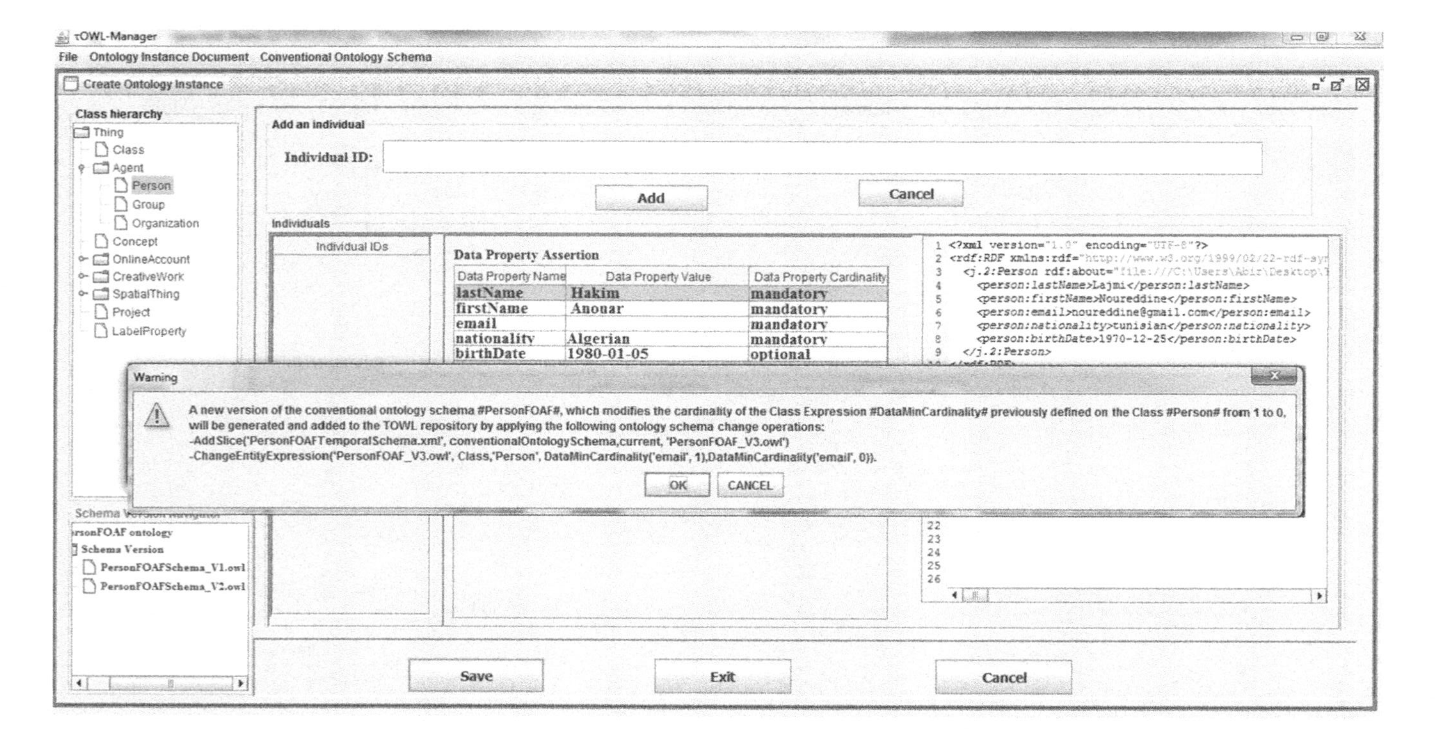

FIGURE 14.4 Step 3 of the non-conservative instance update process session of the example. The system informs the KBA that the addition of the above instance of the class "Person" will give rise to the creation of a new version of the conventional schema of the ontology PersonFOAF, and asks him/her to confirm or to cancel such an addition. Notice that the new conventional ontology schema version will change the cardinality of the class expression "DataMinCardiniality", previously defined on the class "Person", from 1 to 0. Moreover, this ontology schema version will be implicitly created by the system that will apply two schema change operations (triggered by the addition of the new unexpected instance): AddSlice followed by ChangeEntityExpression.

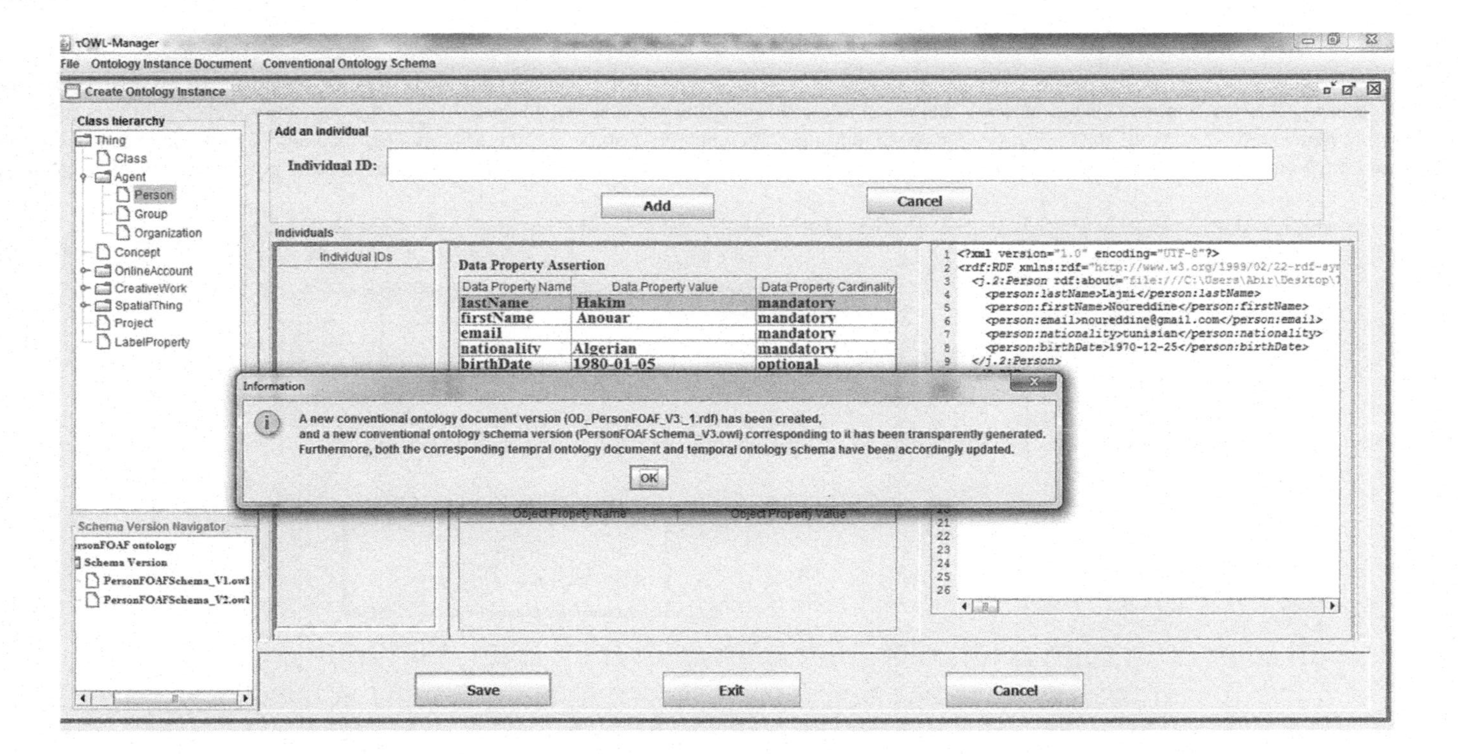

FIGURE 14.5 Step 4 of the non-conservative instance update process session of the example. The system informs the KBA that (after receiving his/her confirmation) the following operations have been executed: creation of a new conventional ontology document version (which stores the new "Person" instance), generation of a new conventional ontology schema version of PersonFOAF, which is associated the new document version, update of the temporal ontology document (to take into account the new version of the conventional ontology document), and update of the temporal ontology schema (to include the new version of the conventional ontology schema).

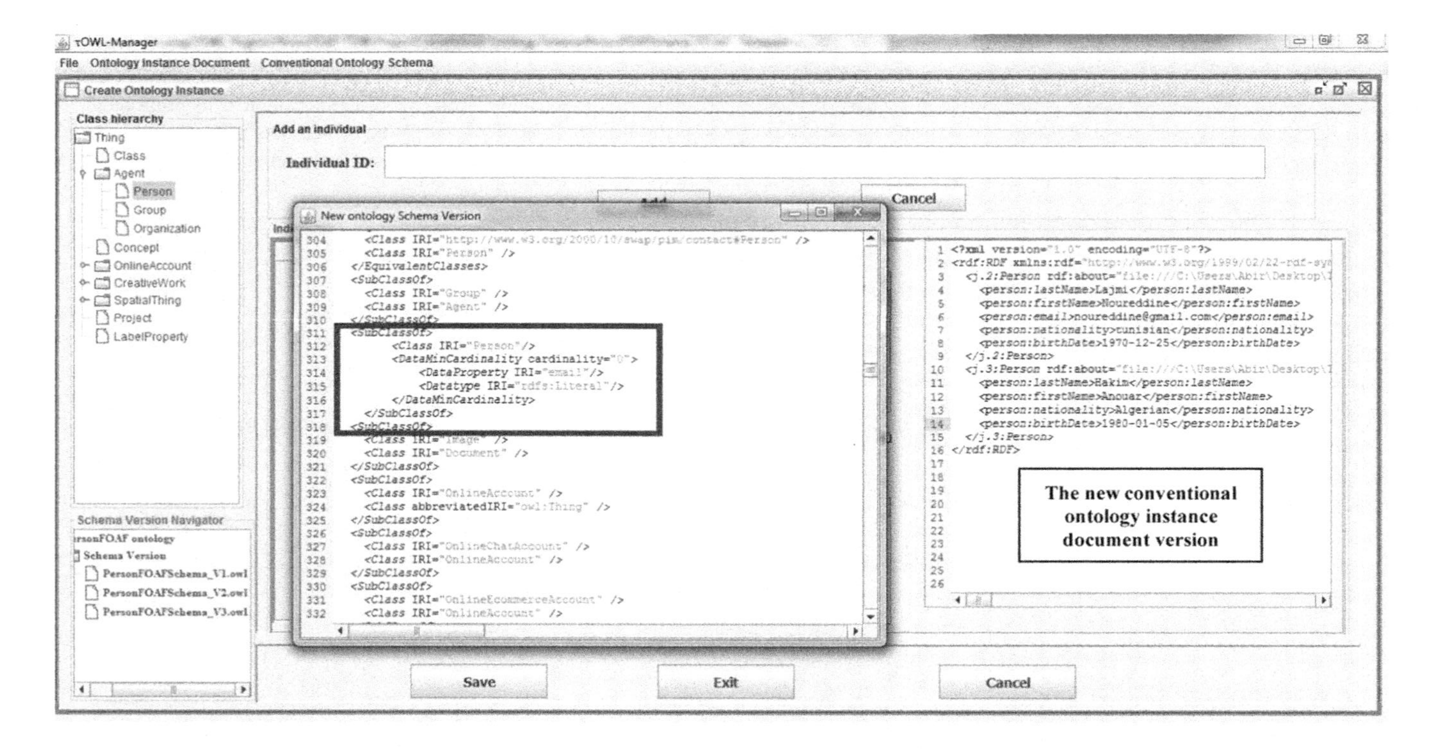

FIGURE 14.6 Step 5 of the non-conservative instance update process session of the example. The system displays (on the left side of the screenshot) the OWL 2 code of the new conventional ontology schema version, in which the minimum cardinality of the "email" data property is equal to 0, and (on the right side of the screenshot) the RDF/XML code of the new conventional ontology document version, which includes the new "Person" instance whose details have been entered above (except the email).

instance of the class "Person" not including a value for a mandatory data property (i.e., "email").

14.6 CONCLUSION

In an IoT-based e-Health system, both data (exchanged between patients, devices, users, etc.) and their structure are evolving over time to reflect changes in such a dynamic environment, in the technologies that are being used or in the application requirements of such a system. Also the specifications of ontologies, which play a crucial role in this type of systems, are time-varying and need to be temporally versioned in order to comply with e-Health systems that are, by nature, temporal and multi-version. In this chapter, we have proposed a new approach for handling ontology instance updates that require ontology schema changes in order to produce a consistent result, in an IoT-based e-Health environment that supports temporal versioning of both ontology data instances and ontology schemas. The proposed approach has been integrated into the τOWL framework, by extending it to support two new functionalities: non-conservative ontology instance updates and implicit ontology schema changes triggered by such instance updates. In order to demonstrate the feasibility of the approach, we have also developed a new release of our τOWL-Manager tool [18] that allows KBAs to perform ontology instance updates that require implicit ontology schema changes. With the use of our tool, non-conservative updates can be executed in τOWL-based IoT repositories, while managing ontology instance and schema changes consistently and guaranteeing the bookkeeping of a full trace of the temporal evolution of the ontology instances and schemata. The involved implicit ontology schema changes are automatically generated and, upon approval by the KBA, executed.

To the best of our knowledge, we are the first to deal with non-conservative updates to ontology instances leading to implicit changes to ontology schemata in an ontology-based IoT environment supporting versioning either at ontology instance level and at schema level. We then applied it to an established temporal semantic framework (τOWL) for managing evolving ontologies and implemented it within a prototype tool (τOWL-Manager). We think that our proposal provides more flexibility in the management of (temporal) ontology evolution and ontology versioning, guarantees safety of the updated τOWL instance documents and the changed τOWL schema documents, and simplifies to KBAs (possibly having no sufficient skills to extricate themselves with devising and applying the otherwise required explicit ontology schema changes) the task of effecting/enforcing non-conservative updates to conventional ontology instance documents. Moreover, in an ontology engineering perspective, the τOWL-Manager provides a practical environment that can be used to support an incremental ontology construction method driven by the gradual availability of instance data.

In our future work, we plan to investigate another interesting scenario for updating ontology instances in batch mode. Moreover, we aim at applying the proposed approach to performing the on-the-fly ontology schema changes which are necessary to the support of high-availability applications (e.g., cloud computing applications), which is an aspect whose study we consider interesting for today's semantic web applications and for which our approach seems promising.

NOTES

1 If the KBA wants to change a property from optional to mandatory, he/she cannot do it through an instance update (e.g., specifying one value for an optional property generates an instance which is valid w.r.t. the current schema). In this case, he/she has to explicitly execute a schema change.
2 If the KBA wants to change a property from generic to functional, he/she has to explicitly execute a schema change.
3 http://xmlns.com/foaf/spec/

REFERENCES

[1] Berners-Lee, Tim, Hendler James, and Lassila Ora. "The Semantic Web." *Scientific American* 284, no. 5 (2001): 34–43.

[2] Guarino, Nicola, ed. *Formal Ontology in Information Systems*. IOS Press, Amsterdam, (1998).

[3] Zablith, Fouad, Antoniou Grigoris, d'Aquin Mathieu, Flouris Giorgos, Kondylakis Haridimos, Motta Enrico, Plexousakis Dimitris, and Sabou Marta. "Ontology evolution: a process-centric survey." *The Knowledge Engineering Review* 30, no. 1 (2015): 45–75.

[4] Artale, Alessandro, Kontchakov Roman, Kovtunova Alisa, Ryzhikov Vladislav, Wolter Frank, and Zakharyaschev Michael. "Ontology-Mediated Query Answering over Temporal Data: A Survey." In *Proceedings of the 24th International Symposium on Temporal Representation and Reasoning (TIME'2017)*, (Sven Schewe, Thomas Schneider, and Jef Wijsen, eds.), 1:1-1:37. Dagstuhl: Schloss Dagstuhl--Leibniz-Zentrum fuer Informatik, (2017).

[5] Taleb, Nora, Tighiouart Bornia, and Laiche Sara. "A method based on OWL schema for detecting changes between Ontology's versions." *Intelligent Decision Technologies* 8, no. 1 (2014): 45–52.

[6] Lambrix, Patrick, Dragisic Zlatan, Ivanova Valentina, and Anslow Craig. "Visualization for Ontology Evolution." In *Proceedings of the 2nd International Workshop on Visualization and Interaction for Ontologies and Linked Data (VOILA 2016)*, pp. 54–67. Aachen: RWTH Aachen University, (2016).

[7] Wang, Jianxin, Lim Ming K., Wang Chao, and Tseng Ming-Lang. "The evolution of the Internet of Things (IoT) over the past 20 years." *Computers & Industrial Engineering* 155 (2021): paper 107174.

[8] Diène, Bassirou, Diallo Ousmane, Rodrigues Joel J. P. C., Hadji E.L. Ndoye M., and Teodorov Ciprian. "Data Management Mechanisms for IoT: Architecture, Challenges and Solutions." In *Proceedings of the 5th International Conference on Smart and Sustainable Technologies (SpliTech 2020)*, pp. 1–6, IEEE, (2020).

[9] Eysenbach, Gunther. "What is e-health?" *Journal of Medical Internet Research* 3, no. 2 (2001): e20.

[10] Jin, Wenquan, and Kim Do H. "Design and Implementation of e-Health System Based on Semantic Sensor Network Using IETF YANG." *Sensors* 18, no. 2 (2018): 629.

[11] Elsaleh, Tarek, Enshaeifar Shirin, Rezvani Roonak, Acton Sahr Thomas, Janeiko Valentinas, and Bermudez-Edo Maria. "IoT-Stream: A lightweight ontology for

internet of things data streams and its use with data analytics and event detection services." *Sensors* 20, no. 4 (2020): 953.
[12] Sanjeevi, P., Siva Kumar B., Prasanna S., Maruthupandi J., Manikandan R., and Baseera A. "An ontology enabled internet of things framework in intelligent agriculture for preventing post-harvest losses." *Complex & Intelligent Systems* (2020). 10.1007/s40747-020-00183-y
[13] Turchet, Luca, Antoniazzi Francesco, Viola Fabio, Giunchiglia Fausto, and Fazekas György. "The Internet of Musical Things Ontology." *Journal of Web Semantics* 60 (2020): paper 100548.
[14] Cosío-León, María A., Ojeda-Carreño D., Nieto-Hipólito J.I., and Ibarra-Hernández J.A. "The use of standards in embedded devices to achieve end to end semantic interoperability on health systems." *Computer Standards & Interfaces* 57 (2018): 68–73.
[15] Rahmani, Amir M., Nguyen Gia Tuan, Negash Behailu, Anzanpour Arman, Azimi Iman, Jiang Mingzhe, and Liljeberg Pasi. "Exploiting smart e-health gateways at the edge of healthcare Internet-of-Things: A fog computing approach." *Future Generation Computer Systems* 78 (2018): 641–658.
[16] Daniele, L., den Hartog Frank, and Roes Jasper. "Created in close interaction with the industry: The smart appliances REFerence (SAREF) ontology." In *Proceedings of the 7th International Workshop Formal Ontologies Meet Industry (FOMI 2015)*, LNBIP vol. 225, pp. 100–112. Cham: Springer (2015). 10.1007/978-3-319-21545-7_9
[17] Li, Hongkun, Seed Dale, Flynn Bob, Mladin Catalina, and Di Girolamo Rocco. "Enabling semantics in an M2M/IoT service delivery platform." In *Proceedings of the IEEE 10th International Conference on Semantic Computing (ICSC 2016)*, pp. 206–213, IEEE, (2016).
[18] Zekri, Abir, Brahmia Zouhaier, Grandi Fabio, and Bouaziz Rafik. "τOWL: A Systematic Approach to Temporal Versioning of Semantic Web Ontologies." *Journal on Data Semantics* 5, no. 3 (2016): 141–163.
[19] Zekri, Abir, Brahmia Zouhaier, Grandi Fabio, and Bouaziz Rafik. "Temporal Schema Versioning in τOWL: A Systematic Approach for the Management of Time-varying Knowledge." *Journal of Decision Systems* 26, no. 2 (2017): 113–137.
[20] W3C. "OWL 2 Web Ontology Language – Primer (Second Edition)." W3C Recommendation, (2012). 11 December 2012. http://www.w3.org/TR/owl2-primer/ (accessed: 2021-04-17)
[21] Snodgrass, Richard T., Dyreson Curtis, Currim Faiz, Currim Sabah, and Joshi Shailesh. "Validating Quicksand: Schema Versioning in τXSchema." *Data and Knowledge Engineering* 65, no. 2 (2008): 223–242.
[22] Rhayem, Ahlem, Mhiri Mohamed Ben Ahmed, and Gargouri Faiez. "Semantic web technologies for the internet of things: Systematic literature review." *Internet of Things* 14 (2020): paper 100206.
[23] Moreira, João, Pires Luís Ferreira, van Sinderen Marten, Daniele Laura, and Girod-Genet Marc. "SAREF4health: Towards IoT standard-based ontology-driven cardiac e-health systems." *Applied Ontology* 15, no. 3 (2020): 385–410.
[24] Sharma, Nidhi, and Aggarwal R.K. "Ontology as a Tool to Enable Health Internet of Things Viable 5G Communication Networks." In *Ontology-Based Information Retrieval for Healthcare Systems*, (Vishal Jain, Ritika Wason, Jyotir Moy Chatterjee and Dac-Nhuong Le, eds.), pp. 293–312, Beverly, MA: Scrivener Publishing LLC, (2020).
[25] Rubí, Jesús Noel Sárez, and Gondim Paulo Roberto de Lira. "Interoperable Internet of Medical Things platform for e-Health applications." *International Journal of Distributed Sensor Networks* 16, no. 1 (2020). 10.1177/1550147719889591
[26] Lucic, Drazen, Caric Antun, and Lovrek Ignac. "Standardisation and regulatory

context of machine-to-machine communication." In *Proceedings of the 13th International Conference on Telecommunications (ConTEL 2015)*, pp. 1–7. New York: IEEE, (2015).

[27] W3C. "Semantic Sensor Network Ontology." W3C Recommendation (2017), 19 October 2017. https://www.w3.org/TR/vocab-ssn/ (accessed: 2021-04-17).

[28] openEHR. openEHR Architecture Overview (2018). https://specifications.openehr.org/releases/BASE/Release-1.0.3/architecture_overview.html (accessed: 2021-04-17).

[29] openEHR. openEHR–an open industry specifications, models and software for e-health (2021). https://www.openehr.org (accessed: 2021-04-17).

[30] Titi, Sondes, Elhadj Hadda Ben, and Chaari Lamia. "An ontology-based healthcare monitoring system in the internet of things." In *Proceedings of the 15th International Wireless Communications & Mobile Computing Conference (IWCMC 2019)*, pp. 319–324. IEEE, (2019).

[31] El-Sappagh, Shaker H., El-Masri Samir, Elmogy Mohammed, Riad A.M., and Saddik Basema. "An Ontological Case Base Engineering Methodology for Diabetes Management." *Journal of Medical Systems* 38 (2014): Article 67.

[32] Peng, Cong, and Goswami Prashant. "Meaningful integration of data from heterogeneous health services and home environment based on ontology." *Sensors* 19, no. 8 (2019): 1747. 10.3390/s19081747

[33] Villanueva-Miranda, Ismael, Nazeran Homer, and Martinek Radek. "A Semantic Interoperability Approach to Heterogeneous Internet of Medical Things (IoMT) Platforms." In *Proceedings of the IEEE 20th International Conference on e-Health Networking, Applications and Services (HealthCom 2018)*, pp. 1–5. IEEE, (2018).

[34] IETF. *YANG – A Data Modeling Language for the Network Configuration Protocol (NETCONF)*, Standards Track (2010), October 2010. https://tools.ietf.org/html/rfc6020 (accessed: 2021-04-17)

[35] Ullah, Kaleem, Shah Munam Ali, and Zhang Sijing. "Effective Ways to Use Internet of Things in the Field of Medical and Smart Health Care." In *Proceedings of the 2016 International Conference on Intelligent Systems Engineering (ICISE 2016)*, pp. 372–379. IEEE, (2016).

[36] Jagadeeswari, V., V. Subramaniyaswamy, R. Logesh, and V. Vijayakumar. "A study on medical Internet of Things and Big Data in personalized healthcare system." *Health Information Science and Systems* 6 (2018): Article 14.

[37] Khamparia, Aditya, Singh Prakash Kumar, Rani Poonam, Samanta Debabrata, Khanna Ashish, and Bhushan Bharat. "An Internet of Health Things-driven Deep Learning Framework for Detection and Classification of Skin Cancer using Transfer Learning." *Transactions on Emerging Telecommunications Technologies* (2020). 10.1002/ett.3963

[38] Kumar, Santosh, Bhusan Bharat, Singh Debabrata, and Choubey Dilip kumar. "Classification of Diabetes using Deep Learning." In *Proceedings of the 2020 International Conference on Communication and Signal Processing (ICCSP 2020)*, pp. 0651–0655. IEEE, (2020).

[39] Svozil, Daniel, Kvasnicka Vladimír, and Pospichal Jiří. "Introduction to multi-layer feed-forward neural networks." *Chemometrics and Intelligent Laboratory Systems* 39, no. 1 (1997): 43–62.

[40] Sharma, Nikhil, Kaushik Ila, Bhushan Bharat, Gautam Siddharth, and Khamparia Aditya. "Applicability of WSN and Biometric Models in the Field of Healthcare." In *Deep Learning Strategies for Security Enhancement in Wireless Sensor Networks*, (K. Martin Sagayam, Bharat Bhushan, A. Diana Andrushia, and Victor Hugo C. de Albuquerque, eds.), pp. 304–329, Hershey: IGI Global, (2020).

[41] Goyal, Sukriti, Sharma Nikhil, Bhushan Bharat, Shankar Achyut, and Sagayam Martin. "IoT Enabled Technology in Secured Healthcare: Applications, Challenges and Future Directions." In *Cognitive Internet of Medical Things for Smart Healthcare*, (Aboul Ella Hassanien, Aditya Khamparia, Deepak Gupta, K. Shankar, and Adam Slowik, eds.). Studies in Systems, Decision and Control, vol. 311, pp. 25–48. Cham: Springer, (2021).

[42] Seylan, İnanç, Franconi Enrico, and de Bruijn Jos. Effective Query Rewriting with Ontologies over DBoxes. In *Proceedings of the 21st International Joint Conference on Artificial Intelligence (IJCAI 2009)*, pp. 923–929, IJCAI Organization, (2009).

[43] Franconi, Enrico, Ibáñez-García Yazmín Angélica, and Seylan İnanç. "Query answering with DBoxes is hard." *Electronic Notes in Theoretical Computer Science* 278 (2011): 71–84.

[44] Etzioni, Oren, Golden Keith, and Weld Daniel S. "Sound and efficient closed-world reasoning for planning." *Artificial Intelligence* 89, no. 1–2 (1997): 113–148.

[45] Heflin, Jeff, and Muñoz-Avila Hector. "LCW-based Agent Planning for the Semantic Web." In *Ontologies and the Semantic Web, Papers from the 2002 AAAI Workshop*, pp. 63–70. Menlo Park: AAAI Press, (2002).

[46] Patel-Schneider, Peter F., and Horrocks Ian. "A comparison of two modelling paradigms in the Semantic Web." *Journal of Web Semantics* 5, no. 4 (2007): 240–250.

[47] Lutz, Carsten, Seylan İnanç, and Wolter Frank. "Mixing Open and Closed World Assumption in Ontology-Based Data Access: Non-Uniform Data Complexity." In *Proceedings of the 2012 International Workshop on Description Logics (DL-2012)*, CEUR Workshop Proceedings vol. 846, paper 17, (2012). CEUR-WS.org

[48] Bajraktari, Labinot, Magdalena Ortiz, and Mantas Šimkus. "Combining Rules and Ontologies into Clopen Knowledge Bases." *Proceedings of the AAAI Conference on Artificial Intelligence* 32, no. 1 (2018): 1728–1735.

[49] Pavlović, Sanja. "Ontology-Enriched Data Management with Partially Complete Data." In *Proceedings of the 13th RuleML+RR 2019 Doctoral Consortium and Rule Challenge*, CEUR Workshop Proceedings vol. 2438, paper 2, (2019). CEUR-WS.org

[50] Brahmia, Zouhaier, Grandi Fabio, Oliboni Barbara, and Bouaziz Rafik. "Schema Change Operations for Full Support of Schema Versioning in the τXSchema Framework." *International Journal of Information Technology and Web Engineering* 9, no. 2 (2014): 20–46.

[51] Brahmia, Safa, Brahmia Zouhaier, Grandi Fabio, and Bouaziz Rafik. "Temporal JSON Schema Versioning in the τJSchema Framework." *Journal of Digital Information Management* 15, no. 4 (2017): 179–202.

[52] Brahmia, Zouhaier, Grandi Fabio, Oliboni Barbara, and Bouaziz Rafik. "Schema Versioning in Conventional and Emerging Databases." In *Encyclopedia of Information Science and Technology* (4th edition), (Mehdi Khosrow-Pour, ed.), pp. 2054–2063. Hershey: IGI Global, (2018).

[53] Roddick, John F. "Schema Versioning." In *Encyclopedia of Database Systems* (2nd edition), (Ling Liu, and M. Tamer Özsu, eds.). New York: Springer, (2018). 10.1007/978-1-4614-8265-9_323

[54] Brahmia, Zouhaier, Grandi Fabio, Oliboni Barbara, and Bouaziz Rafik. "High-level Operations for Creation and Maintenance of Temporal and Conventional Schema in the τXSchema Framework." *Proceedings of the 21st International Symposium on Temporal Representation and Reasoning (TIME'2014)*, pp. 101–110, IEEE Computer Society, (2014).

15 Classification of Text Data in Healthcare Systems – A Comparative Study

Ömer Köksal
Aselsan, Ankara, Turkey

CONTENTS

DOI: 10.1201/9781003189053-15

15.1 INTRODUCTION

Categorizing healthcare text data (for example patients' symptom descriptions) according to diseases using a text classifier is a critical process as well as determining the healthcare procedures to be followed such as online healthcare counseling and information advice. Since decisions in healthcare are crucial and attempt to make up for it later are also very costly at this stage, the most significant factor that will determine the quality of the services to be provided is the high accuracy to be obtained in text classification. This chapter presents and compares the common techniques and classifiers used in healthcare text classification to develop robust healthcare applications with high accuracy.

The main contribution of this study is threefold: we provide a review and comparison of techniques and algorithms to be used in the classification of healthcare text including state-of-the-art approaches. Also, we present a novel methodology to be used for tuning the healthcare text classification process. Further, we provide a case study for healthcare text classification to reveal practical approaches and their effects in the given context.

The rest of this paper is organized as follows: Section 15.2 provides an overview of the related work. Section 15.3 presents the text classification algorithms and methods. Section 15.4 proposes a novel methodology to tune the healthcare text classification process. The details of the data set used in the experiments are given in Section 15.5. Section 15.6 reports the experimental results. Section 15.7 discusses the findings of this study and concludes the paper.

15.2 RELATED WORK

In recent years, artificial intelligence (AI) and Internet of Things (IoT)–based applications are widely used in vast domains as well as in the field of healthcare systems [1–9]. In parallel with the increasing utilization of AI in healthcare, the utilization of NLP applications in healthcare systems is growing. Text classification is an essential task for NLP applications and many studies in the literature have focused on the classification of healthcare text for a long time. In this section, we present an overview of healthcare text classification applications and techniques.

Some researchers published survey papers revealing the improvements and open research areas in healthcare text classification. Shah and Chircu [10] performed a systematic literature review about the usage of IoT and AI in healthcare inspecting 75 journal articles. Yoo and Song [11] provided a survey on biomedical ontologies and text mining techniques used in healthcare. In recent research, Khattak et al. [12] performed a survey for word embeddings in the clinical text. The authors provided clinical text corpora with different types of word representations that are available in pre-trained clinical word vector embeddings, as well as their evaluation, applications, and limitations of these approaches. Similarly, Gupta and Katarya [13] published a survey for a social media–based surveillance system for healthcare.

Apart from surveys, several studies focused on new methodologies and algorithms to improve classification accuracy in healthcare text categorization.

Liu [14] presented a high-quality classifier and reported the results of a case study claiming that high-quality healthcare text classification was seldom in previous studies.

Srivastava et al. [15] developed a system to perform healthcare tweet classification. The authors introduced a feature enhancement methodology that uses an incremental feature selection approach. Using the presented methodology and performing classification tasks on two different healthcare data sets, and categorizing with three different classifiers, the authors claimed that the feature enhancement methodology used in this paper is effective in enhancing classification accuracy.

In their more recent work, Srivastava et al. [16] provided a text classification system and evaluated its performance proposing a concept misrepresentation ratio (MRR) on input data and modeling the performance evaluation criteria to validate their hypothesis. The authors claimed that decreasing the MRR and using the proposed techniques improved classification accuracy up to 6% concerning their previous work.

15.3 TEXT CLASSIFICATION ALGORITHMS AND TECHNIQUES

Text classification is the automated process of categorizing text data depending on its content. Nowadays, text classification is a vital natural language processing (NLP) task widely employed in various domains such as medicine, biology, social sciences, and engineering. Several text classification applications such as document categorization, document summarization, information filtering, sentiment analysis, spam e-mail detection, topic tagging, and intent detection are used in these areas. With the rise of AI, learning-based algorithms have become the most important part of the text classification process. A text classification process has one or more data sets and mainly uses learning-based methods to extract valuable information from data sets. In performance evaluation of text classification processes, various metrics might be used.

15.3.1 Text Classification Framework

This section defines a typical text classification framework, as shown in Figure 15.1. This framework covers almost all the main steps of the text classification process. Some steps of this framework such as pre-processing and correction might be skipped depending on the data and techniques to be used, and application.

The text classification process starts with reading input text data. This input data might be in a structured or unstructured format. It can be accessed via a database or crawled from the Internet. Generally, this input text shall be corrected and pre-processed using the provided rules. Several techniques are used in this step such as removing punctuations and correcting misspelled words with a spell-checker. Then, the text data shall be converted into numbers by vectorization techniques for further processing for classifying. Since the dimension of the vectors is very big to process, the dimension reduction takes place and the features which mostly affect the classification accuracy are extracted. In the classification phase of the framework, text data is classified depending on its contents. The data used for the training process enables obtaining a mathematical classification model. This training data is not reused in the test phase. Instead, new test data is used for prediction and is classified using the classification model obtained. In this step, obtaining interpretable results is crucial. The final step is the evaluation of the whole classification process using appropriate metrics.

15.3.2 Data Correction

In many text classification applications, the input text data has errors. Apart from misspelled words, there might be several forms of intentional or unintentional errors in the text. For example, in sentiment analysis of a product customer feedbacks are

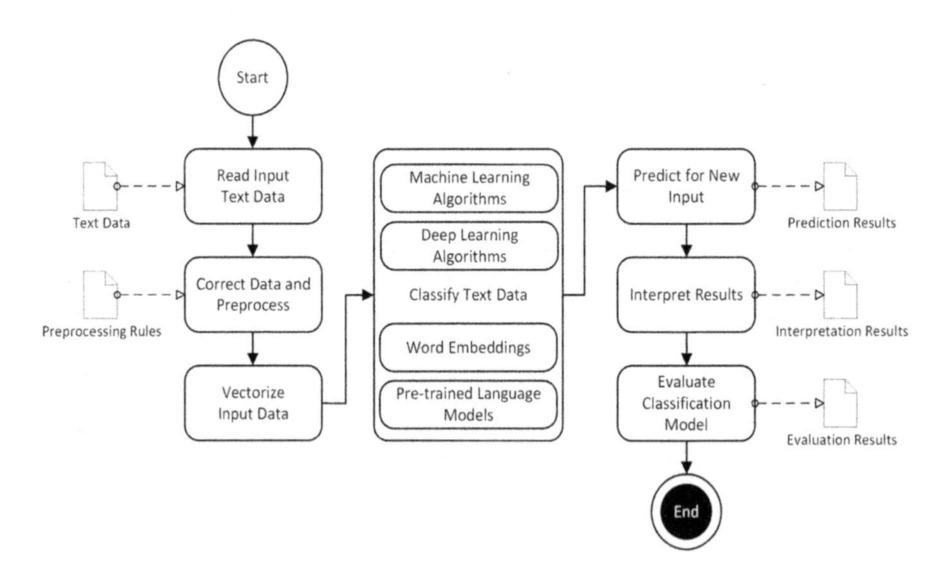

FIGURE 15.1 Text classification framework.

in unstructured format and might include comments with several misspelled words and intentional errors written like "baddd" instead of "bad" and "cmputr" instead of "computer". Several techniques (for example similarity metrics) are used to detect and correct these errors. Although in some applications, spell-checkers are used, and these errors shall be corrected in a context-aware manner not to cause loss of meaning.

15.3.3 Data Pre-processing

Pre-processing is the converting of raw input text data into new representations that are more convenient for text classification. The main object of pre-processing is improving classification accuracy while reducing input data size. Several techniques are used in the pre-processing step: *Tokenization* is the breaking of input text into smaller parts. During the tokenization process all punctuation, delimiters, and extra spaces are removed from the data. The assessed token is a valued part of the unstructured input data. *Lower case conversion* converts all input text to a lower-case format that is one of the most commonly used techniques in the pre-processing phase. This conversion reduces feature dimension and improves the classification accuracy almost in all cases. However, this technique shall be not be applied where the uppercase and lowercase of words have different meanings. For instance, "Opera" is a browser, and "opera" is a kind of music. In such cases, the lowercase conversion process causes the loss of meaning [17]. *Stop word removal* is another commonly used technique in text pre-processing. The most commonly used words in a particular language are called stop words. Stop words are assumed to be irrelevant within the working domain and have no effect on classification. The stop word removal process filters out these words before the classification process. Hence, the stop word removal process provides dimensionality reduction. *Stemming* is can be defined as acquiring the stem or root form of an inflected word by removing the suffix. Stemming is a language-specific process providing a common form for the variants of words. Hence, word frequencies are typically counted after the stemming process in the vectorization process. *Lemmatizing* results in the lemma of an inflected word based on the intended meaning. The lemmatizing process takes morphological information into account whereas stemming just crops the beginning or the end of the word to obtain the root of a word.

15.3.4 Vectorization of Text Data

Text classification requires converting text data into numerical forms to perform further processing. Transforming text data into vector space models is called feature extraction.

15.3.4.1 Bag-of-Words Approach

To vectorize the text input, the bag-of-words (BOW) approach is the characteristic technique used in traditional text classification applications. In this model, input text data is represented as vectors and all terms correspond to features. Put differently, distinct words in documents figure out the dimension of the feature space used.

BOW model does not retain word order in the text; it just distinguishes the existence of a word in the document.

15.3.4.2 Vector Weighting Techniques

To detect the weights of features, diverse methods are utilized in classification. This subsection describes two common methods to determine vector weights.

15.3.4.3 Term Frequency (TF)

TF method takes the terms' frequencies that appear in each text into account. The TF can be expressed as given in Equation 15.1:

$$\mathrm{TF}(t,\ d) = \log(1 + \mathrm{freq}(t,\ d)) \tag{15.1}$$

15.3.4.4 Term Frequency – Inverse Document Frequency (TF-IDF)

TF-IDF is an advanced weighting method that the frequencies in a whole collection take into account. In TF-IDF, the importance of terms is related to their frequencies in the particular document while being inversely proportional to the term's frequency in the batch. The TF-IDF can be expressed as given in Equation 15.2:

$$\mathrm{TF} - \mathrm{IDF}(t,\ d,\ D) = \mathrm{TF}(t,\ d).\ \mathrm{IDF}(t,\ D)) \tag{15.2}$$

where

$$\mathrm{IDF}(t,\ D) = \log(N/\mathrm{count}(d \in D\text{: } t \in d)) \tag{15.3}$$

15.3.5 Word Embeddings

A more recent approach in feature extraction is using word embeddings. Word embeddings acquire the meaning of words or phrases which are mapped to vector representations, enabling a similar grouping of text in a new vector space. Word embeddings might be more efficient than the BOW models. In the BOW models, the broadness of document collection and tagging at the index position causes data sparsity problems. However, word embeddings take the token's surrounding words into account to solve the data sparsity problem. The given text's information is transferred to the model to end up with dense vectors. In this continuous vector space representation, semantically alike words are close to each other. Although several word embedding techniques such as Word2Vec [18] and GLOVE [19] exist in the literature, in this paper, we select to use the Fasttext [20] method for word embeddings. In the following sub-section, we briefly mention Fasttext to justify our selection.

15.3.5.1 Fasttext

Fasttext treats each word as composed of character n-grams as opposed to Word2Vec. For rare words, Fasttext results in better word embeddings. Further, it can generate a vector for an out of vocabulary word that does not exist in the training corpus. This feature is not possible with either Word2Vec or Glove [20].

15.3.6 Sampling Methods

In the text classification, selecting the training and test data sets might dramatically affect the classification accuracy and cause misleading results. So, selecting these data sets to reflect the characteristics of the whole data set is important. Sampling is the process of selecting suitable samples from a data set. In classification tasks, to have reliable predictions several resampling methods such as N-Fold cross-validation, holdout, and bootstrap can be used. In this sub-section, we briefly mention the N-Fold cross-validation sampling method.

15.3.6.1 N-Fold Cross-Validation (N-Fold CV)

N-Fold CV is the most commonly used sampling method in text classification. It randomly partitions the data into 'N' subsets where 'N' experiments are performed. In each experiment, 'N-1' subsets are used for training and the remaining one is used for testing. The CV method is named depending on the number 'N' such as threefold CV or tenfold CV.

15.3.7 Supervised Machine Learning–Based Classifiers

As an essential part of AI, machine learning provides systems to learn without being explicitly programmed. In classification algorithms, features are the input variables, and the output attribute is the predicted class or category [21]. Supervised machine learning algorithms use training data to build a mathematical model that is used to predict the label (classification) or value (regression) of the test data. The following subsections briefly describe the traditional supervised machine learning algorithms. It shall be noted that, since we focus on classification algorithms, the terms 'algorithm' and 'classifier' are used interchangeably throughout the paper.

15.3.7.1 Naïve-Bayes (NB)

As a probabilistic classifier, NB is widely used in classification tasks. NB requires low computation time, and it is interpretable. NB is ground on the Bayes' theorem that assumes a specific feature's value does not depend on other features' value [21] as given:

$$P(Y|X) = P(X|Y) \times P(Y)/P(X) \tag{15.4}$$

The conditional independence between X and Y can be expressed as:

$$P(X, Y|Z) = P(X|Z) \times P(Y|Z) \tag{15.5}$$

NB classifies data computing the posterior probability for each class as:

$$P(Y|Z) = P(Y)\Pi_i(P(X_i|Y))/P(X) \tag{15.6}$$

The independence assumption in Bayes' theorem is not always valid in real life. There are several versions of NB classifiers that are developed to overcome the limitations of NB's independence assumption, such as multinomial NB and Bernoulli NB.

15.3.7.2 Logistic Regression (LR)

LR is another classification algorithm as opposed to what its name implies. Although the mathematical formulation of LR is similar to linear regression, LR performs classification by comparing the logistic function's output with a determined threshold value depending on the problem domain [22]. Denoting the true class label as y_i and the predicted class label as $p(C = y_i \mid U_i)$, LR's objective is to learn the A and b values. The probability of observing label y_i provide a conditional generative model as:

$$p(C = y_i|U_i) = (\exp(\bar{A}.\ \bar{U}_i + b)/(1 + \exp(\bar{A}.\ \bar{U}_i + b)) \quad (15.7)$$

Transforming the previous equation as below shows that LR is a linear classifier since the decision boundary is determined by a linear function of the features [23].

$$\log(p(C = y_i|U_i)/(1 - p(C = y_i|U_i)) = \bar{A}.\ \bar{U}_i + b \quad (15.8)$$

15.3.7.3 Support Vector Machine (SVM)

Since a SVM outperforms other traditional machine learning algorithms in many applications, it is a popular classifier for text classification applications. To classify data, a SVM constructs optimal hyperplanes iteratively to minimize the error. A hyperplane is drawn between the support vectors that belong to the different categories. The closest data points to the hyperplanes are named support vectors. To construct hyperplanes, a SVM utilizes particular kernels. Linear, polynomial, radial basis function, and sigmoid kernels are the most commonly used SVM kernels. Depending on data type and size, a particular kernel might provide higher classification accuracy [22]. In many implementations, RBF is the default SVM kernel that is given in the form:

$$K(x_1, x_2) = \exp(|x_1 - x_2|^2)/(2\sigma^2) \quad (15.9)$$

where $|x_1 - x_2|^2$ is called the squared Euclidian distance of two feature vectors and σ is a free parameter.

15.3.7.4 K-Nearest Neighbors (KNN)

A KNN algorithm is based on feature similarity and has no assumption for data distribution. KNN predicts based on the neighbor data points. 'K' is the only input parameter of the algorithm. The training phase of KNN is fast. KNN is especially important when processing data with no prior knowledge. KNN might use various metrics to calculate distance between neighbors such as the cosine similarity and Euclidian similarity.

The cosine similarity is expressed as:

$$\sin(x_1, x_2) = (x_1 - x_2)/(||x_1||.\ |||x_2||) \tag{15.10}$$

and the Euclidian similarity is given as:

$$\sin(x_1, x_2) = 1/\text{dist}(x_1 - x_2) = 1/\sqrt{\textstyle\sum_i}\left(x_{1i^2}.\ x_{2i^2}\right) \tag{15.11}$$

15.3.7.5 Decision Tree (DT)

DT is a predictive modeling approach that breaks down complex data into more manageable parts using a tree structure. In this structure, internal nodes correspond to tests on attributes, branches represent the outcomes of the tests, and leaf nodes denote class labels. In DT, classification is performed iteratively by initializing at the root node, testing the attributes of the node, and reaching down according to the test's outcome.

15.3.7.6 Random Forest (RF)

RF consists of assemblies of DTs. RF can be presented as ensembles of DTs and generally outperforms them. Having trained all trees in the forest, predictions are determined by voting. RFs are very fast to train text data but they are slower in predictions compared to deep learning–based classifiers.

15.3.8 Deep Learning–Based Classifiers

The deep learning concept is inspired by the functional aspects of human thinking. Deep learning–based classifiers and architectures are widely used in text classification applications with remarkable performances. In the following sub-section, we present artificial neural networks to provide a basis for the architectural structure of deep learning–based classifiers.

15.3.8.1 Artificial Neural Networks (ANNs)

ANNs are devised for learning by multi-connection layers. The architecture of ANNs includes one input layer, one output layer, and one or more hidden layers between these layers.

ANNs' objective is to discover the relationship between these inputs and output with the help of hidden layers. In this structure, each layer acquires the connection from the previous layer. ANN learns by determining a set of weights (w) that minimize the total sum of squared errors as given:

$$E(w) = (1/2).\ \textstyle\sum_i (y_i - \hat{y}_i)^2 \quad \text{where}\, i = 1..\ N \tag{15.12}$$

keeping in mind that

$$\hat{y} = w.\ x \tag{15.13}$$

The input feature space of the text data constitutes the input layer of the ANN. The input layer for text classification can be constructed with feature extraction methods

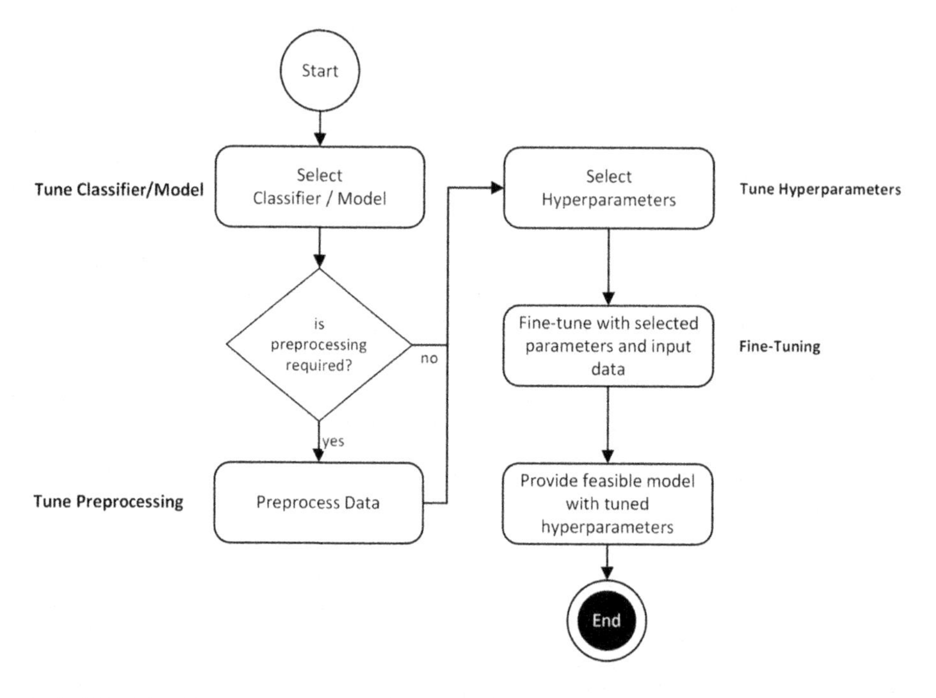

FIGURE 15.2 The proposed research methodology.

like TF, TF-IDF, or word embeddings. The output layer has one node in binary classification and has nodes as much as the number of classes in multi-class classification.

ANN uses a backpropagation algorithm with an activation function. The activation function is sigmoid or RELU functions in many applications. The sigmoid and RELU functions can be defined as shown, respectively:

$$\text{SIGMOID}(x) = 1/(1 + \exp(-x)) \tag{15.14}$$

$$\text{RELU}(x) = \max(0, x) \tag{15.15}$$

In ANNs, the output of the multi-class classification shall be the *Softmax* function. The definition of the *Softmax* function is given in the equation [24].

$$\sigma(Z)_j = \exp(Z_j)/\sum_k (\exp(Z_k)) \quad \text{where} k = 1..\ K \tag{15.16}$$

15.3.9 Pre-Trained Language Models

The use of pre-trained language models is emerging due to their valuable performance in the NLP domain. With the introduction of encoder-decoder models in the transformer architecture, pre-trained language models have seen increasing research interest [25]. Encoder models take input text and generate high-dimensional latent embeddings that do not necessarily belong to a semantic space. Decoder models convert these embeddings back into the natural language to accomplish a language modeling task. Pre-trained language models utilize dynamic representations of words, also referred to as contextual embeddings. The pre-training procedure is carried on using domain-independent large corpora. Deploying such models for downstream applications requires a fine-tuning step that optimizes the model for the task using smaller, domain-specific data.

Due to their success, many pre-trained language models are started to be used, such as ELMO [26], ELECTRA [27], ULMFiT [28], and BERT [29]. However, we select to use BERT models in this paper. In the following sub-section, we present BERT briefly.

15.3.9.1 Bidirectional Encoder Representations from Transformers (BERT)

BERT is a multilayer transformer encoder model. BERT is trained over a large corpus with both a masked language modeling task and a next sentence prediction task simultaneously [29]. It uses an attention mechanism to model long-range dependencies in the input text. The language modeling in BERT is bidirectional, as its name implies. This bidirectional model aims to capture the prediction process's contextual information. The next sentence prediction task samples the next sentence in the input with another sentence at random. It expects the model to predict whether the chosen sentence naturally follows the first sentence. This task enables BERT to develop a broader understanding of natural language by working at the sentence level. BERT brings a compelling basis for a variety of downstream tasks by its fine-tuning feature. The BERT fine-tuning enables to use of additional domain-specific data to adapt pre-trained BERT. For the classification task, the BERT embedding vector for the special "[CLS]" token placed at the beginning of the input sequence is used to encode the entire sequence. An additional fully connected layer maps the sequence embedding to the classification probabilities. BERT has several parameters for improving performance, such as the epoch size, maximum input sequence length, and pre-trained model choice. In the literature, it is shown that BERT outperformed its other pre-trained language models in diverse NLP tasks [29]. BERT can incorporate smaller, task-specific data in the more lightweight fine-tuning process. So it becomes widely adopted for high accuracy gains in a range of downstream tasks [30].

15.3.10 Evaluation Metrics

This section presents several vital metrics used for assessing the classification's performance. Most of the evaluation metrics of classification tasks are built on the confusion matrix concept that reveals the prediction results of the classification model for the test set. In the confusion matrix, the columns present the instances of the predicted classes whereas the rows represent values for the actual classes, as shown in Table 15.1.

TABLE 15.1
Confusion Matrix

	Predicted Positive	Predicted Negative
Actual Positive	True Positive (TP)	False Negative (FN)
Actual Negative	False Positive (FP)	True Negative (TN)

The confusion matrix indicates the ways our model is confused in predicting classes. TP presents the instances that are predicted as positive whose actual classes are positive (i.e., no confusion). Similarly, TN shows the instances that are predicted as negative, which are also true. On the other hand, FP and FN show instances predicted as positive and negative, respectively, which are false.

15.3.10.1 Accuracy

Accuracy can be defined as the division of the sum of correct predictions (TP and TN) to all instances, as given in the equation:

$$\text{Accuracy}(A) = (TP + TN)/(TP + TN + FP + FN) \tag{15.17}$$

15.3.10.2 Precision

Precision shows the accuracy of the positive class. Precision is the division of TP to the total positive predictions (TP and FP) as shown in the following formula:

$$\text{Precision}(P) = TP/(TP + FP) \tag{15.18}$$

15.3.10.3 Recall

Recall (or sensitivity) shows the ratio of correctly detected positive classes, and it is defined as TP divided by the sum of positive classes (TP and FN) as shown:

$$\text{Recall}(R) = TP/(TP + FN) \tag{15.19}$$

15.3.10.4 F-Measure

F-Measure (or F1 Score) compares models having different precision and recall values with a single evaluation measure. F-Measure can be defined as the harmonic mean of precision and recall, as shown:

$$F - \text{Measure}(F1) = 2 * (P \times R)/(P + R) \tag{15.20}$$

15.4 RESEARCH METHODOLOGY

In this section, we propose a methodology to improve the classification accuracy of healthcare text categorization. We consider fundamental phases of the classification process and algorithms' parameters to tune the classification process. The tuning process is generally data-dependent. Hence, the proposed methodology shall be adopted for the data sets used. The proposed methodology is given in Figure 15.2.

The methodology proposed previously starts with the selection of a classification algorithm/model. In this paper, we utilized several classifiers and models to evaluate each technique and checking their improvements on the classification accuracy.

The second step is the application of pre-processing techniques, if required. It shall be noted that different processing techniques are efficient for different data sets. Hence, the processing step shall be applied iteratively on the data set to evaluate the effect of each particular pre-processing technique. Then the hyperparameter selection step takes place. Hyperparameters are the parameters that are not learned by the algorithms, they shall be tuned iteratively as well as parameters of the classifiers iteratively. Then the fine-tuning step takes place. In this phase, selected parameters are tuned with the use of input data. The result of the provided methodology is the feasible model with tuned hyperparameters for the selected data set.

In this paper, we applied this methodology for both traditional machine learning algorithms and pre-trained language models. The results obtained using this methodology are presented and discussed in the later sections.

15.5 DATA SET

To illustrate the effect of selection of classification algorithm and hyperparameter tuning we use a public data set named "Medical Text for Text Classification". In our experiments, we only use the data set's training part that includes five classes and 14,438 samples. The distribution of the samples concerning the categories is given in Table 15.2.

In this chapter, we perform text classification on this data set using supervised machine learning algorithms, word embeddings, and pre-trained language models. The results of these experiments and details of the tests are given in the next sections.

TABLE 15.2
The Distribution of the Samples for Classes in the Data Set

Category	Number of Samples
1	3,163
2	1,494
3	1,925
4	3,051
5	4,805
TOTAL	14,438

TABLE 15.3
Setup Used in the Experiments

Parameter	Value
CPU	Intel Xeon E5 (24 Core)
GPU	Nvidia Quadro M400
GPU-RAM	8 GB
Operating System	Ubuntu 18.04 (64 Bit)
System RAM	64 GB

15.6 EXPERIMENTS AND RESULTS

In this section, we provide experimental results of the classification of the data set presented previously. Firstly, we present the details of the setup used in experiments. Then we provide the results obtained using supervised machine learning algorithms, using word embeddings, and using the pre-trained language models. Finally, we discuss and compare the results obtained using three different classification techniques on the same data set.

15.6.1 Computing Setup

We have used a single board computer for our computations. The details of the experimental setup are as given in Table 15.3. We utilized the given setup in all types of experiments. Please note that the supervised machine learning algorithms are implemented to use Central Processing Unit (CPU); however, the pre-trained language models require GPU.

15.6.2 Experiments Using Supervised Machine Learning Algorithms

In the first part of our experiments, we classified healthcare using traditional supervised machine learning algorithms. We applied the methodology given above in the classification process. We applied data correction first. Then, we iteratively searched the effects of pre-processing techniques: lowercase conversion, stop word removal, stemming, and lemmatizing. Then we perform optimization for the BOW size. After these steps, we performed classification using nine different traditional classifiers using tenfold cross validation. We obtained the best results for the traditional supervised machine learning algorithms using the SVM classifier with the sigmoid kernel. The results of these classifications are given in Table 15.4.

15.6.3 Experiments Using Word Embeddings

In the next step of our experiments, we used word embedding instead of the BOW approaches applied in the previous experiments. As stated in the previous

TABLE 15.4
Classification Results of Traditional Machine Learning Algorithms

Supervised ML Classifier	F1-Measure [%]	Accuracy [%]
Naïve-Bayes	42.07	47.47
SVM-linear kernel	59.30	59.49
SVM-poly kernel	41.98	42.94
SVM-RBF kernel	54.09	54.26
SVM-sigmoid kernel	**61.62**	**61.77**
K-Nearest Neighbor	53.06	54.00
Logistic Regression	60.23	60.60
Decision Tree	41.36	41.28
Random Forest	47.86	48.65

sections, we selected the Fasttext to be used as the word embeddings to be used. We have used Fasttext word weightings trained using huge Wikipedia data, namely 'wiki-news-300d-1M' vector file was used to get term weights. The results of applying Fasttext on traditional machine learning algorithms are given in Table 15.5.

15.6.4 Experiments Using Pre-Trained Language Models

In the final step of our experiments, we utilized pre-trained language models for the healthcare text classification. We selected BERT models as the pre-trained language model to be applied since BERT models generally outperform other

TABLE 15.5
Classification Results of Traditional Machine Learning Algorithms with Fasttext

Classification Model	F1-Measure [%]	Accuracy [%]
Fasttext & Naïve-Bayes	50.61	52.84
Fasttext & SVM-linear kernel	57.02	57.89
Fasttext & SVM-poly kernel	**59.22**	**59.70**
Fasttext & SVM-RBF kernel	58.22	58.83
Fasttext & SVM-sigmoid kernel	50.15	54.88
Fasttext & K-Nearest Neighbor	54.21	55.92
Fasttext & Logistic Regression	56.96	58.28
Fasttext & Decision Tree	31.05	31.28
Fasttext & Random Forest	41.29	41.93

TABLE 15.6
Hyperparameters Used in Classification with BERT Models

Hyperparameter	Value
Maximum Sequence Length	256
Batch Size	16
Number of Epoch	3
Learning Rate	1e-5

pre-trained language models in many domains [29]. There are vast BERT models available to be used for various domains. We have used models available on the Hugging Face web page [31]. So, we selected models trained particularly for healthcare text. We include two general-purpose (base) BERT models and three models particularly developed for healthcare text. Base models are added to construct a baseline and to compare the effects of healthcare models in the healthcare text classification process. The first healthcare model, 'pupcr/clinicalnerpt-healthcare', is modeled in Table 15.6 and is the model developed for general purposes. The second healthcare model 'emilyalsentzer/Bio_ClinicalBERT' is a BERT model particularly developed for the healthcare domain [32]. The third healthcare model used 'simonlevine/biological-roberta-long' is based on Roberta-type BERT models. We tried to perform hyperparameter optimization performing a vast number of experiments on the data set. The best results are obtained using the parameters given in Table 15.6.

The BERT classification results showed that healthcare BERT models provide only slightly better results than generic BERT models for the data set used in this paper. The best results belong to the "simonlevine/biological-roberta-long" model. It shall be noted that these results are valid on the applied data set. To generalize, these models shall be tested on a vast number of data sets. The results of experiments with the BERT models are given in Table 15.7.

TABLE 15.7
Classification Results of BERT Models

Classification Model	F1-Measure [%]	Accuracy [%]
bert-base-uncased	63.87	64.77
bert-base-multilingual	65.60	66.71
pucpr/clinicalnerpt-healthcare	64.42	65.67
emilyalsentzer/Bio-ClinicalBERT	64.40	66.16
simonlevine/biological-roberta-long	**67.02**	**67.89**

15.7 DISCUSSION AND CONCLUSION

In this paper, we presented the details of the algorithms and techniques used in text classification. We presented several traditional machine learning–based classifiers, word embeddings, deep learning–based classifiers, and finally, pre-trained language models that are claimed as state-of-the-art in several NLP tasks. Also, we explained several methods and techniques used in text classification such as text pre-processing, vectorization, N-Gram language models, document similarity models, and sampling techniques. Further, we applied the presented techniques and classifiers on a public healthcare data set to perform a comparative healthcare text classification task. Finally, we have presented the experimental setup and the obtained results in detail.

We observed that traditional machine learning algorithms are only trained with the corpus in the data set. Fasttext model is trained with Wikipedia data, i.e., the data used in the training phase is not particularly specific to the healthcare domain. We have used two base BERT models and three healthcare-specific BERT models that were claimed to be trained particularly for the healthcare domain.

As a result of our experiments, we have seen that the BERT models provided the best results. Even generic models provided better accuracy compared to the previous techniques presented. Further, we have observed that healthcare-specific BERT models resulted in slightly better accuracy compared to the generic BERT models surprisingly.

As future work, we would like to use Fasttext models that were specifically trained for the healthcare domain instead of models trained with Wikipedia data. Further, we would like to test healthcare-specific BERT models on different healthcare data sets.

REFERENCES

[1] Jindal, Mansi, Gupta Jatin, and Bhushan Bharat. "Machine Learning Methods for IoT and Their Future Applications." In *Proceedings – 2019 International Conference on Computing, Communication, and Intelligent Systems, ICCCIS 2019*, 2019-Janua, pp. 430–434, Institute of Electrical and Electronics Engineers Inc, 2019. 10.1109/ICCCIS48478.2019.8974551.

[2] Khamparia, Aditya, Singh Prakash Kumar, Rani Poonam, Samanta Debabrata, Khanna Ashish, and Bhushan Bharat. "An Internet of Health Things-driven Deep Learning Framework for Detection and Classification of Skin Cancer Using Transfer Learning." *Transactions on Emerging Telecommunications Technologies*, May, e3963, 2020. 10.1002/ett.3963.

[3] Köksal, Ömer, and Tekinerdogan Bedir. "Feature-Driven Domain Analysis of Session Layer Protocols of Internet of Things." In *Proceedings – 2017 IEEE 2nd International Congress on Internet of Things, ICIOT 2017*, pp. 105–112, 2017. 10.1109/IEEE.ICIOT.2017.19.

[4] Kumar, Santosh, Bhusan Bharat, Singh Debabrata, and Choubey Dilip Kumar. "Classification of Diabetes Using Deep Learning." In *Proceedings of the 2020 IEEE International Conference on Communication and Signal Processing, ICCSP 2020*, pp. 651–655, Institute of Electrical and Electronics Engineers Inc, 2020. 10.1109/ICCSP48568.2020.9182293.

[5] Panigrahi, Niranjan, Ayus Ishan, and Jena Om Prakash. "An Expert System-Based Clinical Decision Support System for Hepatitis-B Prediction & Diagnosis." In *Machine Learning for Healthcare Applications*, pp. 57–75, Wiley, 2021. 10.1002/9781119792611.ch4.

[6] Paramesha, K., Gururaj H.L., and Jena Om Prakash. "Applications of Machine Learning in Biomedical Text Processing and Food Industry." In *Machine Learning for Healthcare Applications*, pp. 151–167, Wiley, 2021. 10.1002/9781119792611.ch10.

[7] Pattnayak, Parthasarathi, and Jena Om Prakash. "Innovation on Machine Learning in Healthcare Services–An Introduction." In *Machine Learning for Healthcare Applications*, pp. 1–15, Wiley, 2021. 10.1002/9781119792611.ch1.

[8] Sharma, Nikhil, Kaushik Ila, Bhushan Bharat, Gautam Siddharth, and Khamparia Aditya. "Applicability of WSN and Biometric Models in the Field of Healthcare." In, 304–329, 2020. 10.4018/978-1-7998-5068-7.ch016.

[9] Goyal, Sukriti, Sharma Nikhil, Bhushan Bharat, Shankar Achyut, and Sagayam Martin. "IoT Enabled Technology in Secured Healthcare: Applications, Challenges and Future Directions." In *Studies in Systems, Decision and Control*, 311, pp. 25–48. Springer Science and Business Media Deutschland GmbH, 2021. 10.1007/978-3-030-55833-8_2.

[10] Shah, Rushabv, and Chircu A. "IoT and AI in Healthcare: A Systematic Literature Review." *Issues in Information Systems* 19 (2018). 10.48009/3_iis_2018_33-41.

[11] Yoo, Ill-Hoi, and Song Min. "Biomedical Ontologies and Text Mining for Biomedicine and Healthcare: A Survey." *Journal of Computing Science and Engineering* 2 no. 2, (2008): 109–136. 10.5626/jcse.2008.2.2.109.

[12] Khattak, Faiza Khan, Jeblee Serena, Pou-Prom Chloé, Abdalla Mohamed, Meaney Christopher, and Rudzicz Frank. "A Survey of Word Embeddings for Clinical Text." *Journal of Biomedical Informatics: X*. Academic Press Inc, 2019. 10.1016/j.yjbinx.2019.100057.

[13] Gupta, Aakansha, and Katarya Rahul. "Social Media Based Surveillance Systems for Healthcare Using Machine Learning: A Systematic Review." *Journal of Biomedical Informatics*. Academic Press Inc, 2020. 10.1016/j.jbi.2020.103500.

[14] Liu, Rey Long. "Text Classification for Healthcare Information Support." In *Lecture Notes in Computer Science (Including Subseries Lecture Notes in Artificial Intelligence and Lecture Notes in Bioinformatics)*, 4570 LNAI, pp. 44–53, Springer Verlag, 2007. 10.1007/978-3-540-73325-6_5.

[15] Srivastava, Saurabh Kumar, Singh Sandeep Kumar, and Suri Jasjit S. "Effect of Incremental Feature Enrichment on Healthcare Text Classification System: A Machine Learning Paradigm." *Computer Methods and Programs in Biomedicine* 172 (April) (2019): 35–51. 10.1016/j.cmpb.2019.01.011.

[16] Srivastava, Saurabh Kumar, Singh Sandeep Kumar, and Suri Jasjit S. "Chapter 16 - A Healthcare Text Classification System and Its Performance Evaluation: A Source of Better Intelligence by Characterizing Healthcare Text." In *Cognitive Informatics, Computer Modelling, and Cognitive Science*, (G.R. Sinha and Jasjit S Suri, eds.), pp. 319–369. Academic Press, 2020. 10.1016/B978-0-12-819445-4.00016-3.

[17] Işık, Muhittin, and Dağ Hasan. "The Impact of Text Preprocessing on the Prediction of Review Ratings." *Turkish Journal of Electrical Engineering and Computer Sciences* 28, no. 3 (2020): 1405–1421. 10.3906/elk-1907-46.

[18] Mikolov, Tomas, Chen Kai, Corrado Greg, and Dean Jeffrey. "Efficient Estimation of Word Representations in Vector Space." In *1st International Conference on Learning Representations, ICLR 2013 - Workshop Track Proceedings*. International Conference on Learning Representations, ICLR, 2013. https://arxiv.org/abs/1301.3781v3.

[19] Pennington, Jeffrey, Socher Richard, and Manning Christopher. "GloVe: Global Vectors for Word Representation." In *Proceedings of the 2014 Conference on Empirical Methods in Natural Language Processing (EMNLP)*, pp. 1532–1543, Doha, Qatar: Association for Computational Linguistics, 2014. 10.3115/v1/D14-1162.

[20] Joulin, Armand, Grave Edouard, Bojanowski Piotr, and Mikolov Tomas. "Bag of Tricks for Efficient Text Classification." In *Proceedings of the 15th Conference of the European Chapter of the Association for Computational Linguistics: Volume 2, Short Papers*, pp. 427–431, Valencia, Spain: Association for Computational Linguistics, 2017. https://www.aclweb.org/anthology/E17-2068.

[21] Alpaydin, Ethem. *Machine Learning: The New AI*. The MIT Press, 2016. https://www.amazon.com.tr/Machine-Learning-New-Ethem-Alpaydin/dp/0262529513.

[22] Köksal, Ömer. "Tuning the Turkish Text Classification Process Using Supervised Machine Learning-Based Algorithms." In *2020 International Conference on INnovations in Intelligent SysTems and Applications (INISTA)*, pp. 1–7, IEEE, 2020. 10.1109/INISTA49547.2020.9194669.

[23] Aggarwal, Charu C., and Zhai Cheng Xiang. "A Survey of Text Classification Algorithms." In *Mining Text Data*, 9781461432 pp. 163–222, Springer US, 2012. 10.1007/978-1-4614-3223-4_6.

[24] Kowsari, Kamran, Meimandi Kiana Jafari, Heidarysafa Mojtaba, Mendu Sanjana, Barnes Laura E., and Brown Donald E. "Text Classification Algorithms: A Survey." *Information (Switzerland)* 10 (4) (2019). 10.3390/info10040150.

[25] Vaswani, Ashish, Shazeer Noam, Parmar Niki, Uszkoreit Jakob, Jones Llion, Gomez Aidan N., Kaiser Łukasz, and Polosukhin Illia. "Attention Is All You Need." In *Advances in Neural Information Processing Systems*, 2017-Decem, pp. 5999–6009. Neural information processing systems foundation, 2017. https://arxiv.org/abs/1706.03762v5.

[26] Peters, Matthew E., Neumann Mark, Iyyer Mohit, Gardner Matt, Clark Christopher, Lee Kenton, and Zettlemoyer Luke. "Deep Contextualized Word Representations." In *Proceedings of the 2018 Conference of the North American Chapter of the Association for Computational Linguistics: Human Language Technologies, Volume 1 (Long Papers)*, 1, pp. 2227–2237, New Orleans, Louisiana: Association for Computational Linguistics, 2018. 10.18653/v1/N18-1202.

[27] Clark, Kevin, Luong Minh-Thang, Le Quoc V, and Manning Christopher D. "ELECTRA: Pre-Training Text Encoders as Discriminators Rather Than Generators." *ArXiv* (2020) abs/2003.1.

[28] Howard, Jeremy, and Ruder Sebastian. "Universal Language Model Fine-Tuning for Text Classification." *ACL 2018 - 56th Annual Meeting of the Association for Computational Linguistics, Proceedings of the Conference (Long Papers)* 1 (January) (2018): 328–339. http://arxiv.org/abs/1801.06146.

[29] Devlin, Jacob, Chang Ming-Wei, Lee Kenton, and Toutanova Kristina. "BERT: Pre-Training of Deep Bidirectional Transformers for Language Understanding." In *Proceedings of the 2019 Conference of the North American Chapter of the Association for Computational Linguistics: Human Language Technologies, Volume 1 (Long and Short Papers)*, pp. 4171–4186, Minneapolis, Minnesota: Association for Computational Linguistics, 2019. 10.18653/v1/N19-1423.

[30] Ambalavanan, Ashwin Karthik, and Devarakonda Murthy V. "Using the Contextual Language Model BERT for Multi-Criteria Classification of Scientific Articles." *Journal of Biomedical Informatics* 112 (December), (2020). 10.1016/j.jbi.2020.103578.

[31] "Hugging Face." n.d. Accessed April 26, 2021. https://huggingface.co/models.

[32] Alsentzer, Emily, Murphy John, Boag William, Weng Wei-Hung, Jindi Di, Naumann Tristan, and McDermott Matthew. "Publicly Available Clinical." In *Proceedings of the 2nd Clinical Natural Language Processing Workshop*, pp. 72–78, Stroudsburg, PA, USA: Association for Computational Linguistics, 2019. 10.18653/v1/W19-1909.

16 Predicting Air Quality Index with Machine Learning Models

G. Abirami, Anindya Das, and Navneeth Sreenivasan
SRM Institute of Science and Technology (SRMIST), Kattankulathur, Tamil Nadu, India

R. Girija
Vellore Institute of Technology (VIT) Chennai, Tamil Nadu, India

CONTENTS

16.1 INTRODUCTION

Fresh and pollutant-free surroundings exist as important for species' all-round development [1]. The air everybody inhales assumes a compelling job in the natural as well

DOI: 10.1201/9781003189053-16

as the mental advancement of the bodies possessed by human beings. Open air provides oxygen that helps our brain to function properly cleans our lungs, assistances within the transportation of blood, in addition to many other aids. Many earlier humans or tribes practiced this in order to comprehend this fact and protect our natural ecosystem. They would worship the rivers and plants as well as many other natural resources. However, from the time of the age of industries and human modernization began the concern aimed at our environment started to decline pretty ghastly. Deforestation [2–4] began at a huge scope so as route for making place on behalf of innovative businesses. Through the development in the range of the quantity of ventures the percentage of poisons being transmitted in the direction of the air moreover extended, and through the amount of timberlands decreasing there weren't sufficient trees to acclimatize these toxins and convert them in the form of oxygen in addition to supplementary natural materials. This lopsidedness prompts air contamination.

The presence or on the other hand presentation of unsafe substances towards the outdoor air is branded by way of air contamination [5,6]. It occurs when substances like carbon dioxide (CO_2), carbon monoxide (CO), chlorofluorocarbons (CFC), etc. are presented towards world's air at an excessive quantity. This can cause sensitivities, ailments, in addition to losses of people; it could likewise make hurt other living beings, for instance, creatures and nourishment crops, and thus going on. WHO's 2018 report states that around 6 to 7 million general public die every single 12-month period owing to diseases caused by outside air toxic waste. Therefore, it remains highly vital toward screening and foreseeing the stages of toxins in the atmosphere. In this application we appraise various ML procedures to discover which method predicts the air quality index best. The novelty of the work is to predict the quality of air using various effective attributes of benchmark data set which has taken from open government data (OGD). The data set has been run on different ML models. Moreover, the missing data information is rectified by finding the mean and average value of the respective attribute column. By this way, the data has been processed to provide an accurate prediction of AQI.

Nowadays, ML approaches play a vital role in detection and classification of skin cancer [7–10]. Wearable healthcare systems, sensors, security and privacy are based upon IOT [11]. Biometric models play a good role in the field of healthcare [12]. There are various machine learning methods for IOT [13]. Diabetes are well analysed in ML approaches [14]. Not only in medical field, machine learning also played a major role in many fields such as image processing, security and trust-based access control [15]. Encrypting images using Walsh-Hadamard transform [16], fractional Hartley transform was reported with a very good accuracy [17,18]. The trust-based access control using machine learning for classify the trust value of each person according to the parameters namely performance, direct observation, feedback and expected trust [19–21].

This chapter is organised as follows: Section 16.2 talks about the introduction of the chapter and all the related surveys are shown in Section 16.3. Section 16.4 and Section 16.5 speak about model selection and regression models and Section 16.6 provided implementation, respectively. Data collection and missing value processing are discussed in the Sections 16.7 and 16.8. The feature sections are given in Section 16.9. In Section 16.10, the data transformation and feature scaling are provided. Results are analysed and discussed in 16.11, 16.10. Section 16.10 is the conclusion.

16.2 RELATED WORK

Liu Bo et al. saw that RFR played out the greatest with Mean Absolute Error (MAE) and RMSE [22,23]. The evidence utilized contained clamour which could have brought around a poor showing of support vectors. However, the solid equipment reliance of neural systems attached to the processor besides the obscure time term of BPNNs made this less proficient. Decision trees stand quicker in addition to the fact of being extra interpretable than BPNNs. Soh et al. [24] functioned with the maximum relevant spatial-temporal relations and a mixture of numerous neural networks together with ANN and CNN in addition to a long-short term memory toward abstracting spatial-temporal relations. It also uses dynamic time warping and long-short term memory besides it similarly includes trends from multiple locations. But this scheme contains evidences of missing data, absent memory, unsupervised learning and overfitting owed to their usage of CNN (convolutional neural network). It furthermore stays much slower and extra complicated associated to further ML prototypes such as per decision tree models, which don't cause any problems in the circumstances of misplaced statistics.

Sankar et al. [25] used air quality index which hinges on the attention of impurities like SO_2, NO_2, CO_2, etc. It uses ML models such as SVR and LR. It gives means as well as ways for refining the outcomes of ML representations which has not accomplished fit. But it uses comparatively less number of training and testing data in case of Delhi. This work has only considered a portion of records from Delhi, one of the most polluted cities of the world. In comparison, almost 10,000 more records of information from Houston was taken for this work.

Ying Zhang et al. [26] indicated an upgraded air superiority expectation strategy dependent based with the LightGBM type to anticipate the PM2.5 fixation on 35 air quality checking stations at Beijing during an assortment of 24 h. Light GBM is fast and may deal by way of the enormous magnitude of information and takes lower memory to run. But still, in our undertaking which nearly utilizes 1,000 columns, it isn't fitting to utilize LGBM since they stand delicate to overfitting and will, without a lot of stretch overfit little information. It moreover inputs a great number of factors while coding.

Z. Ghaemi et al. [27] utilized a spatio-fleeting framework, planned utilizing a LaSVM-considered online calculation. Execution of this framework is assessed by contrasting the expectation aftereffects of the AQI through that of a conventional SVM calculation. At this juncture, the preparing time altogether diminishes by expelling the non-bolster vector tests at the preparation step, and without diminishing the exactness. Be that as it will, the data records employed in this above-mentioned undertaking is imbalanced which doesn't enable the design to exist appropriately. Timothy et al. [28] utilized five prescient models, k-closest neighbours (KNN), support vector machine (SVM), Naïve-Bayesian classifier, irregular woodland, and neural system. The error metrics utilized were CV execution, confusion accuracy, and ogloss execution. Though they got good outcomes in lieu of neural networks, the utilization of neural system can prompt a more slow reaction taking place at a bigger scale, which we have exploited inside our information.

Yu Zheng et al. [29] have used LR, neural networks, a dynamic aggregator and inflection predictor. Indirectly, [2] derived from this. They assessed their design by means of information from 43 cities. Their use of neural networks has made it much slower and further complicated related to other ML methods such as DTR models. Hable-Khandekar et al. [30] have placed to light various big data perspectives by considering various heterogeneous data sources and factors affecting the air condition. It has also explored recent tools meant for contemporary air quality monitoring. However, they had uncertainty and non-linearity within the system.

Vito et al. from the National Agency of New Technologies [31], have found a system that considers LR, SVR, neural networks, DTR and Lasso regression. But since Lasso encourages shrinking of coefficients to 0, i.e. dropping those variates from model, Lasso regression is measured as unreliable. Sang Hyun Sohn et al. [32] have foreseen an ozone development utilizing neural systems. In this work, they confirmed that by means of the assistance of various strategies for handling information, the custom of machine learning practices towards air quality expectations performs sensibly well. Similar to [1], the solid equipment reliance of neural systems attached to the processor plus the obscure time term of BPNNs have made this less proficient.

K.P. Singh et al.[33] have used principal component analysis within this work, using single decision tree, decision tree forest, decision tree boost and support vector machines. They established that both DTF as well as DTB have outperformed SVM. However, the designs are very complex to generate beside the point that it could require a long amount of time.

Dragomir et al.'s effort on air quality forecast utilizing K-closest neighbour calculations [34] is interrelated with [7], as they also have worked with a similar sort of algorithm, though on different scenarios. This catalogue is used to categorize the effluence quantity and on the road to inform the populace about some possible episodes of pollution. Nonetheless, the training data set of the prototype takes a huge amount of period to work. Chaloulakou et al. worked on forecasting the subsequent 24-hour period's maximum every 60-minute stretch ozone absorption in the Athens basin [35] using LR and neural networks, finding the neural networks as providing improved outcomes than linear regression. Neural networks may take ample time to process and could require a good deal of hardware dependence.

Vlachogianni, A et al. [36] have used LR, ANN and DTR to compare the air quality index in Greece. They established that ANN accomplishes improved performance to discover the day-to-day AQI and LR performs best to catch the hourly AQI. Keller et al. showed that the random forest algorithm allowed them to forecast better as soon as the awareness change of atmospheric species because of chemistry devoid of the necessity to invoke the chemical integrated [37]. They predicted the prototype consuming standard chemistry model and ML designs and displayed that 50% of these concentrations predicted by means of ML consist of an error not as much as 1 ppb their work included a sparse data set which has partial memory and restricted processing power which makes the system run very slow. DTR and RFR are faster to train matched with the use of a sparse data set. The comparative analysis of various machine learning techniques have been given in Table 16.1.

TABLE 16.1
Review of Machine Learning Models in Various Areas

Category	Authors	Description
RFR	Liu Bo et al. [22,23]	Apply different ML strategies for forecasting AQI.
ANN and CNN	Soh et al. [24]	Forecast air quality for 48 h using a combination of ANN, CNN and a long short term memory to extract spatial-temporal relations.
SVR and LR, stochastic gradient descent	Sankar et.al.[25]	This work has considered a portion of records from Delhi for predicting the air quality index.
LGBM	Ying Zhang et al. and Ameer et al. [26]	The 35 air quality checking stations at Beijing during an assortment of 24 h have been installed.
Density-based spatial clustering of applications with noise	Z. Ghaemi et al. [27]	The output clusters of VDCT have been compared to those of DBSCAN.
Deep distributed fusion network	Timothy et al.[28]	Online air pollution air prediction sytems.
KD and data mining	Yu Zheng et al. [29]	Demonstrated the DeepAir beyond baseline models
ML techniques	Hable-Khandekar et al. [30]	It summarizes the air quality forecasting models as well as real-time monitoring tools.
Pattern recognition	Vito et al. [31]	Results show that e-noses could be used as first line low-cost NDT tool in aerospace CFRP assembly and maintenance scenarios.
ANN	Sang Hyun Sohn et al. [32]	ANN was trained by using hourly pollutant and meteorological data that resulted in complex patterns of ozone formation.
Principal components analysis (PCA)	K.P.Singh et al. [33]	The DT and SVM models discriminated the seasonal air quality rendering misclassification rate (MR) of 8.32% (SDT); 4.12% (DTF); 5.62% (DTB), and 6.18% (SVM), respectively, in complete data.
K-nearest neighbor	Dragomir et al. [34]	Uses the class of KNN to classify the new instance and predicting the AQI.
Multiple linear regression models	Chaloulakou et al. [35]	Performance measures are calculated based on a wide set of forecast quality.
Multiple linear regression	Vlachogianni, A et al. [36]	Applied and used various statistical evaluation parameters to analyse the performance of the models, and inter-compared the performance of the predictions for both cities.
Random forest algorithm	Keller et al. [37]	Forecasting the change of atmospheric species due to chemistry devoid of the necessity.

16.3 MODEL SELECTION

There exist various categories of ML models for instance regression models, classification models, clustering models, etc. Each ML model solves a very definite kind of problem. There remain features that ought to be looked upon while selecting the appropriate ML designs such as, requirement or required output on behalf of the problem, category of data, availability of absorption and production data (as in supervised learning), and so on and so forth.

In this chapter, a data set has been used that already consists of absorption data and production data, and to practice supervised learning. The supervised learning is again partitioned into two types: regression and classification. The regression method is meant for foretelling numerical values on behalf of a prearranged input value (which stays by the same token a numerical value) in addition to the classification method, which is used toward foreseeing the class or category for a specified input value. Since the product of our data set exists as a numerical value (AQI value) we will be using regression models intended for our calculations.

16.4 REGRESSION MODELS

There remain various types of regression models; however, only limited forms of regression models stay present widely. In this application, we have adopted some widely used regression models, for example multiple linear regression (MLR), decision tree regression (DTR), support vector regression (SVR) and random forest regression (RFR).

16.4.1 Multiple Linear Regression

Multiple linear regression (MLR), in a like manner is alluded to similarly as multiple regression, is an arithmetical procedure that practices a limited autonomous variables to clarify or foresee the consequence related to a variable. The aim of MLR is to demonstrate the linear connection amongst the (independent) variables as well as response (dependent) variable.

Mathematically, a MLR model could be represented by means of the subsequent equation 16.1.

$$y_i = \beta_0 + \beta_1 x_1 + \beta_2 x_2 + \ldots + \beta_n x_n \tag{16.1}$$

where y_i is the measured variable, β_0 is the y-intercept, $x_1, x_2, x_3, \ldots, x_n$ are the independent features and $\beta_1, \beta_2, \ldots \beta_n$ are the weights of the individual independent features.

16.4.2 Decision Tree Regression

A decision tree means a decision-production device that works with a flow chart–like tree structure. A decision tree is made of vertices and boundaries associating vertices with each other. These inward nodes speak toward a condition with respect to the quality, every single branch speaks toward the outcome of the condition and every single leaf edge speaks towards a class name or consequences aimed at an agreed subset of foundations of facts. The DTR model is viewed as truly outstanding and for the maximum part, utilized directed learning methods. Tree-based systems empower judicious models with extraordinary accurateness, adequacy and straightforwardness of interpretation.

16.4.3 Random Forest Regression

Random forest regression remains a more advanced and robust system of DTR algorithm. In DTR, only one decision tree is generated which stays responsible in lieu of expecting the outcome. In RFR, arbitrary K data points are selected belonging to training set. By means of the selected K data points a decision tree is produced. This procedure is repeated for N amount of times, resulting in N distinct decision trees. The average forecast of the N decision trees stands the random forest forecast. RFR process can envisage for both continuous (real-valued) and categorical data.

16.4.4 Support Vector Regression

The support vector regression (SVR) utilizes indistinguishable standards from the support vector machines (SVM) for arrangement, with only a pair of minor contrasts. Like SVM, SVR also selects data points belonging to the data sets and attempts toward fitting the residual data points founded on these selected points. These are called support vectors.

16.5 IMPLEMENTATION

In this experiment, a scikit-learn library has been used. Scikit-learn is a library in Python that offers numerous built-in unsupervised and supervised learning procedures. The succeeding section does a profounder discussion on the prevailing methods, and the procedure followed in this chapter.

16.6 DATA COLLECTION

India consists of 28 states with 8 union territories and has a populace of roughly around 1.37 billion. The data set we used intended for the aforementioned experiment has AQI data collected from 19 different states. This data set is available from Open Government Data (OGD) Platform India. This site provides real-time national AQI outputs from varied observing places from corner to corner of India. The toxins observed are sulphur dioxide (SO_2), nitrogen dioxide (NO_2), particulate matter (PM_{10} and $PM_{2.5}$), carbon monoxide (CO), ozone (O_3) and so forth. This site provides the informational index by means of a XML record. In this manner, before changing the XML document into a CSV record, it had the accompanying sections in our informational index: state, city, station, date, time, centralization of contaminations, say, $PM_{2.5}$, PM_{10}, NO_2, NH_3, SO_2, CO, O_3, AQI esteem and predominant matter.

16.7 MISSING VALUE PROCESSING

As of dissimilar reasons, missing qualities in the informational index are very common in meteorological informational collections. The lost data might reduce the excellence of the application created through ML algorithms. At present, there exist various methods for working around lost information. Deleting entire rows that have absent data is a unique method. However, the aforementioned method is not suitable when the extent pertaining to the data set is small. Doing so in a minor data set could result in the damage of vital facts as well as the design produced using the machine learning algorithms might never be accurate. Moreover, we cannot delete records in a data set that contain sensitive data.

A different technique for the treatment of the absent information may be completed by replacing the omitted points with the mean (average), median or else mode of that particular column. It is worked with a similar technique aimed at this experiment. In the aforementioned experiment, the lost records have been replaced with the mean (average) in equation 16.2 of that column in lieu of a specific state. The ensuing formulation is aimed at calculating the average as well as processing absent data.

$$(mean)_s = \frac{\sum_1^n (Z_i)_s}{n_s} \qquad (16.2)$$

where Z_i is the impurity concentration on behalf of a state s, n is the the entire number of records for a state s and s signifies a unique state.

16.8 FEATURE SELECTION

As per stated previously, the data set of Table 16.2 involves the features, namely *state, city, station, date, time,* $PM_{2.5}$*,* PM_{10}*,* NO_2*,* NH_3*,* SO_2*,* CO*,* O_3*, AQI value* and *predominant matter*. Feature selection is important for generating accurate models. In feature selection, a feature or an independent variable is nominated if this one contains an arithmetically important consequence on the consequent variable.

TABLE 16.2
Estimation of p-Values for Concentration of Pollutant

Feature	p-Value	Outcome
$PM_{2.5}$	0.00	Significant
PM_{10}	0.00	Significant
NO_2	3.91e - 84	Significant
NH_3	4.09e - 109	Significant
SO_2	6.61e - 07	Significant
CO	1.70e - 53	Significant
O_3	4.90e - 08	Significant

This numerical import is determined through the *p-value.* In general, assuming that the *p-value* aimed at a feature is less than 0.05, then it can be said that the feature has a noteworthy influence with the result variable, and therefore it is possible to predict that the feature is *arithmetically important.*

Hence, it is easily understood that the whole of the contaminations significantly affect the result variable (AQI). Thus, all of the contaminant features will stand measured within our feature set. Additionally, towards these features, are furthermore supplied *state, city* and *station* columns in the feature set. The reason behind this stands that the normal AQI result of an agreed state or place stays almost constant with only a few minor fluctuations. Even by way of use of these fluctuations the air quality index value almost stays pretty close to its average value. For instance, ponder the states of Chennai and Delhi. Their average AQI index is around 93 and 164, respectively. Thus, on some specified day, their AQI indexes could be closer towards their normal values like 91 and 166 for Chennai and Delhi, respectively.

Therefore, our closing feature set consist of the columns of *state, city, station* and all *pollutant matters.*

16.9 DATA TRANSFORMATION AND FEATURE SCALING

The given feature set comprises both numeric data (concentration of pollutants) and non-numeric data (state, city, station) and has been shown in Table 16.3. Since regression procedures are built with a numerical model, it uses numeric facts intended for its computation and model generation. Thus, it cannot directly have use of our feature set on account of non-numeric data.

Therefore, it is essential to alter the data set by converting the string values (non-numeric data) into integer values (numeric data). This may be completed in a limited number ways. The chief method is to allocate a unique arithmetic value to every non-numeric values. For example, give value 1 to state Andhra Pradesh, value 2 to Assam and consequently until the final state is allocated. Follow this identical procedure aimed at the city and station column. Check the subsequent table meant for an improved implication.

This methodology may look right but there is a chief problem in this technique. This technique will make a regression design that will provide upper position en route for the state having larger value (*West Bengal with assigned value 19*) in

TABLE 16.3
Value Assigning to Each State

State	Numeric Equivalent
Andhra Pradesh	1
Assam	2
....	....
West Bengal	19

TABLE 16.4
Data Set Sample before Transformation

State	.....	$PM_{2.5}$
Andhra Pradesh	.....	68
Assam		141
...	...	...
West Bengal	.....	133

Table 16.4 and lower position to the state having a smaller value (*Andhra Pradesh with assigned value 1*) are shown. Thus, it may cause inaccurate predictions. Another process intended for changing the non-numerical data to mathematical data could be accomplished by making a different new section for every single non-numeric values. Generate an innovative column for every single non-numeric data and allot the data 1 in case the row contains that non-numeric data else assign 0 if otherwise. Contemplate the subsequent instance for better understanding.

The above data set is converted to the succeeding data set (*new feature set*), which is shown in Table 16.5.

Thus, the regression model generated by means of the newfangled feature set will give equal status to every state as well as make further correct predictions.

Once it has been attained, our new transformed data set its time on behalf of feature scaling. Feature scaling is a system that is used with normalizing the independent features existing in the data set in a permanent range. It is realistic as soon as the free variables differ in the direction of magnitudes from further free variables. It essentially aids to normalize the information inside a precise series and it likewise benefits in hastening the arithmetic in a procedure. To achieve feature scaling, the *Standard Scaler* class exists in the *sklearn. preprocessing* module.

Thus, afterwards, execution of the entire data transformation in addition to the feature scaling on our data set, the new data set obtained contains about 334 columns and more than 1,500 rows. After that the feature set has been divided into two parts, creating training data set and testing data set. The size of the testing data set was 25% of the training data set.

TABLE 16.5
Data Set Sample after Transformation (New Data Set)

Andhra Pradesh	Assam	.....	West Bengal	......	$PM_{2.5}$
1	0	.....	0	......	68
0	1	.....	0	.....	141
..	..	.....	..	.....	..
0	0	.....	1	.....	133

16.9.1 Error Metrics

Coefficient of Determination:

$$R^2 = \frac{\Sigma(y_{predict} - y_{mean})^2}{\Sigma(y - y_{mean})^2} \tag{16.3}$$

Root Mean Square Error:

$$RMSE = \sqrt{\frac{\Sigma(y_{predict} - y_{real})^2}{n}} \tag{16.4}$$

Mean Absolute Error:

$$MAE = \frac{1}{n}\Sigma|y_{predict} - y_{real}| \tag{16.5}$$

Root Mean Squared Logarithmic Error (RMSLE):

$$RMSLE = \sqrt{\frac{1}{n}\Sigma(\log(y_{predict} + 1) - \log(y_{real} + 1))^2} \tag{16.6}$$

16.10 RESULTS AND DISCUSSION

The outcomes were gained by contrasting the working of various ML techniques (mentioned earlier) and also through judging their presentation on numerous error metrics.

Tables 16.6 and Table 16.7 display the presentation of the machine learning models on both the training data set as well as the testing data set. We understand that DTR performed extremely well on the training data set but didn't achieve that good on testing data set. The reason behind this might be that the DTR model was learning the values and its results by heart (i.e. over-fitting) from the training data set. Thus, when shown the exact training data set, it predicted very accurately, but

TABLE 16.6
Model Performance on the Training Set

Models	R^2	RMSE	MAE	RMSLE
MLR	0.9965	5.9334	3.2952	0.0595
DTR	1.0000	0.0000	0.0000	0.0000
RFR	0.9996	2.0237	0.7106	0.0195
SVR	0.9494	22.628	16.076	0.1423

TABLE 16.7
Model Performance on the Testing Set

Models	R^2	RMSE	MAE	RMSLE
MLR	0.9965	5.4973	3.4796	0.0517
DTR	0.9955	6.2370	2.354	0.0563
RFR	0.9982	3.8577	1.7016	0.0422
SVR	0.9164	27.0025	19.0722	0.1686

when fed with new information (testing data set) it could not accomplish that well. On a further case, RFR achieved really well on the training data set as well as the testing data set. This may be explained owing to the added healthy nature of RFR. As cited before, RFR generates N number of decision trees from K-selected data points and the mean calculation of the above-mentioned N decision trees is the random forest prediction. Thus, while generating a design, the bad predictions done by a few decision trees (over-fitted trees) are outnumbered through the good predicting decision trees because of the mean prediction. We likewise observe that MLR performed quite well on both training data set and testing data set, but then not as good as RFR. Ever since the MLR generated a direct model built on training points, it produced less error while predicting the training data set, but overall it had the identical outcome on a training data set and testing data set. At last, it is found that SVR performed the least well in evaluation with all the former regression models. This might be because of the multifaceted nature of SVR. Unlike other regression models, where the error rate is minimized, support vector regression attempts to contain the error by a certain threshold by appropriating the hyperplane that consists of the maximum number of data points amongst the boundary lines.

The subsequent diagrams express the contrast of various ML models on the training data set and the testing data set. Figure 16.1, Figure 16.2, Figure 16.3 and Figure 16.4 shows the comparative analysis of various ML model for predicting AQI.

The subsequent diagram (scatter plots) indicates the presentation of various regressions for expecting the testing data. AQI values are taken on the y-axis, besides the impurity concentration in the x-axis. The testing data is represented through the blue dots and then the expected values remain represented through the orange dots.

On behalf of the MLR model in Figure 16.5, because the R^2 value is 0.9965, it has been observed that most of the forecast readings overlap the real values. Thus, the prototype gives a more precise fit.

Figure 16.6 and Figure 16.7 display the presentation of DTR and RFR, respectively. From the figures, it is well understood that the two designs have predicted accurately. Almost the entire forecast points overlap by means of the testing data points. Thus, they have high R^2 value in addition to fewer errors.

Figure 16.8 signifies the presentation of the SVR model. It is understood that this design didn't do well because the forecast points stand far away from their actual point (test data). Thus, it consists of a low R^2 score and high error values.

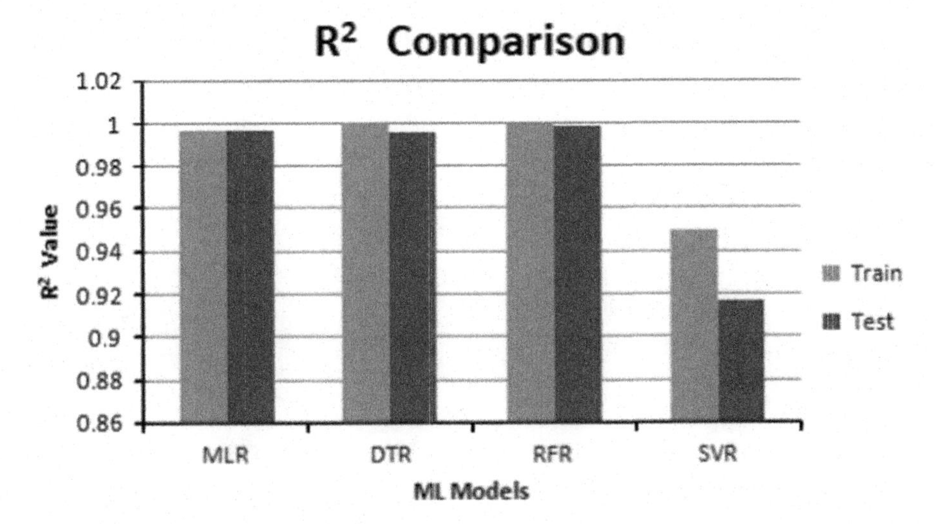

FIGURE 16.1 Comparison of R^2 on various ML models.

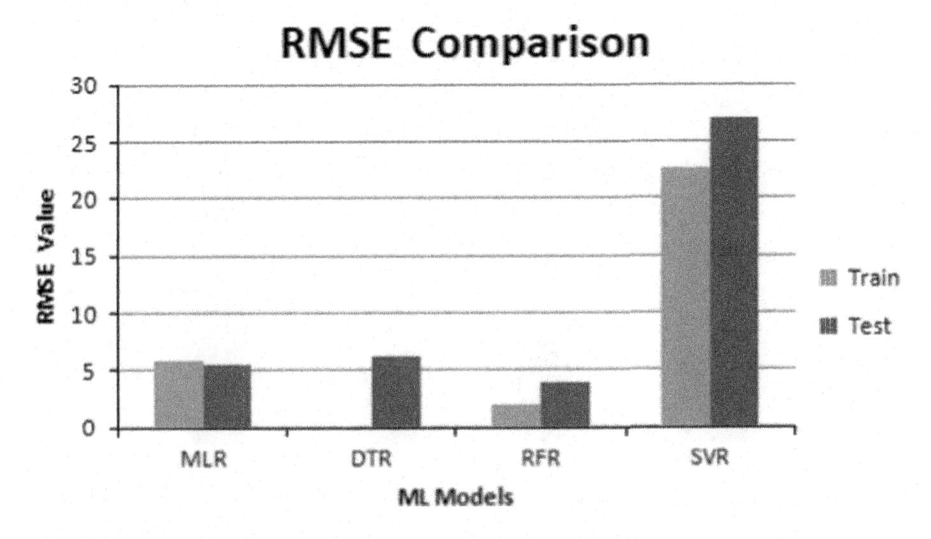

FIGURE 16.2 Comparison of RMSE on various ML models.

The ensuing reasons might be a conceivable explanation for a better outcome by RFR:

- Since RFR creates many small decision trees, it might be possible that the amount of decision trees providing correct results outdoes the amount of decision trees, providing incorrect results.
- Random forest algorithm is superior even if the data set has outliers in them.

Random forest can generalize data easier and it doesn't need feature scaling.

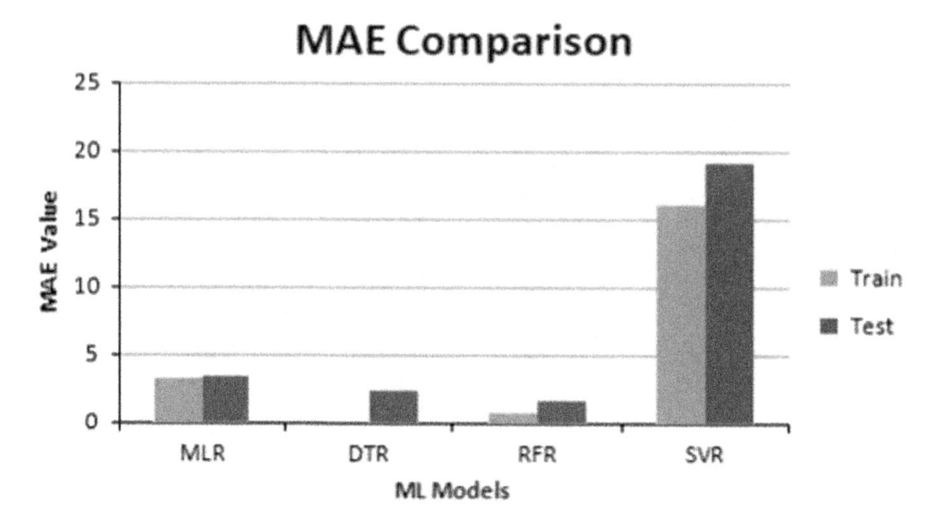

FIGURE 16.3 Comparison of MAE on various ML models.

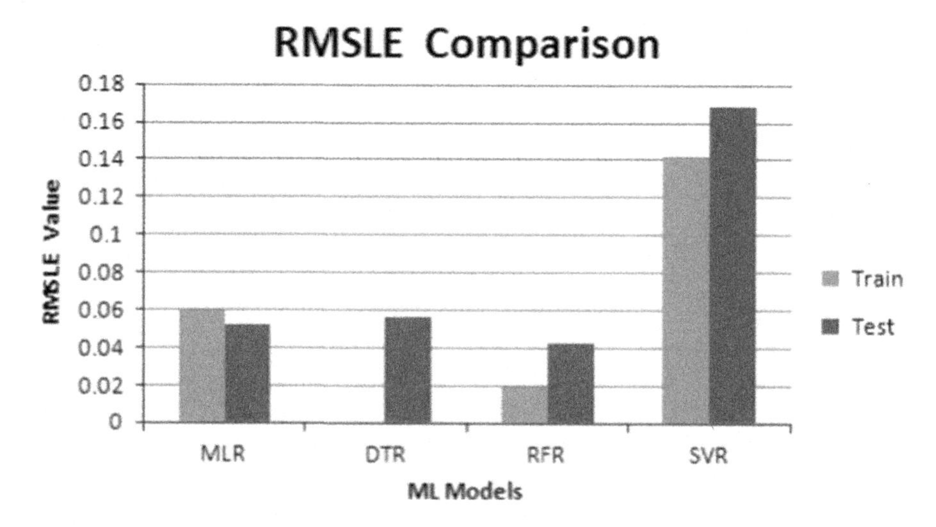

FIGURE 16.4 Comparison of RMSLE on various ML models.

16.11 CONCLUSION

A detailed comparison made for four ML designs, MLR, DTR, RFR and SVR, and their presentations were discussed in detail. As of the outcomes obtained, it is settled that random forest algorithm performed the greatest compared to other models, and SVR performed the poorest. MLR model data did equally well on both training set and testing data set, thus creating the second-best ML model. The presentation exhibited by the DTR model was satisfactory.

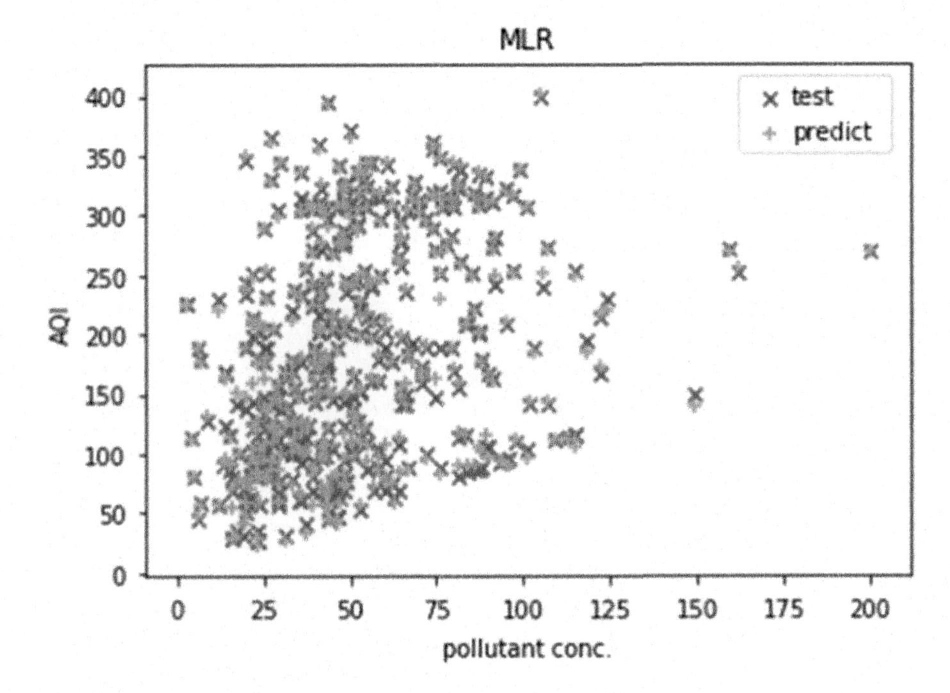

FIGURE 16.5 Performance of MLR.

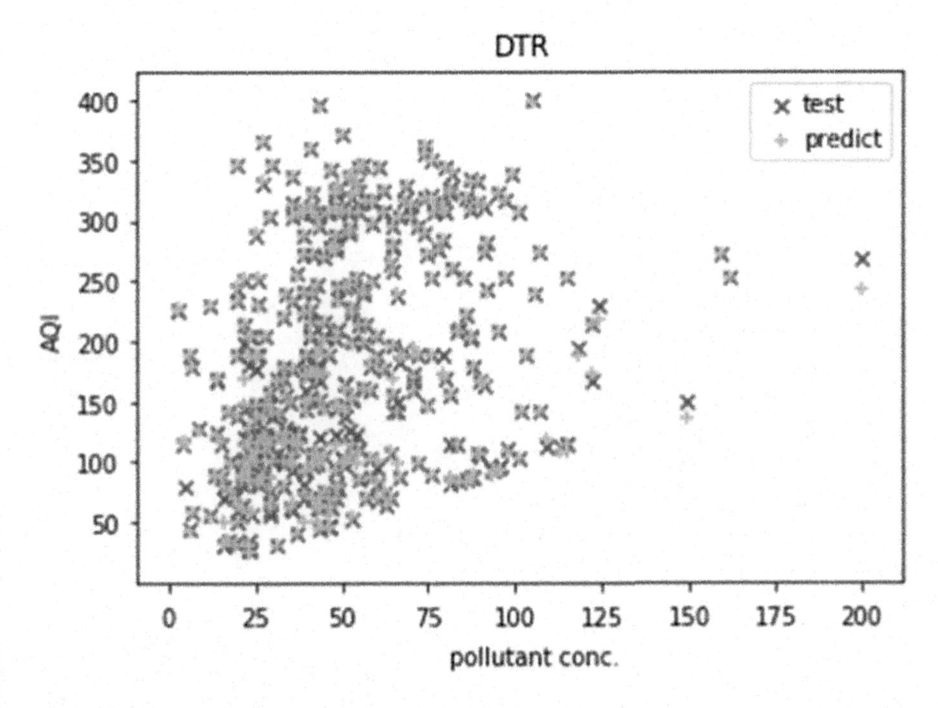

FIGURE 16.6 Performance of DTR.

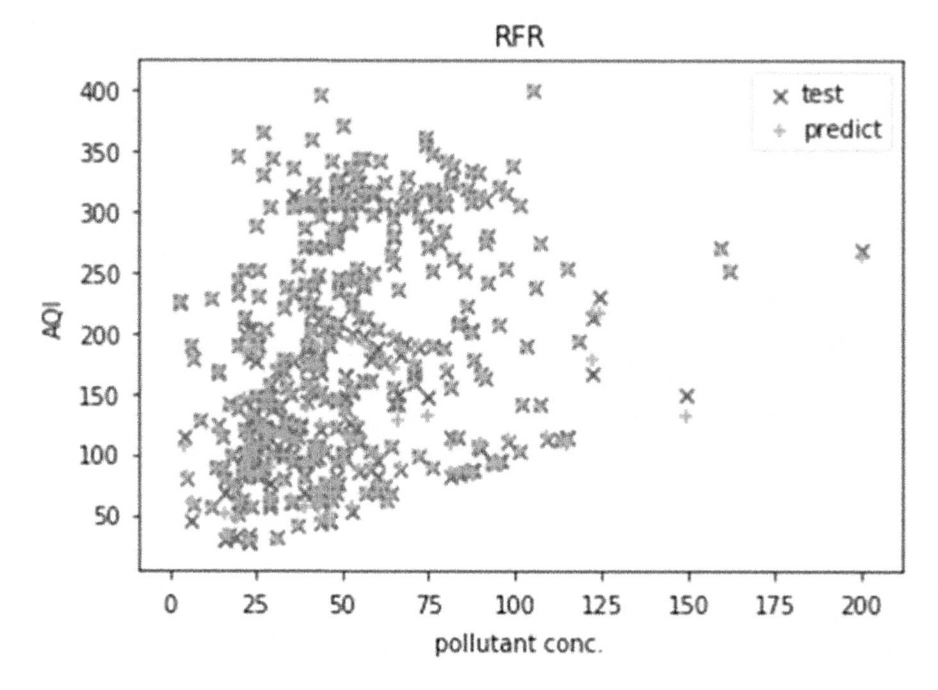

FIGURE 16.7 Performance of RFR.

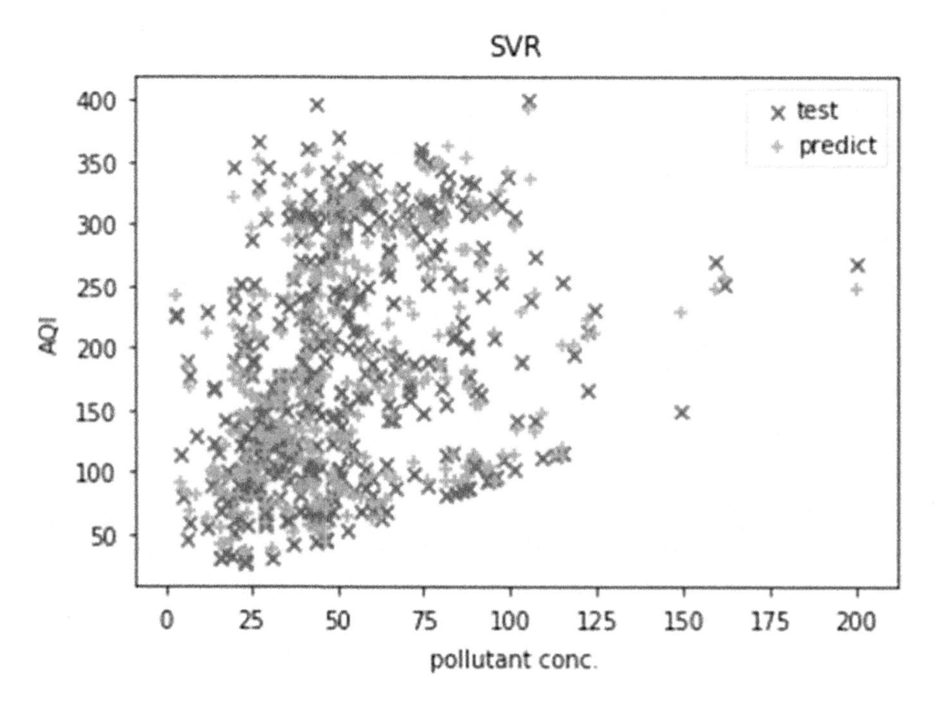

FIGURE 16.8 Performance of SVR.

REFERENCES

[1] Manisalidis, Ioannis, Stavropoulou Elisavet, Stavropoulos Agathangelos, and Bezirtzoglou Eugenia. "Environmental and health impacts of air pollution: a review." *Frontiers in Public Health* 8 (2020).

[2] Angelsen, Arild, and Kaimowitz David. "Rethinking the causes of deforestation: lessons from economic models." *The World Bank Research Observer* 14, no. 1 (1999): 73–98.

[3] Allen, Julia C., and Douglas F. Barnes. "The causes of deforestation in developing countries." *Annals of the Association of American Geographers* 75, no. 2 (1985): 163–184.

[4] Laurance, William F. "Reflections on the tropical deforestation crisis." *Biological Conservation* 91, no. 2-3 (1999): 109–117.

[5] Lebedev, A.T., Polyakova O.V., Mazur D.M., Bol'shov M.A., and Seregina I.F. "Estimation of contamination of atmosphere of Moscow in winter." *Journal of Analytical Chemistry* 67, no. 14 (2012): 1039–1049.

[6] Liu, Shuzhen, Tao Shu, Liu Wenxin, Liu Yanan, Dou Han, Zhao Jingyu, Wang Luguang, Wang Jingfei, Tian Zaifeng, and Gao Yuan. "Atmospheric polycyclic aromatic hydrocarbons in north China: a winter-time study." *Environmental Science & Technology* 41, no. 24 (2007): 8256–8261.

[7] Khamparia, Aditya, Singh Prakash Kumar, Rani Poonam, Samanta Debabrata, Khanna Ashish, and Bhushan Bharat. "An internet of health things-driven deep learning framework for detection and classification of skin cancer using transfer learning." *Transactions on Emerging Telecommunications Technologies* (2020): e3963.

[8] Panigrahi, Niranjan, Ayus Ishan, and Jena Om Prakash. "An Expert System-Based Clinical Decision Support System for Hepatitis-B Prediction & Diagnosis." *Machine Learning for Healthcare Applications* (2021): 57.

[9] Paramesha, K., Gururaj H.L., and Jena Om Prakash. "Applications of Machine Learning in Biomedical Text Processing and Food Industry." *Machine Learning for Healthcare Applications* (2021): 151.

[10] Pattnayak, Parthasarathi, and Jena Om Prakash. "Innovation on Machine Learning in Healthcare Services—An Introduction." *Machine Learning for Healthcare Applications* (2021): 1.

[11] Goyal, Sukriti, Sharma Nikhil, Bhushan Bharat, Shankar Achyut, and Sagayam Martin. "Iot enabled technology in secured healthcare: applications, challenges and future directions." In *Cognitive Internet of Medical Things for Smart Healthcare*, pp. 25–48. Springer, Cham, 2021.

[12] Sharma, Nikhil, Kaushik Ila, Bhushan Bharat, Gautam Siddharth, and Khamparia Aditya. "Applicability of WSN and Biometric Models in the Field of Healthcare." In *Deep Learning Strategies for Security Enhancement in Wireless Sensor Networks*, pp. 304–329. IGI Global, 2020.

[13] Jindal, Mansi, Gupta Jatin, and Bhushan Bharat. "Machine learning methods for IoT and their Future Applications." In *2019 International Conference on Computing, Communication, and Intelligent Systems (ICCCIS)*, pp. 430–434, IEEE, 2019.

[14] Kumar, Santosh, Bhusan Bharat, Singh Debabrata, and Choubey Dilip kumar. "Classification of Diabetes using Deep Learning." In *2020 International Conference on Communication and Signal Processing (ICCSP)*, pp. 0651–0655, IEEE, 2020.

[15] Abirami, G., and Venkataraman Revathi. "Attribute Based Access Control with Trust Calculation (ABAC-T) for Decision Policies of Health Care in Pervasive Environment." *IJITEE* 8 (2019).

[16] Girija, R., and Singh Hukum. "A new substitution-permutation network cipher using Walsh Hadamard Transform." In *2017 International Conference on Computing and Communication Technologies for Smart Nation (IC3TSN)*, pp. 168–172, IEEE, 2017.

[17] Girija, R., and Singh Hukum. "Triple-level cryptosystem using deterministic masks and modified gerchberg-saxton iterative algorithm in fractional Hartley domain by positioning singular value decomposition." *Optik* 187 (2019): 238–257.

[18] Girija, R., and Singh Hukum. "An asymmetric cryptosystem based on the random weighted singular value decomposition and fractional Hartley domain." *Multimedia Tools and Applications* (2019): 1–19.

[19] Abirami, G., and Venkataraman Revathi. "Performance Analysis of ABAC and ABAC with Trust (ABAC-T) in Fine Grained Access Control Model." In *2019 11th International Conference on Advanced Computing (ICoAC)*, pp. 372–375, IEEE, 2019.

[20] Abirami, G., and Venkataraman Revathi. "Attribute based access control policies with trust (ABAC-T) mechanism in pervasive computing". *Journal of Advanced Research in Dynamical and Control Systems*: (2019).

[21] Abirami, G., and Venkataraman Revathi. "Performance analysis of the dynamic trust model algorithm using the fuzzy inference system for access control." *Computers & Electrical Engineering* 92 (2021): 107132.

[22] Liu, Bo, Shi Chao, Li Jianqiang, Li Yong, Lang Jianlei, and Gu Rentao. "Comparison of different machine learning methods to forecast air quality index." In *International Conference on Frontier Computing*, pp. 235–245. Springer, Singapore, 2018.

[23] Ameer, Saba, Shah Munam Ali, Khan Abid, Song Houbing, Maple Carsten, Islam Saif Ul, and Asghar Muhammad Nabeel. "Comparative analysis of machine learning techniques for predicting air quality in smart cities." *IEEE Access* 7 (2019): 128325–128338.

[24] Soh, Ping-Wei, Chang Jia-Wei, and Huang Jen-Wei. "Adaptive deep learning-based air quality prediction model using the most relevant spatial-temporal relations." *IEEE Access* 6 (2018): 38186–38199.

[25] Ganesh, S. Sankar, Modali Sri Harsha, Palreddy Soumith Reddy, and Arulmozhivarman P. "Forecasting air quality index using regression models: a case study on Delhi and Houston." In *2017 International Conference on Trends in Electronics and Informatics (ICEI)*, pp. 248–254, IEEE, 2017.

[26] Zhang, Ying, Wang Yanhao, Gao Minghe, Ma Qunfei, Zhao Jing, Zhang Rongrong, Wang Qingqing, and Huang Linyan. "A predictive data feature exploration-based air quality prediction approach." *IEEE Access* 7 (2019): 30732–30743.

[27] Ghaemi, Zeinab, and Farnaghi Mahdi. "A varied density-based clustering approach for event detection from heterogeneous twitter data." *ISPRS International Journal of Geo-Information* 8, no. 2 (2019): 82.

[28] Amado, Timothy M., and Dela Cruz Jennifer C. "Development of machine learning-based predictive models for air quality monitoring and characterization." In *TENCON 2018-2018 IEEE Region 10 Conference*, pp. 0668–0672, IEEE, 2018.

[29] Zheng, Yu, Yi Xiuwen, Li Ming, Li Ruiyuan, Shan Zhangqing, Chang Eric, and Li Tianrui. "Forecasting fine-grained air quality based on big data." In *Proceedings of the 21th ACM SIGKDD international conference on knowledge discovery and data mining*, pp. 2267–2276, 2015.

[30] Hable-Khandekar, Varsha, and Srinath Pravin. "Machine Learning Techniques for Air Quality Forecasting and Study on Real-Time Air Quality Monitoring." In *2017 International Conference on Computing, Communication, Control and Automation (ICCUBEA)*, pp. 1–6, IEEE, 2017.

[31] Vito, Saverio De, Miglietta Maria Lucia, Massera Ettore, Fattoruso Grazia, Formisano Fabrizio, Polichetti Tiziana, Salvato Maria, Alfano Brigida, Esposito Elena, and Francia Girolamo Di. "Electronic noses for composites surface contamination detection in aerospace industry." *Sensors* 17, no. 4 (2017): 754.
[32] Sohn, Sang Hyun, Oh Sea Cheon, Jo Byung Wan, and Yeo Yeong-Koo. "Prediction of ozone formation based on neural network." *Journal of Environmental Engineering* 126, no. 8 (2000): 688–696.
[33] Singh, Kunwar P., Gupta Shikha, and Rai Premanjali. "Identifying pollution sources and predicting urban air quality using ensemble learning methods." *Atmospheric Environment* 80 (2013): 426–437.
[34] Dragomir, Elia Georgiana. "Air quality index prediction using K-nearest neighbor technique." *Bulletin of PG University of Ploiesti, Series Mathematics, Informatics, Physics, LXII* 1, no. 2010 (2010): 103–108.
[35] Chaloulakou, Archontoula, Saisana Michaela, and Spyrellis Nikolas. "Comparative assessment of neural networks and regression models for forecasting summertime ozone in Athens." *Science of the Total Environment* 313, no. 1–3 (2003): 1–13.
[36] Vlachogianni, A., Kassomenos P., Karppinen Ari, Karakitsios S., and Kukkonen Jaakko. "Evaluation of a multiple regression model for the forecasting of the concentrations of NOx and PM10 in Athens and Helsinki." *Science of the Total Environment* 409, no. 8 (2011): 1559–1571.
[37] Keller, Christoph A., Evans Mathew J., Kutz J. Nathan, and Pawson Steven. "Machine learning and air quality modeling." In *2017 IEEE International Conference on Big Data (Big Data)*, pp. 4570–4576, IEEE, 2017.

Index

D

E

F

G

H

I

N

O

P

T

U

V

W

X

Y

Z

Printed in the United States
by Baker & Taylor Publisher Services